50 FOODS

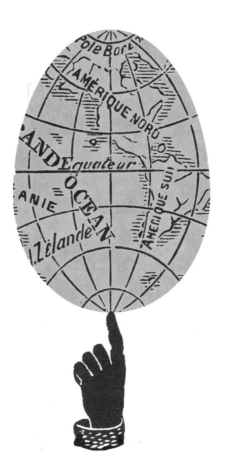

50 FOODS

THE ESSENTIALS OF GOOD TASTE

WITH NOTES ON WINE

Edward Behr

THE PENGUIN PRESS

NEW YORK

2013

THE PENGUIN PRESS
Published by the Penguin Group
Penguin Group (USA) LLC
375 Hudson Street
New York, New York 10014

USA · Canada · UK · Ireland · Australia
New Zealand · India · South Africa · China

penguin.com
A Penguin Random House Company

First published by The Penguin Press, a member of Penguin Group (USA) LLC, 2013

Portions of this book appeared in different form in the magazine *The Art of Eating.*

Excerpt on page 183 from *Simple French Food* by Richard Olney.
Reprinted by permission of the publisher, Grub Street, London.

LIBRARY OF CONGRESS CATALOGING-IN-PUBLICATION DATA

Behr, Edward, 1951-
50 foods : the essentials of good taste / Edward Behr.
pages cm.
title: Fifty foods
Includes bibliographical references and index.
ISBN 978-1-59420-451-7
1. Gastronomy. I. Title. II. Title: Fifty foods.
TX631.B387 2013
641.01'3—dc23

Printed in the United States of America
1 3 5 7 9 10 8 6 4 2

DESIGNED BY AMANDA DEWEY
ILLUSTRATIONS BY MIKEL JASO

For those who produce these great foods

Contents

Preface

This is a book about taste—a guide to deliciousness. I've tried to tell the things that will turn the reader into an instant connoisseur, which is a contradiction in terms, of course. It can't be done. But I hope to give a good head start.

My choices may provoke arguments over which are the top fifty foods, but I don't claim that mine are the absolute best and most delicious. The world has too many great foods for anyone to settle on a mere fifty. I chose them because I know and love them and they provide a broad sensory range. Most are raw materials, but some—ham, bread, cheese—have been fermented or otherwise transformed. In fact, six of the fifty are cheeses, and you may wonder: why so many? The answer is that cheese is probably the best food, just as wine is the best drink, and even six doesn't cover all the wonderful basic kinds.

I've tried to present clear, simple, practical information about buying, using, preparing, and enjoying. I focus on aroma, appearance, flavor, and texture. For each food, I tell what the "best" means, when that's clear—often there's more than one "best." I tell where the foods come from and the methods used to make them. I give the signs of top quality—indications of freshness and ripeness, best season, top varieties, proper aging. I tell things to avoid and provide questions to ask. If the food can be stored, I tell how, even how to mature certain soft cheeses. This isn't a cookbook, but if the way to prepare, serve, or eat something isn't well-known, I explain it—how to open an oyster, why the best way to cook green beans is boiling, how to clean a whole salted anchovy, when to eat and when to discard the rind of a cheese. I name the complementary flavors.

50 Foods has plenty of advice and opinions, but most of my conclusions are dictated by facts. During the more than twenty-five years I've been writing about food, I've often made wrong assumptions, and I've learned to be skeptical of both received wisdom and my own ideas. I try to be clear when I offer pure prejudice—in favor of tart apples over sweet, green asparagus over white, classic baguettes over modern sorts, young skinny French-style green beans over fatter kinds, dry-aged beef over meat sealed in plastic.

I strongly believe that food tastes more delicious when it's closer to nature, something that after years of careful tasting seems to me obvious. By closer to nature, I mean made using simpler processes, generally lower technology, and without deceptive additions.

Yes, some MSG or a trace of artificial flavoring may possibly improve the taste of something in an absolute sense. But even if that's true, how can we fully enjoy a food if we don't know where the flavor comes from and understand just how good nature can be on its own?

Industrial processing tends to simplify flavor. Advanced technology creates vast quantities of low-cost food for a mass market, while its cost-cutting and controls eliminate the extremes of both bad and good. *Skilled* traditional methods are almost always superior. Generally they're simpler and less powerful, and they leave more flavor intact. If there is a catch, it's that low-technology food is more seasonal and variable, coming in a much wider range of quality, sometimes the highest of all but now and then just awful. Traditions evolve, of course; sometimes we can improve them. With scientific insight, artisans can understand what really works, refine old methods, and achieve more consistent high quality.

I've included notes on wine because there's no better drink with food. Wine provides counterpoint, refreshment, and relaxation. Almost any simple wine without defects will do that, assuming it's somewhat light—light in body and flavor, low to moderate in alcohol, and low in tannin. It helps if the wine also has a pleasing acidity. Lighter wines tend to go with a wider range of foods, and with them it matters less whether the color is white, pink, or red. If you want, stick to light, simple everyday wines and ignore my sometimes expensive recommendations. They're not essential, although their more particular flavors go better with the food in question, and a few combinations really soar.

You can't always have the best food, but with the information in this book you will eat better every day. Knowing good food is part of a complete understanding of the world—part of a full enjoyment of nature, a full experience of the senses.

50 FOODS

1 ANCHOVIES

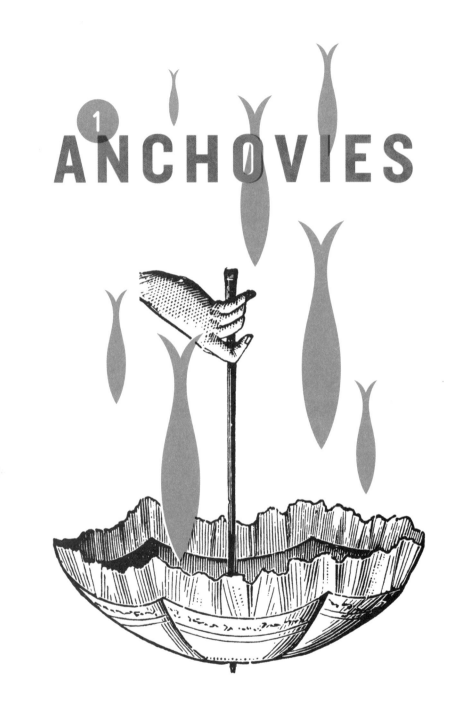

I. ANCHOVIES

A cured anchovy represents the very essence of a big taste—strong if you use a lot of anchovies (and why not?)—a timeless flavoring used by rich and poor, by those living near the water and those far inland. The taste is freshest and best when the anchovy is taken straight from the salt and cleaned just before use. The flesh is red, not brown like that of an anchovy from a can. The salt and complicated, emphatic flavor make anchovies highly useful. The combinations are as simple as an anchovy mashed into garlic-rubbed, olive oil–coated toast or chopped anchovies in a tomato or beet salad. Cured anchovies often boost flavor in the same way as a piece of dry-cured ham, fermented soy, or Southeast Asian fermented fish paste or sauce (the last two being based on anchovies). And just a few minutes' cooking over low heat reduces a cured anchovy to a paste and the flavor to something so subtle that in a sauce, such as for braised beef, it can hardly be identified. It's an umami underlining.

The narrow fish with their silver sides and green or blue-green backs, which quickly turn gray out of the water, are also delicious when just caught. Full of oil and quick to turn, they're cooked on the day they're caught, often within hours. The taste is rich but delicate. The fresh fish are so cheap and plentiful that they don't often appear in cookbooks. Around the Mediterranean, they're cooked in simple ways, such as dusted with flour, deep-fried, and served with salt and a sprinkling of vinegar or lemon juice. In Turkey along the Black Sea, *hamsi,* fresh sardines, are cleaned on the boats on the way back to port and then, still on the boats, grilled over hot charcoal with bay leaves; customers eat them right there, squeezed with lemon. "It's insane when you get *hamsi* like that. The smell is different, the taste is different," a Turkish friend of mine says. Widely popular in the Mediterranean are *boquerones,* to use the Spanish name: raw anchovy filets marinated in salt and vinegar for a few hours and up to overnight, until the dark flesh turns white, then dressed with olive oil, garlic, and parsley, to make a form of ceviche that's an excellent opening to a meal.

Dozens of species in oceans around the world are called anchovy, but the center of appreciation is the Mediterranean. The fish in question is the European anchovy, *Engraulis encrasicolus,* which feeds largely on plankton. Certain places are known for cured anchovies, like Collioure in France, where the fish come from the Gulf of Lion. In Campania, south of Naples, the anchovies cured in the little port of Pisciotta are caught using the ancient net called the *menaica* (these anchovies—*alici di menaica*—are said to be more delicate because they bleed in the net). Outside the Mediterranean, many excellent anchovies are cured in Cantabria in northern Spain, where the fish come from the Bay of Biscay.

The cure—there's almost nothing to it—probably hasn't changed for centuries. As soon as the fish arrive, with their skins still shining, the heads are pulled off, bringing the entrails with them. In Spain in the Costa Brava town of L'Escala, I watched as the anchovies were covered in sea salt. They mature in it and their own liquid. The length of the cure depends on the time of the year. In that spot, the anchovies caught from April through July, and thus cured during the heat of July and August, are ready by September. The ones caught in September aren't ready until the following April or June.

The anchovies packed in oil in jars and cans were first cured in salt, then the filets were removed from the bone and cleaned. Their texture is more firm and floury, and their taste is simpler, sharper, and saltier. Those you take directly from salt have the texture of fish. Their taste is curiously less salty, fuller, and fresher.

Among cured anchovies' many uses, anchovy butter, which may be due for a revival, is just soft butter mixed with mashed anchovies and put through a sieve, then melted on lean or not so lean grilled steak. In Liguria, *acciugata,* a mix of anchovy and olive oil, goes on "boiled" (gently simmered) meats and boiled vegetables. Provençal *anchoïade,* for toasted bread, is made by pounding salted anchovies with raw garlic in a mortar (or mashing them with the tines of a fork) and mixing in olive oil and black pepper, a little parsley, and a few drops of vinegar. For Piedmont's *acciughe col bagnet verd* (called *salsa verde,* "green sauce," in Italian), the cleaned salted anchovies are layered in a sauce of parsley, oil, and hot pepper and eaten as an antipasto or a snack. Also in Piedmont, in fall and winter anchovies are highly traditional in *bagna caoda,* the warm anchovy- and garlic-filled sauce for dipping bell peppers and cardoons. Cured anchovies are a key component of the complicated French *salade niçoise,* along with tomatoes, bell peppers, red onions, olives, and more.

HOW TO BUY AND PREPARE FRESH AND CURED ANCHOVIES: If you're in the right fishing port, look for shiny anchovies sold as soon as possible after they were caught, certainly on the same day. (Fresh anchovies used to be utterly ignored in the US; now, very exceptionally, you can find them.) Cook them within hours and in the meantime keep them as cold as possible, ideally on ice. Scale them with a dull blade, remove the head, clean them, and, for most purposes, filet them by pulling the backbone toward the tail.

Buy cured anchovies packed in salt rather than oil. With a cured anchovy, there's no danger of spoilage, but after a year they're firmer and the flavor is less good. If you live near a shop that sells them "loose" from a tin or bucket, buy only as many as you need for immediate use, since they lose flavor and color to the air. If you love anchovies enough to buy an entire tin to have on hand, keep them refrigerated so they don't turn mushy. To prepare cured anchovies for use, rinse off the salt and scrape away the skin with a dull table knife. Using your thumbnail, separate the two filets from the backbone, pulling away the fins and tail, and rinse and dry the filets. Use them promptly.

COMPLEMENTS TO ANCHOVIES: The best complements to a cured anchovy may be olive oil, garlic, parsley, and black pepper (which come together in *anchoïade* for toast), then lemon juice, orange juice, vinegar, capers, fresh tomato salad with hard-cooked eggs, beets (in vinaigrette), broccoli and cauliflower, eggplant (baked, with chopped garlic and basil and alternating slices of tomato). Top complements to fresh anchovies, as to the cured, are olive oil, garlic, parsley, black pepper, lemon juice. The opening to a Spanish meal frequently sets the salt of cured anchovies against sweet, cooked red bell pepper. Among red meats, for one example, cured anchovies go with cooked garlic in a sauce for roast lamb made from the juices in the pan. Anchovies are mashed with olives and capers in tapenade (olive paste). They're key to Green Goddess dressing—anchovies, garlic, capers, parsley, chives, tarragon, lemon juice, all in a medium of mashed avocado.

NOTES ON WINE: With fresh anchovies, drink a traditional Mediterranean rosé, meaning not too strong, or a light white wine—nearly any clean light white without too much character. A good Muscadet, which does have character, also goes, and along the Roussillon coast of France, where anchovies are caught and cured, a light example of the local red Collioure is drunk with fresh anchovies as well as other fish. With the cured anchovies in tapenade, one option is Fino or Manzanilla sherry. With Piedmont's *bagna caoda,* regional options are red Freisa and Barbera, as well as Nebbiolo. Cured anchovies aren't at all difficult with wine when a few filets are melted into a sauce, but in quantity they're difficult. The salt exaggerates the bitterness of red wine's tannin, which in turn underlines the fishiness and can produce a metallic effect. Go with a simple white.

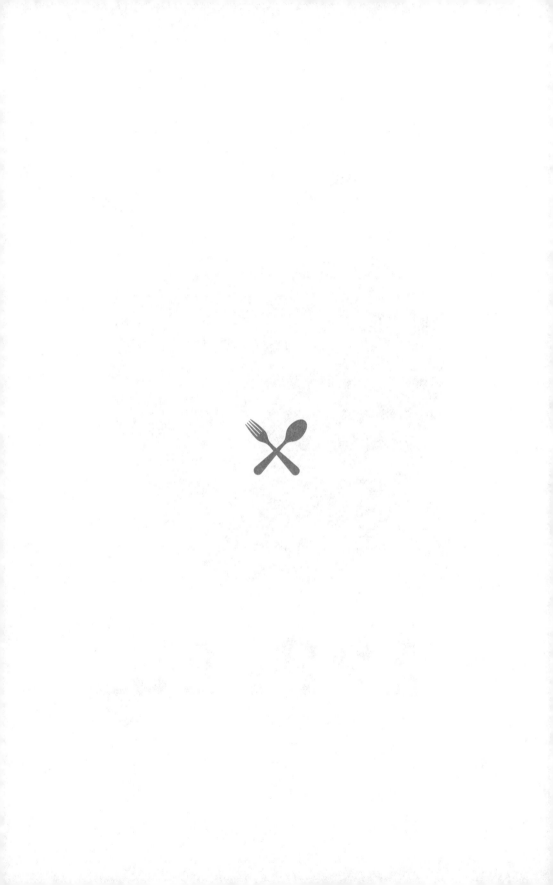

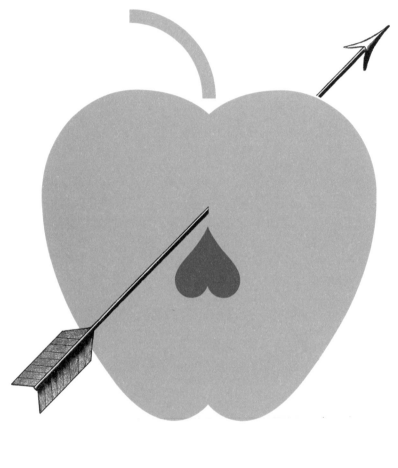

APPLES 2

2. APPLES

T he best apples have a generous acidity, a sweet-sour intensity with aromatic high notes. Good apples are grown in many places, but in my experience all the best are northern. I may be prejudiced because I live in a northern place, where fruit tends to be acidic; to me a purely sweet apple is distasteful. (Some apples are of course too sour—picked too early, taken from a wild tree, coming from a cold year when the fruit struggled to ripen.) There's a moment in fruit when flavor rises, acidity declines, sugar rises, and in the best varieties everything comes into a ripe balance, achieving a rightness that can be a matter of taste. Apple flavors often recall those of other fruits, of nuts, sometimes spices. There might be strawberry, raspberry, quince, pineapple, a wininess, a fennel-anise spice, and almost always there is something that might be essence of apple. Each variety has its peak. The very first apples of summer last hardly a day before they lose all acidity and turn insipid; the last to ripen in fall tend to hold their good qualities for weeks or longer in the cellar or in controlled-atmosphere storage. From year to year, apples, like wine grapes, show the effects of vintage. The concentrated flavor, sugar, and acidity of the best eating apples also make them excellent cooking apples, though to support the added sugar an apple needs especially strong acidity, which a cooking variety supplies. Apple desserts are some of the surest successes with great sweet wines.

New conventional plantings have the trees in hedgelike rows. Machines head down between them, pruning in some cases with very rough saw cuts, spraying, and finally harvesting. Maybe there's nothing inferior about the taste of apples raised in a hedge. But wide, mature, freestanding, standard-size apple trees have all the grace. Beautiful-looking apples are hard to grow by any means, and they're especially hard to grow organically, though it can be done. Organic growers sometimes plant newer varieties that are resistant to disease, and some of those have moderately good flavor. Mostly, the growers focus on avoiding problems by building the health of the soil and the tree.

The genetic variability of the apple easily gave rise to varieties adapted to different places, possibly eight thousand varieties around the world. A few hundred of those might be really good, and some dozens might be called best, though they don't necessarily succeed in the supermarket. Curiously, a few of the top commercial varieties are antiques. The number-one apple grown in the US is Red Delicious, from a tree found in 1881 by a farmer in Iowa. A good one is juicy but has no special flavor. Number three is the unrelated Golden Delicious, from a volunteer tree that sprouted in West Virginia in the 1880s. But now those varieties take the form of sports: trees propagated from mutated shoots that bear redder or bigger apples or have other desired qualities unrelated to taste. Both kinds of Delicious to me have insipid flavor and weak acidity. They're the antithesis of a northern apple. Granny Smith, roughly tied for fourth place, originated in Australia and was bearing by 1868. It's reliably crisp with some acidity, but the Granny Smiths in stores are devoid of interest. McIntosh, number six, comes from a wild seedling discovered by John McIntosh on his farm in Ontario in 1796.

The leading commercial varieties do change, however slowly. Apple trees don't start to bear overnight, and then for a number of years they're monitored for growth, productivity, and other qualities, including taste. Varieties that have become popular in the US in the last decade or two—Gala, now the number-two US-grown apple (New Zealand, 1934); Fuji (Japan, 1930s), in fourth or fifth place, depending on the year; Braeburn, number ten (New Zealand, 1952); and Honey Crisp, not yet on the charts (Minnesota, 1960, released 1991)—all have clear fruit flavor, crisp texture, and the ability to hold those qualities for a time even in warm conditions. They're not bad, but none are among the great apples.

Superior old kinds have been widely revived in North America, though they're generally available only in limited quantities in the fall. The old apples have more varied textures, flavors, and seasons, and unlike more popular varieties, some of the best are entirely russeted—covered with a flat golden brown not far in appearance from rust. Some apples, especially cider varieties, have an astringent dryness. France isn't a prime source of great eating varieties, although Normandy is a province of apples and a producer of good cider and of Calvados, the great apple brandy. I was shocked when I first realized that the common French idea of a good apple is the completely boring and generic Golden Delicious.

Roxbury Russet, with its fine, firm texture, is one of the oldest as well as best American apples. Duchess of Oldenburg is a good eating apple, and a Vermont nurseryman once described it to me as "the best cooking apple." Other respected old apples are Red Astrachan, sprightly Esopus Spitzenburg and Newtown Pippin, Northern Spy, Mother (often praised; I've never tasted it), and Gravenstein. The Api, or Lady Apple, is very old, a pretty, small, flat, red apple, often admired, though I've never had a great one. From California comes Sierra Beauty (nineteenth century). Albert Etter, an inspired early twentieth-century northern California breeder, sought concentrated flavor and sweet-sour taste, producing many varieties of fruit (a number of them saved from extinction by the current nursery-man Ram Fishman), including the juicy apples Wickson Crab and Pink Pearl, the latter with red-stained flesh. Among English varieties, I especially like Ashmead's Kernel, a smallish apple in a russet skin, great for both eating and cooking.

The McIntosh family of apples probably descends from trees brought from France to Quebec in the seventeenth century. The fruits have a slightly elastic skin over snowy white flesh—whose softness means they bruise easily—and they have a particular apple flavor sometimes called "vinous." Even a couple of weeks outside refrigeration eliminates their fine acidity and good fruit flavor and starts to turn them mealy. Others in the family are the Fameuse, or Snow Apple (Quebec, eighteenth century or earlier); the Saint-Laurent, or St. Lawrence (probably descended from Fameuse); the McIntosh itself; and the best of them all, the Macoun (McIntosh crossed with Jersey Black, introduced in 1923). Empire, another Mac cross, is always disappointing, and the variety Early McIntosh has only a fraction of the flavor of a normal October Mac. The best territory for McIntosh may be the Champlain Valley of Vermont and New York, because of its combination of a cold climate, which slows the ripening while increasing the aroma, with certain clay-loam soils, which also increase aroma.

England, with its cool, moist, ocean-tempered climate, is an old center of apple connoisseurship. (Apples are surely an English taste transferred to North America, where only crab apples are indigenous.) Edward Bunyard, the great English fruit nurseryman before the Second World War, focused on taste, meaning the best varieties. In his relaxed book *The Anatomy of Dessert,* the longest chapter is about apples (only the one about pears comes at all close). He praises Irish Peach, Lady Sudeley, James Grieve, Ellison's Orange, Egremont Russet, Allington Pippin, Pitmaston Pineapple, and more. "In December we reach the apogee of the apple season," he writes, "Cox's Orange, Margil, being at their best, and Blenheim Orange and Orleans Reinette just coming into ripeness." He cites flavors of anise, pineapple, strawberry, musk, honey. If you have a place to grow and store apples, he says, you can have them for all but two months a year. As certain English ones evolve in the cellar, they gain spicy flavors. (The nutty dry varieties go with Port.) "A Cox's in October is a little too acid," writes Bunyard, "but as the acid gradually fails, the aromatic ethers develop, and the end of November and early December see them at their height. It then slowly declines, very slowly if properly stored, and even in May, after a sunny summer, it is still worthy." Cox's, he says, is "the Château Yquem of apples."

Unlike Europeans, North Americans didn't develop separate varieties for eating, cooking, and cider (hard cider). Most of our apples are meant for both eating and cooking. (A new generation of American cider makers has focused on cider varieties, generally from Europe.) For eating, you need juiciness, varied textures, good fruit flavor, and sweetness. For cooking, an apple needs enough acidity to stand up to added sugar, a flavor that, transformed by heat, is good, and it's usually appealing that an apple holds its shape rather than turns to fluff. Specifically for cooking, there are Belle de Boskoop (Dutch), Bramley's Seedling (English), Calville Blanc d'Hiver (French), and varied crab apples (especially from North America). There's flavor next to the skin, and the skin helps hold a baked apple together. If you make sauce with apples in their red skins, they'll stain the sauce pink.

It's a more northern habit to eat fruit with meat, cooked medium to well—sweet fruit isn't a natural companion to rare meat. I grew up eating pork invariably with sweet applesauce, and the combination is good. But on the rare occasions I now eat meat with fruit, I like the fruit to be tart, with little or no added sugar, which allows the food to go better with a glass of dry wine. (Traditionally, sweet wine came only from rare sugary grapes, sometimes left to concentrate further on the vine or indoors. Dry wine was almost all anyone drank. What kept sweetness to a minimum in the savory dishes of classical French cooking was surely the necessity to go with great dry wine.) In Normandy, apples, cream, and Calvados are combined with chicken, pheasant, and veal. Apple slices sautéed in butter are the best partner to blood sausage (*boudin noir*).

You can bake sliced apples with butter and sugar, uncovered if they're moist, and eat them that way or use them as a filling for a pie or a tart. Or you can cook the slices on the stove in butter and sugar (two tablespoons butter per pound of fruit, sugar to taste), turning them gently with a wooden spatula so as not to break them. To fill a raw tart shell, slice the apples very thin so they'll be done at the same time as the pastry. Cut-up apples, in place of the traditional cherries, make an excellent clafoutis (cook the apples in butter in a cast-iron pan, pour over them a sweetened York-shire-pudding batter, and bake in a very hot oven). Pie might be the best apple dessert, and nothing is better than the single-crust *tarte Tatin,* cooked upside down so the apples caramelize on the bottom and the crust is almost inevitably crisp. An old-school charlotte is baked in its own particular mold, lined with buttered toast and filled with apples. Apple fritters, battered and deep-fried, require very flavorful apples. Apple sorbet is good boosted with Calvados. Apples are good in homey bread pudding.

One particular old American apple product has come back into fashion: boiled cider, which can replace sugar in applesauce, baked apples, pies, or any other apple dessert. The freshly pressed sweet juice is simmered, without any burning that would give a caramel taste, until it's reduced to a syrup. That's it. I like the intensity of a syrup so thick that, when cooled, it's gelatinous. One gallon of juice makes roughly three cups of syrup like that (three liters make about 400 milliliters). About half that amount of syrup will sweeten roughly three pounds of fruit, for the purest, most intense apple taste.

HOW TO PICK AND BUY APPLES: Don't *pull* an apple from the tree, which may rip off a fruiting spur with it, reducing next year's crop. Rather, lift and twist—the stem of a ripe apple readily separates from its branch. Most varieties keep best if they're picked in a ripe or near-ripe state and then held in a controlled atmosphere (cold plus an absence of oxygen). The apples for sale in supermarkets have sometimes picked up off-flavors in storage, and as a rule they're coated with an ugly, shiny wax meant to hold in moisture. In nature, the skin of an apple has a dull, whitish bloom. In a display, you can only go on appearance. Riper apples, like ones going by, have a more yellow background color for the variety, if by nature the variety isn't entirely red or russeted. When you cut an apple open, physiological ripeness is shown by a dark brown seed (though some wild apples taste best before that). Often the apples for sale have been out of storage and in the warmth for too long, and they're overripe. Firm, acidic varieties, including the old cooking ones, tend to store better.

For cooking, among the varieties that turn to "snow" are the McIntosh family—even their skins tend to burst. Some that hold their shape are Braeburn, Granny Smith, Northern Spy, Golden Delicious, Rhode Island Greening, and Yellow Newtown, as well as the classic European cooking varieties. If you're uncertain about a variety, gently cook some slices in butter to see whether they hold together.

COMPLEMENTS TO APPLES: A fresh ripe apple needs no particular complement. The lead one for cooked apples, in savory or sweet uses, is butter, followed by cream. Sautéed unsweetened apples go with pork, fresh and cured, goose, and wild boar. Apples go with onions and red cabbage. More elaborate is the trio of apples, cream, and Calvados, with pork or veal. In dessert, cinnamon makes sense with apples, but it's used so often in such great quantity that it's not at the top of my list. As often as quince is suggested with apple, each fruit is much better on its own. Calvados gives a heightened flavor, though equally it can hide the flavor of the apples at hand. Apples are complemented by cow's-milk cheeses, not least cheddar, by walnuts or chestnuts, and by all the ingredients of a rich mincemeat. Golden buttered toast complements apples in a charlotte. Caramel hides some of the fruit flavor, but I place it ahead of all other sweet complements to apples—a good *tarte Tatin* is one of the best desserts in the world.

NOTES ON WINE: A fresh apple needs no wine. Cooked apples with meats require a rich white, including one with some sweetness if the apples are cooked with sugar. The bottle might be, for example, an Alsace Pinot Gris or a Loire Chenin Blanc. A cooked apple dessert, especially one containing cream and buttery pastry, may be the safest choice with a glass of sweet white wine, including one enhanced by "noble rot" (botrytis), which might be a Beerenauslese ("selection of berries"), a Trockenbeerenauslese ("selection of dried berries"), a Jurançon, a Coteaux du Layon, a great aged Sauternes. The inflexible rule is that the dessert must be less sweet than the wine, or the wine will taste tart and simple, and its good flavors be hidden, in proportion to the excess sugar in the dessert.

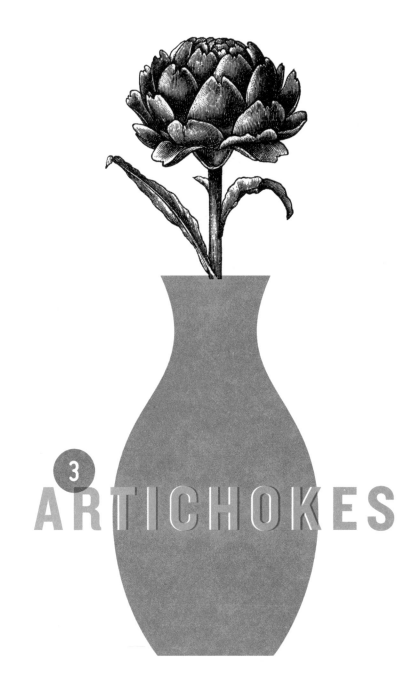

3 ARTICHOKES

3. ARTICHOKES

T he artichoke, that most Italian vegetable, is a thistle. More narrowly, it's a descendant of the cardoon, a vegetable rarely seen in North America but valued for its mild-flavored stalks. (It's little grown here partly because of the labor required: for the best cardoons, the plants are hilled up with soil, which deprives them of sun, making them delicate, tender, and white.) Artichoke plants are perennials that grow up to five feet tall, with long, untidy, frondlike leaves. The part we eat is the bud, and its leaves are properly called bracts. A single big artichoke grows at the top of the plant, while smaller ones form among the leaves lower down. Harvested young, they don't have the furry inner choke, which is unpleasant to eat but harmless. With a little trimming, they're tender enough to eat whole. A raw artichoke heart has an astringent immediacy; it's perfect sliced in thin crescents and dressed with only fresh olive oil and salt. Cooked, the heart turns soft and rich and gains a vegetable-nutty flavor. The heart runs partly into the stem, which trimmed to its center can be as good as the heart.

Almost all US artichokes are grown in California, specifically around Castroville, which calls itself "The Artichoke Center of the World." The area lies next to the cool Pacific Ocean, and average summer highs reach only into the 60s F (no more than 21 degrees C). They receive full sun, they thrive in the coolness, and there's no danger of damaging frost. Artichoke season very much reflects climate: in California it's spring and fall, while in Italy it runs from about December through March. Italians say that artichokes from older plants are tougher and have bigger chokes; they raise them only on year-old plants. Different varieties can be round, long, conelike, green, violet-tinged, purple, with or without thorny tips, and they have different flavors. Conventional US artichokes belong to the bulbous

Green Globe variety. A French one that gardeners in various countries cite for flavor is Gros Vert de Laon. Italian markets offer many choices, often purplish ones, including the dominant round Romanesco and the elongated Violetto.

A Venetian once said to me that, like other vegetables, artichokes used to flood the Rialto market at the peak of the season and the price would fall. Everyone bought artichokes then because they were inexpensive and at their best. They appeared at meal after meal. Families grew tired of them. Cooks—mothers—responded by preparing artichokes in many ways, not all of which were ideal. That's why, the Venetian said, there are so many recipes. These days the season for artichokes and most other vegetables has been stretched through breeding early and late-season varieties, through greenhouse production, and through shipping from places with warmer climates and different seasons. The concentrated peaks have all but disappeared. At US farmers' markets, there's rarely a flood of anything (and the price never seems to tumble far).

Cooks cut off the top quarter or third of a mature artichoke with a knife to get rid of the spines and for the same reason clip the tips of the remaining leaves with scissors. You can serve a whole mature artichoke, eating the meat at the base of the leaves and then the heart, or you can trim it to leave only the heart. That can be stuffed with mushrooms, ham, tuna. Even small young artichokes must be trimmed of outer leaves, tips, and tough surfaces.

Three well-known preparations from Rome are among the best. Tender artichokes are prepared *alla giudia,* Jewish-style: trimmed and pressed to flatten and open them, and fried whole in olive oil, pressing with a fork, to a deep golden color. *Carciofi alla romana* are filled with a mix of the trimmed, chopped stems with garlic, parsley, and the mint *mentuccia* (*Menta pulegium*), then braised in olive oil and water. *Carciofi con i piselli* are stewed in lard or olive oil with onion, prosciutto, and, toward the end, peas.

Similarly, Italians cook a risotto with artichokes and peas or fava beans. Tender artichokes are battered and fried for a *fritto misto.* Cooked artichokes sometimes go in a frittata and often in a Genoese *torta pasqua-lina,* combining greens, egg, and cheese in a thin yeast-leavened crust.

HOW TO BUY ARTICHOKES AND PREPARE THEM FOR COOKING: They lose quality from the moment they're cut from the plant. The stem, a telltale part, should look freshly cut and should be thick, not thin, in proportion to the bud. Artichokes should be heavy for their size and the leaves tightly closed (not about to open into a flower), though elongated kinds are by nature more open. The leaves should be full and firm, not withered or rubbery—when the artichoke is pressed, it squeaks.

Snap off the leaves by pulling them backward toward the stem, taking some of the strings. Trim away the tough upper and outer portions; even a small young artichoke has some. According to the preparation, either re-move the stem or leave about an inch and a half of it. Once cut and exposed to air, artichoke flesh quickly turns gray. To avoid discoloration, rub the trimmed artichokes with lemon or put them in water acidified with lemon juice or vinegar or, to avoid an acid taste, coat them with olive oil; don't use reactive metal (old-fashioned high-carbon-steel knives or aluminum pots); and add a little acid to your water if it's alkaline. It's more convenient to eat a whole artichoke if you remove the choke, either before or after cooking, using a melon baller or a sharp-edged teaspoon, then fill the center of the cooked artichoke with a warm sauce or a cool vinaigrette.

COMPLEMENTS TO ARTICHOKES: They're easy with other food, going well with peas and other vegetables, olive oil, butter (in hollandaise sauce), lemon, vinaigrette, garlic, onion, bay laurel, black peppercorns, ham, an-chovies, tuna, mushrooms, herbs, grating cheese, eggs (in frittata), and meats generally, including beef and lamb stews.

NOTES ON WINE: Over and over it's been said that artichokes don't go with wine. They contain the chemical cynarin, which makes any liquid con-sumed immediately afterward taste sweet. Yet only a minority of people perceive the effect, and not all of them are equally sensitive. (I experience only a mild sensation.) If you're concerned about the danger, you can override the effect by braising artichokes in flavorful stock, or you can compensate for the cynarin sweetness by choosing a somewhat acidic, very dry wine. Many Rieslings qualify, as do many cooler-climate Sauvignon Blancs, Muscadet, a no-oak Chardonnay such as Chablis, and Champagne. Also good are Fino and Manzanilla sherry and a more traditional (more salmon-colored) dry rosé.

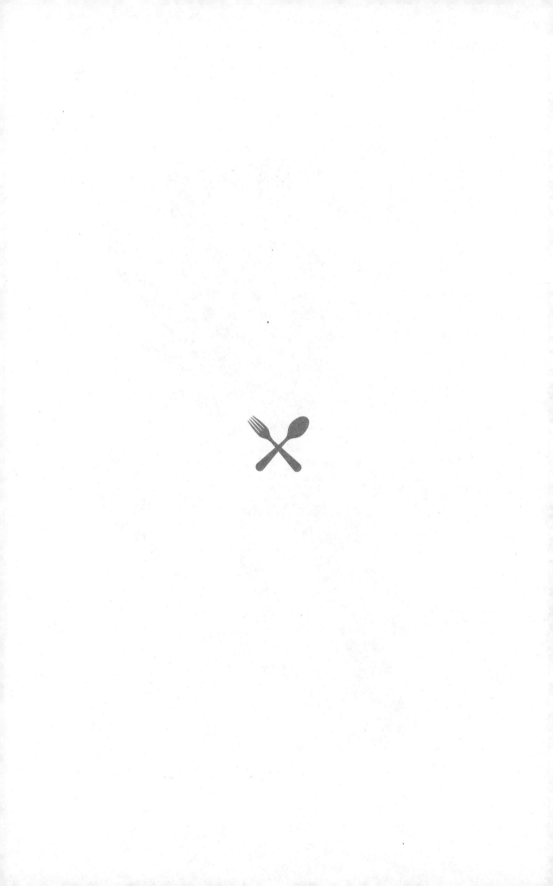

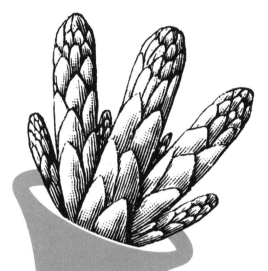

ASPARAGUS

4

Just cut green asparagus—the joy of a vegetable garden in spring—with its touch of bitterness and astringency, tastes clean, fresh, green, sweet. On the warmest days when the soil is moist, the spears push upward with uncanny speed, rising half a foot or more in a day. Once cut, they immediately start to change. Supermarket asparagus, so many days having passed, has muddy, unclean, nearly human flavors. For maximum freshness, I sometimes put the water on to boil before going out to the garden with a knife. Although I enjoy white asparagus, I, like most Americans and Italians and many French, prefer green for its stronger, more vegetable flavor.

The spears of white asparagus (preferred by Germans, Dutch, and Belgians, along with many French and Spanish) can be very thick and succulent, meaty, although in flavor they're more reserved than the green and can be more noticeably bitter. White asparagus costs more because it requires more labor. Before the season starts, to block sunlight that would otherwise turn the spears green, the soil is hilled up around the crowns or the plants are sealed off with black plastic. In fact, the blanched spears come in two versions: all-white and violet-tipped. It's said that in origin the all-white spears were picked at dawn, while the violet-tipped ones were picked in the evening, their tops having poked up through the soil during the day and acquired a little more flavor and color from the sun. Raw white asparagus is more brittle than the green, and its surface is more fibrous, becoming still more so as time passes after cutting. For that reason, white asparagus is always peeled.

To understand the appeal of white asparagus, you must eat it at its very best. If the spears weren't just harvested, then in the field they must have been plunged immediately into very cold or iced water and afterward held at just above freezing. Green asparagus deserves the same treatment, but white demands it. Otherwise, the white soon has a cardboard flavor. Rarely do New World growers of white asparagus give it such care, though a little promptly chilled white asparagus is flown to North America from Europe.

And then there's purple asparagus, such as the US variety Purple Passion, selected from the Italian Violetto di Albenga, which has become a rarity even in its home territory in Liguria. In my limited experience of Purple Passion, the flavor isn't special. Violetto di Albenga is cut when the spear is still mostly underground, so it's half or more white. But the top is emphatically purple, and the color survives a quick, full cooking. Purple is the sweetest, mildest, tenderest asparagus, to the point of being creamy in both flavor and texture.

Asparagus is always said to prefer sandy soils, which are easier for the farmer to work and warm more quickly in spring than clay soils. In Holland, different flavors are said to come from different sandy soils.

Gathering the thin, willowy shoots of wild asparagus is a rite of spring in many countries. *Asparagus officinalis,* the cultivated species, grows wild all over Europe, in northwest Africa, and as far east as Iran. We have it in North America, too, but here it escaped from cultivation only after it was brought over by European settlers, so our wild and cultivated asparagus are more similar. In some parts of the world, what is called wild asparagus belongs to other stronger-flavored species (one or two of them quite bitter), including a few that are completely unrelated to the cultivated kind. Wild asparagus shoots are delicious but not as refined and sweet.

HOW TO BUY OR HARVEST AND STORE ASPARAGUS: In the store as in your own garden, the tips should be smooth and tight, not starting to open. Like other vegetables, truly fresh asparagus looks as though it were still growing—no part should appear dry. You can check the bases for a recent clean cut, although they are often kept in water and might have been recut. Buy asparagus from a chilled display, or go early in the day to a farmers' market. Avoid white asparagus unless you believe it has been continuously chilled since harvest.

If you have your own, harvest the spears just before you cook, not first thing in the morning. I cut them at eight to ten inches, using a knife and leaving an inch or two behind, but it's fine to snap them off with your fingers a little higher up. The season is six to eight weeks—stop harvesting when summerlike heat arrives and the shoots of weaker plants are pencil thin. The remaining spears will grow into tall fronds that send strength back to the crowns for next year.

With green asparagus, both fat and thin spears have their partisans, although in my garden I don't notice any difference in flavor. In the supermarket pipeline, however, a fat green spear stays fresher longer and is possibly less stringy. And lovers of white asparagus all agree that fat white spears are sweeter, juicier, and hold their good qualities longer.

Cook asparagus on the day that you pick or buy it. While the spears wait, if they must, wrap them in plastic to hold in moisture, and refrigerate them.

HOW TO PREPARE AND SERVE ASPARAGUS: Although a raw spear tastes pleasant, asparagus gains character with cooking. If you haven't done so in harvesting, break the stalks where the tough and tender portions meet— the point where they break easily—and discard the tough bases. I peel green asparagus, and with the white, since it's more fibrous, you have no choice. A vegetable peeler works well; French cooks often use a small knife, cutting so the diameter of each spear is the same top to bottom. For adding to scrambled eggs, an omelette, or a frittata: cut them in ⅛- to ¼-inch diagonal slices, leaving the tips whole, and cook them gently in butter, stirring, until tender.

Is peeling green asparagus worth it? Emphatically, *yes*. Peeling reduces the stringiness that exists to some extent even in green asparagus, and it eliminates any grit lurking behind the shieldlike bracts on the stems. Because the strongest flavor lies in the skins, peeled asparagus tastes sweeter and more delicate. Peeling also eliminates much of the crude taste of store-bought green asparagus, making it too seem sweeter. And peeling reduces the danger that the tips, because they cook faster than the rest, will fall apart if cooking goes on too long. They're least likely to overcook if you boil the spears upright in a tall asparagus pot, with a removable metal basket, so the tips peek out of the water.

With whole spears, boiling is best. (Steaming is somewhat slower, and because there isn't plentiful water to wash away the vegetable's acidity, the green color is less bright. Grilling fresh asparagus is barbaric—it destroys all the good taste.) If you have a mix of fat and thin spears, sort them by thickness into two or three groups to be dropped into the pot in sequence, so none will overcook or undercook. It's useful to tie them in bundles about two inches across (not much more or the inside spears will cook more slowly than the rest), which can be retrieved from the pot all at once.

Use plenty of well-salted, vigorously boiling water. Put the vegetable in and replace the lid for a minute while the water returns to a boil, then uncover the pot so you can keep an eye on the contents. Asparagus quickly becomes too soft and the tips fall off, but for flavor it's better to slightly *over*cook than *under*cook. Thin spears are done in two to three minutes, the fattest green spears, if just picked, in no more than four to five, the precise time depending on the heat of the stove, the quantity of boiling water, even its pH and the amount of salt (see "Green Beans").

Drain the spears well, wrap them in a towel to absorb remaining water and keep them hot, and serve them in the same towel or a cloth napkin. For eating cool, it's often said that, to stop the cooking, asparagus should be put immediately into ice water. But the water rinses away flavor, and I notice no improvement in color or taste, so I spread the spears on a towel instead.

COMPLEMENTS TO ASPARAGUS: Most flattering is butter. (Place melted butter, lemon wedges, and salt and pepper on the table for each person to make a pool of seasoned butter into which to dip the warm spears. It's easy to add too much lemon, and if the asparagus and plates aren't hot, the butter will congeal. If that's a danger, use olive oil instead.) The most re-fined forms of butter for asparagus are *sauce hollandaise* (butter held by egg yolk in a lemon-flavored emulsion), *sauce béarnaise* (hollandaise with tarragon), and above all classical *sauce maltaise*—hollandaise with fresh blood-orange juice. Asparagus was born for *sauce maltaise,* which originally had no other purpose.

After butter comes sweet, fruit-tasting olive oil—*sweet* because the bitterness of much of the best olive oil shows baldly against the sweetness of asparagus. The oil can be mixed in a vinaigrette, and for flavor sherry vinegar is best. Beware that an acid dressing left too long on the spears will discolor them. Optionally, also sprinkle on raw shallots (finely chopped just before serving) and hard-cooked egg (sliced, finely chopped, or pushed through a coarse strainer to make *mimosa*) or both. Or serve asparagus with mayonnaise flavored with extra lemon juice or fines herbes (chervil, chives, parsley, and tarragon).

Asparagus goes well with eggs, especially scrambled. Excellent for dipping spears is a sauce of hot soft-cooked egg, one per person in individual cups, mixed with a tablespoon of butter and salt and pepper. In another direction, good strong-flavored complements to asparagus are paper-thin slices of dry-cured ham, chopped tarragon with fried bacon, and sautéed morels or boletes.

NOTES ON WINE: It used to be said that asparagus doesn't go with wine—and red wine is certainly impossible—but asparagus goes well with an array of white wines. I'm fascinated by the possibilities. Served with butter, especially, or with plain sweet olive oil, asparagus likes a clean, floral white wine with refreshing acidity, as long as the wine is also just slightly sweeter than the vegetable, or in proportion to the difference the wine will taste tart and its good flavors will disappear. Best of all with asparagus is Condrieu, made from Viognier grapes in the northern Rhone Valley. In particular, the flavors of young Condrieu—smooth peach, a suggestion of vanilla, and something like the caramel of browned butter—merge seamlessly with those of buttered green asparagus in a union unlike almost any other in food and wine.

(The wine most often recommended with asparagus is Sauvignon Blanc, on the theory that its green-leaf and herbal flavors will echo those of the vegetable. But even the best, ripest Sauvignon from the Loire Valley is too dry for any green asparagus, and good Sauvignon has little or no such green-leaf or herbal character and none of the cat-pee aroma—no euphemism will do—that sometimes goes with it. Better than pure Sauvignon is a Bordeaux blend with Sémillon, but that still doesn't interact much with asparagus.)

Apart from the special success of Condrieu, I like not-quite-dry Loire Valley Chenin Blanc, whose aromas of delicate flowers, acacia honey, beeswax, and vanilla are coupled with a mineral taste. (Appellations include Anjou, Jasnières, Savennières, and Vouvray—the *demi-sec* is too sweet. Fully dry Chenin is less useful—with so many wines, it's frustrating not to be able to tell the sweetness from the label; you have to open the bottle and taste.) Very good *cru* Chablis, although dry and somewhat acidic, has a minerality and an aromatic richness that go well with asparagus. Riesling, the great wine grape that is overall best suited to vegetables and most widely adapted to food in general, normally has the acidity needed with green asparagus and often also the floral side, whether the bottle comes from Germany, Austria, or Alsace. The difficulty is finding a Riesling with the right low level of sugar, such as a Mosel Halbtrocken. Less common wines in the mold of floral-plus-slightly-sweet are Jurançon *sec* from southwest France and Cour-Cheverny from the central Loire. More strongly floral and also suited to asparagus are the rare examples of very ripe but only slightly sweet Alsace Pinot Blanc and Pinot Gris. Grüner Veltliner from Austria, often suggested, isn't bad, but it's not special.

My exploration has been almost entirely with green asparagus from my garden and rarely with the milder flavor of white, where one concern is to cover any bitterness. Most provocative with any kind of asparagus, and coming from deep in the realm of flowers, is dry or nearly dry Muscat and, almost as good, Gewürztraminer, both from Alsace. The rose perfume of the two wines speaks to the sweetness of just-picked asparagus, although the flavors of the wine and the vegetable don't truly interact. A still more unusual choice with asparagus, which works well for some tasters (not so much me), is the utterly dry and definitely acidic *vin jaune,* from the Jura region of France, which speaks to the slightly bitter side of green asparagus. Good Fino sherry has a similar effect.

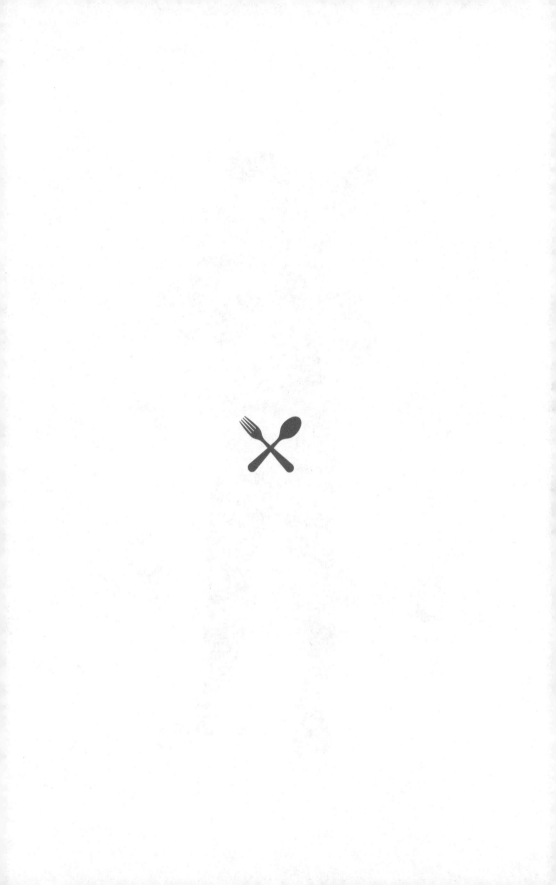

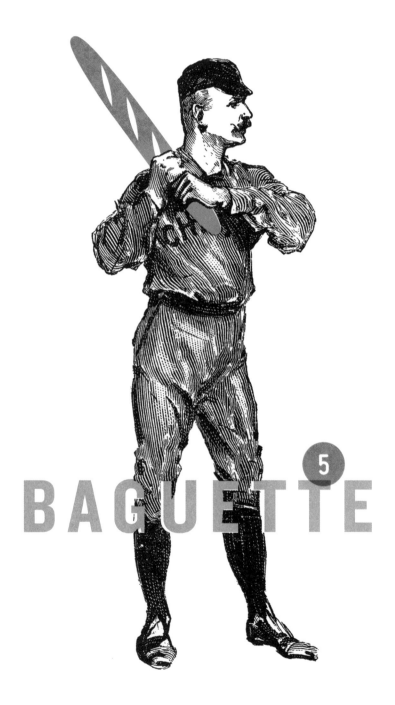

BAGUETTE 5

5. THE BAGUETTE—LONG, NARROW BREAD

Baguette means "stick." The long, narrow shape creates a high proportion of crisp, delicious, golden-brown crust, so there's crust and tender
interior in every bite. The five to seven precise slashes cut in the top
have opened in the oven and filled with crust, a phenomenon essential to
the baguette. Related French shapes—*pain parisien, bâtard, petit pain, flûte,
ficelle*—have different ratios of crust to interior. The smaller sizes react
more quickly to the oven's heat, expanding more, gaining more crust, cooking more thoroughly, each one achieving a slightly different taste. Judging
by the baguette's popularity, for most people it has the best balance between crust and interior. As you bite in and pull the bread away from your
mouth, it pulls back just a little. The cream-colored interior is well bubbled
and open—*bien alvéolé,* French bakers say. Where the crust is nutty, the
inside is buttery, eggy, subtly wheaty. But the lightness and generous
amount of crust cause the baguette to dry out and lose aroma quickly. That,
too, you might say, is part of the point. The baguette was originally a luxury; to have it at its best, you must buy it freshly baked, once, twice, three
times a day.

The dough for a classic baguette contains just white flour, water, commercial yeast, and salt—nothing else—and the method is outwardly simple.
Yet tiny differences in amounts, timing, temperature, and handling make
huge differences in flavor. The classic baguette is a test of the baker's skill,
an essay in the delicate flavor that can be drawn from white flour.

Born in Paris just after the First World War, the baguette, although
a luxury, quickly became popular. It combined a series of innovations
going back to the nineteenth century and before: efficient milling to create
plentiful white flour, commercial yeast, machine-kneading (as opposed to

hand-kneading in troughs), ovens with injected steam, the long shape, and *fermentation directe.* Those last words mean that the water, yeast, salt, and flour were mixed together all at once, a big savings in time. Previously, bakers had built up their doughs gradually, the way sourdough is still made. The baguette, urban in its lightness and refined flavor and in requiring immediate consumption, was soon copied in other French cities. But it was slow to penetrate France's towns and villages, as I was told long ago when I asked in such places, not reaching parts of the countryside until the 1970s.

There are plenty of bad baguettes—bloated, cottony, dead white inside, and filled with fine, even bubbles. Their bit of flavor comes almost entirely from the browning of the crust and vanishes within a few hours. The popularity of such cheap, airy baguettes in France peaked in the 1970s and early 80s. Then came the revival of good bread and, in the 1990s, even an official definition of *pain de tradition française.*

As every novice bread baker knows, when flour is mixed with water, the protein forms an elastic web of gluten that captures and holds the gas from fermentation: the bubbles inflate and the dough rises. North American bakers for a long time tended to believe that flour with more protein—wheat can reach 14 percent and higher—makes better bread. But if you use the more traditional methods that give the best flavor, then higher-protein flour makes tighter, more rubbery dough and denser, tougher bread. (Yes, wonderfully flavorful bread comes from high-protein durum, or semolina, flour, from its own species of wheat, but that flour behaves differently.) The relatively low-protein wheat flour traditional in France makes softer, looser dough with better flavor and texture. Softer flours are also sweeter, including those from US winter wheat and more so certain French wheats. A range of 9.5 to 10.5 percent protein might be ideal.

Some people believe that the baguettes in France are superior because French flour is superior, and that's partly right. Much bread in the US is made of bleached flour, with its doubtful advantage of whiteness. It has been artificially matured with one or another chemical to make it more elastic in bread baking (saving the two to three weeks required for the maturation to occur naturally). But bleached flour is hopelessly lacking in flavor, and it's illegal in France. Unbleached flour retains the nutty flavors associated with the yellow carotenoid pigments. Beyond any question of bleaching, both flavor and amount of protein are influenced by the variety of wheat, the growing conditions, and the milling. North American mills work faster and rougher, and slightly more bran ends up ground into the white flour, hiding its fine flavors with a subtle, almost imperceptible bitterness. Big mills in many countries divide the wheat into different streams of white flour coming from different parts of the wheat berry and having different amounts of protein, different flavors, and other qualities. In North America, those flours are sold separately, with a rather high-protein white one normally going for bread. French flour is more carefully milled, and the streams are typically combined in a single softer, more flavorful white flour. The best French flour makes baguettes with nearly cakelike aromas.

Good bread is often credited to the kind of water, but barring a few mineral extremes, the *kind* of water in truth has little effect. The *amount* does matter; the most flavorful dough contains a lot of water. The extra water doesn't create more flavor, but the looser dough stretches more easily, forming bigger bubbles that hold more aroma. Because so much flavor is trapped in the bubbles of the baked loaf, some professionals judge aroma by slicing off a section of baguette and squeezing as if they were pumping a bellows. In the pursuit of optimum texture, some bakers have adopted a nontraditional, very wet, hard-to-handle dough for baguettes, and the results can be excellent. To make this flaccid dough spring up in baking, however, they use an extra-hot oven, which can give distracting flavors. The finished baguettes tend to be more moist, so they may stay fresh a little longer.

More kneading develops more gluten, which gives a more substantial texture. But kneading also exposes the dough to air, which takes away flavor. The more you knead, the less flavor there is, and the air in the dough becomes more evenly distributed in tiny bubbles. Good kneading used to be seen as a logical compromise between a loss of flavor and a gain in interesting texture—a lighter interior, a crisper crust. But during fermentation the stretching that occurs throughout the mass of dough accomplishes much the same thing, and now many good bakers mix their dough minimally, some only enough to make sure all the flour is wet.

A relatively long, cool fermentation like that originally used in the 1920s produces more flavor, and skill really comes into play. (Only sour rye competes in difficulty, the rye process being less precarious but more complicated.) Complex transformations affect flavor as enzymes in the flour turn the starch into sugar, which the yeast turn into carbon dioxide and alcohol, and secondary fermentations produce further substances, including acids. Most mills add to their flour a little malt, a benign substance whose extra enzymes ensure the transformation into sugar. In *fermentation directe,* dough at 71 to 75 degrees F (22 to 24 degrees C) is at its peak and ready for the oven after about five hours.

(These days some misconceived baguettes are made of sourdough. The long, narrow shape doesn't allow sourdough to swell enough in the oven, and the high proportion of crust is a disadvantage, because sourdough crust tends to be tough. Sourdough is much better in a big round or oblong shape.)

Almost all baguettes today are shaped by machines that forcefully flatten the dough before they roll it up into a limp snake. The loss of aroma from squeezing out all but the smaller bubbles isn't huge, but to keep more aroma, a few French bakers take the time to shape some baguettes in the old way, by hand. Once the loaves have risen for the final time, just before they go into the oven, the tops are slashed with an extremely sharp blade.

At this moment, if all has gone well, fermentation is at its peak, with maximum sugar being created for the rapidly reproducing yeast. Inside the oven, steam—from the dough itself and from steam pipes activated by the baker—condenses on the relatively cool raw dough. The moisture speeds the penetration of heat and keeps the surface of the dough flexible long enough for the insides to expand fully, and the moisture contributes to a glossy golden crust. The penetrating warmth stimulates a final burst of fermentation, until the yeast are overcome by heat. The gas in the bubbles warms and expands, and the bread bursts outward in what's called "oven spring." As the temperature of the interior reaches almost boiling, the crumb sets. By the end of baking, complex reactions on the surface have darkened the crust, creating rich flavors in it. As the bread cools, these migrate inward, contributing a large part of the interior flavor.

In making certain foods—in roasting coffee, ripening cream, raising bread—elusive ideals of time and temperature, variable especially according to the weather, produce a leap of flavor. A baker must have a keen sensual awareness in order to know when the dough is exactly right, and no baker produces great bread every time. That comes from steady vigilance and an accumulation of items from large to very small, everything from the qualities of flour to the gentleness of the baker's touch and the exact minutes of rising. When everything comes together perfectly, you no longer perceive flour but only a transcendent taste of bread.

HOW TO BUY A BAGUETTE: Even before you smell or taste, you can predict the quality of a baguette with fair accuracy using clues of appearance. But first, if the baguettes are self-serve, pick one up and squeeze lightly to be sure it's crisp and neither light nor heavy for its size.

Shape. A flavorful baguette is somewhat swollen, but it's not a tense, airy balloon. The slashes have opened wide, almost covering the top and forming a neat interlocking row. No dough has poured like lava through a break in the crust because the dough was underrisen or there was too little steam in the oven or both. Beyond that, look for a baguette that was baked not in a perforated or wire-mesh mold but instead directly on the hearth. That allows free expansion and better bottom crust: a cross-section of the loaf shows an oval shape, and the baguette arcs and sometimes twists a little.

Crust color. A well-fermented baguette baked at just the right point of liveliness acquires a sheen and an amber color with reddish tints. The crust in the slashes is slightly paler than the rest, while the curl of the wave that forms along one side of each well-made cut is fully brown. (Sometimes you can peer beneath this edge, called *la grigne,* and see whether the texture is properly bubbled within.) Many people opt for pale crust, and some bakers undercook to please them, as well as to keep the loaves from drying out too much and to steer clear of burned ones. A slightly browner crust gives more flavor, but too much browning hides the delicate wheat and fermentation flavors that largely define the baguette.

Crust texture. A good crust shows little or no trace of flour and is visibly crackled, a result of the interior of the loaf shrinking slightly as it cools, pulling on the rigid exterior. North American baguettes and other loaves are often covered with small blisters, which come from shaping the loaves ahead and holding them under refrigeration overnight (so the baker can get some sleep). In France, the blisters are seen as a defect, though they do no harm. Once you buy and break open the loaf and see inside, an erratic mix of small to large holes doesn't guarantee full flavor, but you can't have it without them.

HOW TO STORE A BAGUETTE: A great classic baguette keeps much of its fresh flavor for half a day—you're blessed if you find such bread—but it's best eaten soon after it cools, within two or three hours. Meanwhile keep it at room temperature, either unprotected or inside the paper bag it may have come in. Slice it or any fresh bread no more than ten minutes before it will be eaten.

COMPLEMENTS TO A BAGUETTE: Bread, as good as it is on its own, almost magically makes other food taste better. It completes such foods as fresh and briefly aged cheeses and meat terrines. It reins in the intensity of cured meats and strong, mature cheeses, making them easier to taste. It improves soups and meats; it usefully gathers up sauce, making it, too, taste better. Darker bread is sometimes the best choice, but white bread, not least the baguette, is less likely to compete. While the baguette is *the* bread for the *haute* and *bourgeoise* French cooking it originally went with, it goes well with nearly every sort of savory Western food and much food from places beyond. (For decades, fine baguettes have been made and appreciated in Japan.) Butter, for reasons of texture as much as flavor, deliciously complements a baguette, but a great one is best appreciated without it.

NOTES ON WINE: Eating bread, especially white bread, with other food makes even difficult items go more easily with wine.

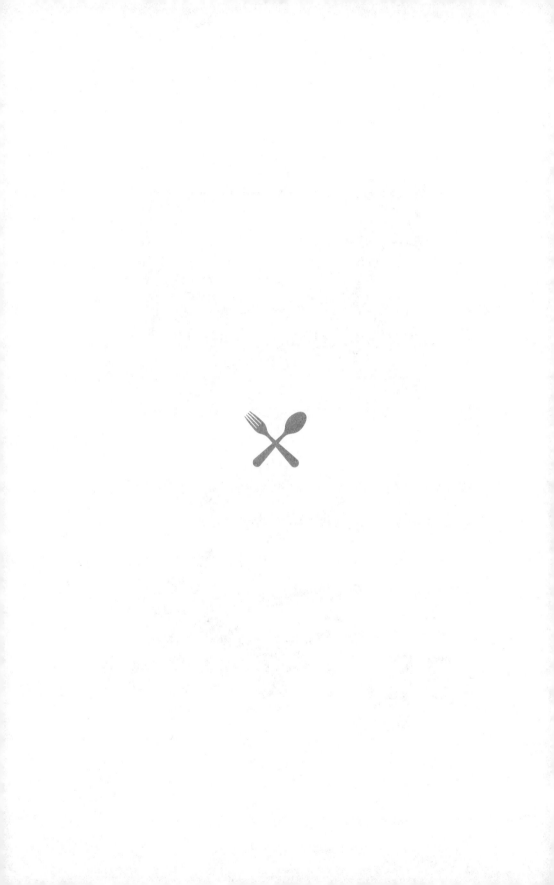

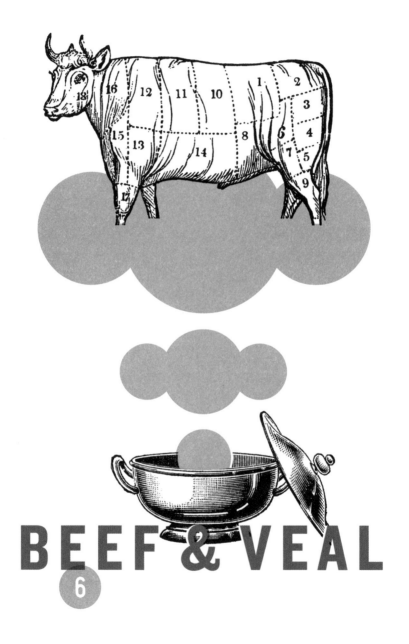

BEEF & VEAL

6

6. BEEF AND VEAL

Beef always used to be placed ahead of all other meats and by most people may still be. It provides some of the best meat flavor and most satisfying, succulent textures—in a grilled rib-eye (Delmonico) steak, a sirloin strip steak (with its varying North American names), a standing rib roast, braised oxtail, grilled hamburger, pot-au-feu, bœuf bourguignon, and Texas-style barbecued brisket. Since the 1950s, North American beef cattle, after being raised on pasture or range, have been transferred to feed-lots to fatten intensively on corn. Under the old American prime grade, the rib eye used to be intermingled with white fat and surrounded by another vast quantity of it. French chefs often used to admire American beef. Fat carries flavor; it's mainly fat that enables us to tell one kind of meat from another. Marbling tends to make beef taste beefier, it gives an impression of juiciness, and it often coincides with tenderness. Sometimes held up as the model of extreme beef goodness is the highly fatty, very marbled Wagyu beef from Japan, now also produced elsewhere, from cattle fed a very rich diet of grain and sometimes even beer. The four breeds that make Wagyu beef naturally have a high proportion of soft, unsaturated fat. (The meat is also called Kobe beef, which strictly means Wagyu beef produced in Kobe prefecture.) But if all we wanted to eat was fat, we could eat just that and ignore the lean. The fat really acts as a complement to the lean, and some lean cuts—flank steak, skirt steak, and hanger steak, to cite a trio—are highly flavorful, just as very lean game can have too much flavor. And fat isn't automatically flavorful.

The most delicious beef might be something very different from Wagyu or the old American prime meat. A timeless ideal would be tender beef, with some marbling, but much leaner overall. The cattle would be finished solely on permanent grass in a place with enough rainfall to produce fields or range heavy in nutritious plants. Cattle have stomachs with four compartments so they can digest forage. Pure grain isn't their natural food, although they tolerate it in moderation. Compared with grain, grass is easier to raise organically and sustainably (it eliminates the North American difficulty of avoiding genetically modified corn). But grass-fed beef is often lean and tough and has been criticized for having strong herbal, even gamy flavors, which professionals call "grassy," "cowy," or "milky" because they're associated with beef from dairy cows rather than beef cattle. Grass-fed beef can be terrible, but sometimes it's great. And it takes more skill to raise tender, flavorful beef on grass than it does in a feedlot.

North American beef used to taste reliably beefy, but the quality of commodity meat in supermarkets has declined. It doesn't taste like much, and to me it doesn't taste healthy. There's not much reason to care about USDA grades these days, because mass-market beef doesn't taste good no matter what. A couple of decades ago, the amount of marbling required for each of the old supermarket grades, prime, choice, and good, was reduced. "Good" was renamed "select" to promote leaner meat, and the beef in supermarkets became dramatically leaner. Now growth promotants—hormones and a muscle relaxant called beta2-adrenergic agonist—are given to the cattle to make them grow bigger faster, and they're given antibiotics to enable them to eat large amounts of corn, these days GMO corn, that would otherwise make them sick. There's now much more meat per animal, and yet the taste is meager and to me unclean. The age of a cow or steer at slaughter also makes a big difference. A century ago in France, sought-after beef was as much as five and even seven years old. In the US in the 1950s, beef from two-year-old animals was common; now it can be as little as a year old. There's no ideal, but twenty months might be a minimum for a distinct beefy taste.

Meanwhile, North Americans have been eating less beef.

Happily, new butcher shops have been opening across the United States, specializing in meat from particular farms. We're seeing a revival of careful cutting. Different countries cut their meat differently, sometimes dividing between muscles more precisely than we do in the US and creating many more cuts. In the small new butcher shops, the meat isn't graded. A customer goes by appearance but mainly on experience with the shop, what it sells, and whatever information is offered about how the meat was raised and handled. Still, we have a long way to go to achieve anything like the varied appellation and Label Rouge meats of France.

Besides the quality of the farming, the breed of cattle makes a difference, although sometimes there's more difference between individual animals than particular breeds. Some more or less familiar names are Angus, Devon, Galloway, Hereford, Highland, Piemontese, Belgian Blue, Shorthorn, Simmental, Tarentaise, and Texas Longhorn, and I've had excellent beef from most of them.

For me and many people the best beef is dry-aged, though wet-aging has been the norm since perhaps the 1970s, when butcher shops and meat counters stopped commonly receiving whole sides or quarters and instead received smaller primal cuts vacuum-sealed in plastic and shipped in cardboard boxes. Any aging takes place during the time between slaughter and retail sale. In just a few days, the meat becomes much more tender, but the changes continue after that and dry-aging can last three weeks or longer. It helps if the sides and quarters literally hang, so the muscles stretch and don't tighten. Only relatively large pieces protected by fat can be dry-aged; small pieces would dry out. Enzymes produce the tenderness, while a host of other changes heighten flavor. The changes take place faster at higher temperatures, but to avoid too much microbial growth, the meat coolers are usually set at just above freezing. In dry-aging, the meat loses a lot of moisture and weight, and depending on whether humidity is low or high, the surface either hardens or (beneficially) molds, and the outside must be trimmed and discarded. Dry-aged beef tastes nuttier and beefier. But inside the plastic, there's no loss of moisture and no waste, and some people prefer the taste of wet-aged beef, which is often described as more metallic. Other people prefer very fresh meat; Argentinians, known for their beef, don't age theirs at all.

Beef begins with a calf, which means veal. The goal in the past was to have the fat and lean of veal as close to white as possible and as tender as possible. The tactics were cruel, including separation from the mother and confinement in crates, and cruel practices continue at some producers.

Good veal, like all good meat, results from kind treatment and tends to come from organic and sustainable methods. Ideally, veal is seasonal, raised in the field during the warm months "under the mother," though outdoor exercise makes the meat a little less tender. The calves consume mostly milk and are slaughtered only when they start to eat a significant amount of grass. The meat is naturally pale, gaining color in proportion to the amount of grass the calves eat. Most of today's humane "veal," however, comes from calves that have eaten a high proportion of grass, and their meat is very pink and even red, not far from beef. Calves have been slaughtered as young as six weeks, but they are naturally weaned only when the mother is ready to bear the next calf, which may be nine months or more, and meat up to that point, if the color is light enough, may qualify as veal. Pale perfectionist veal raised "under the mother" is rare—I'm not sure I've ever had it.

Veal's utter blandness keeps it from being one of the great meats. But it's gratifyingly tender and provides a strong base for added flavors—herbs, onions, other aromatic vegetables; acidity from lemon, wine, or sorrel. A group of dishes, described in English as "veal birds," are thin scallops surrounding some sort of stuffing. Saltimbocca (though sometimes cooked flat) is one of them: the tender scallop is rolled up with a paper-thin slice of prosciutto and half a sage leaf, browned briefly in butter or olive oil, with white wine added to finish the cooking more gently and provide a sauce. Milanese osso buco, "bone with a hole," refers to the hind-shank marrow-bone and the meat around it. It's slowly braised to tenderness and served with *risotto alla milanese* (saffron risotto), along with the sauce it was cooked in (aromatic vegetables, stock, wine, optionally tomato) combined with a sprinkling of *gremolata* (grated lemon rind, parsley, and garlic). Italian-American veal parmigiana is made by dipping veal scallops in grated cheese, then egg, then breadcrumbs, and frying them, and serving the meat while the surface is crunchy.

Veal seems drier than other meats because there's no fat in the lean, but compared with them it contains more of the substance collagen, which readily dissolves into gelatin. That and the blandness make veal stock the base of all the classic French sauces for meat. Veal gives excellent sweetbreads and liver. Most calf's liver in North America is red, but the best is beige-pink. Like chicken liver, it's fried in fat, often butter, until it's colored on the surface but no more than medium-rare within, tender, having lost no juices. (The more it's cooked, the stronger it tastes.)

Increasingly, meat is reduced to retail cuts at the slaughterhouse, which eliminates the need for any skill at the butcher counter. In the United States as a rule, meat on the bone is trimmed with a power saw very close, so a rib roast looks as if it were swelling out of the bones, like a large man in a small suit. Sometimes there's so little bone that the meat topples over. And the saw leaves a white paste of bone smeared over the surface. The meat of a chop should be cut with a knife and the bone finished with a blow from a cleaver, its thickness being determined by the space between the ribs. Long ago, just before he became for a time the most famous butcher in the world, I visited the shop in Tuscany of Dario Cecchini. It was a gray November day, the shop was empty, and we asked for Chianina steaks (porterhouses, from the region's Chianina breed). Cecchini brought out a whole intact side of beef and extracted the steaks with a large knife. It was like watching two wrestlers; Cecchini was badly outweighed, but he had the advantage of skill.

Grilling over charcoal or hardwood (the latter gives a lighter taste) is hot and fast—too fast to melt tough connections or penetrate large items—and it gives smoke. (Roasting before a fire, at the front of the hearth, is slower and gives a more refined taste with no more than a hint of smoke.) The cuts of meat for grilling are tender and somewhat thin, so the inside is done before the outside burns.

Most of these tender cuts come from the less-exercised muscles of the back. They start with rib eye and sirloin strip steak (also called shell steak, New York strip, Kansas City strip) and move to other parts of the sirloin, including T-bone and porterhouse steaks. The flat-iron steak, cut from the top blade in the shoulder, is exceptionally tender and highly marbled. Generally I avoid steaks from the flavorful chuck, because some of the mixed muscles are tough and they're not equally tasty. Flank steak, skirt steak, and hanger steak are all full of flavor but tough; they're sliced thin so they seem more tender. A collection of smaller pieces, called *pièces du boucher* in French, never used to be sold on their own in the United States; *poire, merlan,* and *araignée* are set apart for special customers in France because there's only one per side.

With lean grass-fed beef, there's not enough fat to disguise dry, tough overcooking. Cooking requires close attention and careful use of heat. You begin with high-heat browning and then switch to slow cooking, so the doneness you're looking for doesn't slip by.

The many cuts of beef run further to the cheek, short ribs, and oxtail, all of them rich in fat and flavor. An oxtail is ideal for braising (and then sometimes it's cooled, breaded, and slowly grilled). A "pickled" (brined) tongue is one of the best, tastiest pieces of all. There are the several forms of beef tripe, often today made so clean that they taste almost neutral. The strong flavor of beef stock is at home in onion soup and with chicken in a pot-au-feu. Beef kidney fat has often been considered the best for frying (though there are other candidates for that).

One of the best of all beef dishes is bœuf bourguignon, especially when made with oxtail and served with the classic *bourguignon* garnish of little onions, mushrooms, and *lardons.* I always marinate the meat in red wine, though I never include raw onion. Half an hour after onions are sliced, their flavor turns crude, even in a marinade. You have to cook or serve them promptly. (It's not the exposure to air that changes them; it's breaking the cell walls so that rank sulfur compounds form.) Shallots and chives aren't as bad, but among alliums only crushed garlic belongs in a marinade.

A pot-au-feu is a fundamental dish of French family cooking; it contains mixed cuts of beef with different textures simmered in a broth of carrots, onion, celery, turnips, leeks, parsnips, and perhaps cabbage. When done, the same big pot gives soup, meat, and vegetables. The soup is served first with toasted bread and, optionally, grated cheese; then come the meat and vegetables, moistened with a little of the remaining liquid and served with potatoes, cooked separately, and with coarse salt, mustard or horse-radish, and pickles.

HOW TO BUY BEEF AND VEAL: It's best to buy beef from the farmer or rancher who raises it, or from one of the small butcher shops specializing in well-raised meats. Such a shop is likely to dry-age its beef for at least a short time. Look for beef that's at least twenty months old, finished mostly or entirely on grass. Especially in fall, look for pale veal raised outdoors with its mother on pasture.

Fresh meat is ideal, but freezing allows you to buy from a good small producer that doesn't offer fresh meat. There's some loss of juice and freshness, and the meat was probably frozen before any aging took place, but much less harm is done by freezing than by overcooking. (According to USDA research, you can thaw a one-inch-thick steak in eleven minutes in water at 102 degrees F, or 39 degrees C, and there's no more loss of juice or tenderness than if you thawed it for eighteen to twenty hours in a refrigerator.)

COMPLEMENTS TO BEEF AND VEAL: Some of the very many complements to veal are onions, shallots, garlic, olive oil, lemon juice, white wine, Marsala, fresh mushrooms, cream, green peas (which go with cream sauces in general), tomatoes, and Parmigiano-Reggiano. Excellent canned tuna goes with veal in *vitello tonnato;* saffron risotto and *gremolata* go with veal in osso buco.

Hot roast beef needs no flavoring apart from salt and pepper; it goes with accompaniments of green beans, root vegetables, and Yorkshire pudding. Cold roast beef goes with mustard, horseradish, and pickled black walnuts. Beef in general is complemented by mushrooms, black pepper, onions, garlic, parsley, anchovies, mustard, tomatoes, walnut oil, and red bell peppers. Steak goes with tarragon in béarnaise sauce; a black-pepper steak (*steak au poivre*) goes with an old-school sauce of flamed Cognac and cream. Steak goes with creamed spinach, red wine (in a pan sauce), garlic, blue cheese (mixed into butter), and plain butter on lean, unmarbled steak (actually, it's good even on marbled steak). When braised, beef goes with red wine, prunes, balsamic vinegar (added to the sauce for a braise just before serving), and hints of spice, such as in *brasato al Barolo* (with its frequent juniper, clove, and cinnamon).

NOTES ON WINE: With the mild flavor of veal, everything depends on the sauce or other accompaniments; many flavorful whites and light reds are possible. Beef almost invariably calls for red wine. (An exception is one of the concentrated Friulian or Slovenian "orange" wines, made from white varieties, which can have enough flavor and acidity to stand up to red meat.) Usually a young red wine goes with a grilled steak, something middle in weight with a braise, and a more mature bottle with roast beef. When grass-fed beef has stronger flavors that seem gamey, it suits the earthier wines often put with game, such as more substantial Burgundy and older Bordeaux, gamier bottlings of Syrah, including Australian Shiraz, traditional red Rioja, and traditional Nebbiolo.

With a grilled steak, choose medium-weight red Burgundy, such as a Volnay or other wine from the Côte de Beaune, or a predominately or entirely Merlot wine, such as Saint-Émilion or Pomerol. Clear oak flavor generally isn't flattering to food, but a grilled steak holds moderate oak in check. (The old idea was that the char of grilling would hide the bitter tannin of a young Cabernet Sauvignon, so the wine's fruit would stand out, but red wines with bitter tannin like that are all but extinct. And the survivors are good and special enough that they deserve to be aged.) The sweet-sour component of hamburger with ketchup throws off the balance of a dry wine; go with a simple, fresh fruity red with good acidity and sweet fruit—Beaujolais, a Loire Gamay, Zinfandel.

Roast beef shows off special bottles of older red wine—Bordeaux, Napa Cabernet, Burgundy, Brunello di Montalcino, traditional Rioja, and substantial mature wines from many places. In the face of the more complicated flavors inherent in most braises, especially those made with red wine, a common response is to match strength with strength and serve a big, flavorful red, such as Châteauneuf-du-Pape, Barolo, or Amarone, but those pairings turn into competitions. Better to let the braise take the lead and choose a moderate-quality, moderate-strength red, such as a Pinot Noir from Burgundy, Sancerre, Jura, or Oregon, or a Syrah from Australia, a Côtes-du-Rhône-Village, Crozes-Hermitage, or Saint-Joseph.

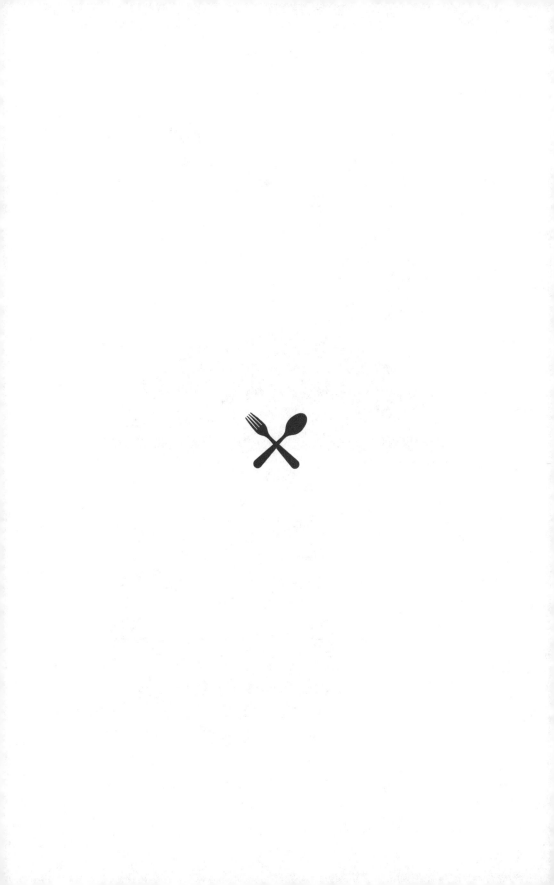

BOLETES 7

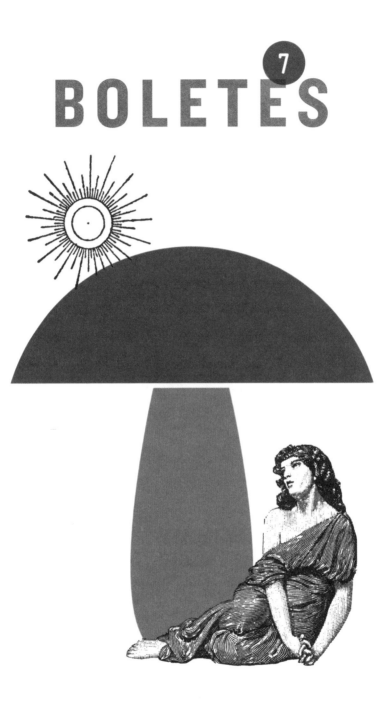

7. BOLETES

The wild *Boletus edulis,* with its bulbous cartoon shape, is the essential fungus of Western cooking—large, meaty, full of deep, earthy, woodsy flavor. It's the king bolete, sometimes known in English by the French name *cèpe* and often by the plural Italian one *porcini.* Other mushrooms are rarer or more prized, but none is more valued for adding essential mushroomness to dishes. Boletes are among the most deliciously flavorful mushrooms when fresh, and drying curiously doesn't just concentrate their flavor but intensifies it. King boletes carry their thick, wide, fawn-colored caps on fat white stems marked with irregular vertical lines, like pencil marks on coarse paper. Exceptionally in Europe, a cap reaches eight inches (twenty centimeters) across. Boletes are fairly common, popping up in the woods ten days after a rain. Some appear in spring and summer, but the big display comes in fall. Often a bolete has been nibbled by slugs and insects. The underside of the cap doesn't have the radiating gills of most mushrooms; instead, a bolete has pores, really tiny tubes, which have a spongy feel. The cap has firmer texture and better flavor; the fresh stem is just slightly stringy. Boletes are often eaten raw in salad, although even the safest mushroom is safer and more digestible when cooked.

Boletes earned their reputation in Europe, but we have them in North America, too. Ours are good, but their flavor is only a shadow of the European's. A few years ago, the California king bolete was classified more narrowly as *Boletus edulis* var. *grandedulis,* referring to its large size—the cap can be more than twice as wide as that of the European. I know the northeastern king bolete better, and it's not the best local mushroom—morels, parasols, and bearded hedgehogs (lion's mane) rank much higher. There may be more bolete potential from South America: I used to find imported ones, species unnamed, that were wonderfully flavorful and smoky, presumably dried over a fire. The world, by one count, holds nearly three hundred *Boletus* species (and there are perhaps five hundred more in other genera of the Boletaceae family), yet a mere handful are valued for their taste. In Europe four rise to the top, and in North America, where the species are less firmly identified and named, maybe five or six. On either continent, some mushroom lovers place one or two other species above the king. Then there's the influence of just where the boletes grow, including beneath what sort of tree.

Like other mushrooms that spring from the soil (as opposed to grow-ing on decaying wood), boletes live in symbiosis with the roots of certain trees, and some tree-mushroom combinations yield a much better taste. The fungi we eat are merely the fruiting bodies, the visible signs, of large perennial underground networks: mycelia, threadlike structures that digest organic matter. They coat tree roots but extend well beyond them. The mycelia provide nutrients to the trees, including nitrogen and minerals, as well as water, and in return they receive sugars from the roots. Mycelia are so important to soil and plants, not least those we eat, that some of the best farmers and gardeners no longer turn their soil unless doing so is required to sow a crop. Plowing breaks the threads of the mycelia (and damages the soil structure); in your garden, shallow hoeing to eliminate weeds is enough.

No bolete is commonly fatal, but some—such as the white-capped *B. satanus,* with its red pores and stem—can make you very ill. If you bruise certain boletes, including a few edible ones, they turn a disconcerting blue. When in doubt about species, mushroomers often slice a bolete cleanly in two, top to bottom, to see whether the white interior changes color; the blue of some spreads like a stain from the underside of the cap down the stem.

Often within a language, a species has more than one common name, even many names. You can tell something by color, but generalizations have exceptions, and colors darken as a bolete matures. The complicated bolete family tree is still evolving, including the relationships of similar European and North American species. And in different regions of North America, apparently similar species may not be identical. On either side of the Atlan-tic, experts are unsure about many details of habitat, distribution, and season. Boletes sold as *edulis,* knowingly or unknowingly, may belong to other, similar species.

By consensus, the four tastiest European boletes are:

The summer cèpe, *B. reticulatus* (formerly *aestivalis,* in Italian *porcino estivo,* in French *cèpe d'été*), has a light brown cap and stem. The pores beneath the cap, as in other top boletes, are white when the mushroom is young, then cream-colored, and as the mushroom goes into decline they darken further, eventually becoming olivey. The summer cèpe grows variously under oaks, beeches, chestnuts, and other trees. Of the top European boletes, it is usually considered to have the least interesting flavor, yet that may depend on the part of Europe where it grows.

The pine bolete, *B. pinophilus* (in Italian *porcino rosso,* in French *cèpe des pins*), has a browner cap than the king. The stem, much lighter than the cap, is typically more swollen than that of the king. The pine bolete, commonly found under pines, is rarer than *edulis* and not as good.

The king bolete, *B. edulis* (in Italian *porcino,* in French *cèpe de Bordeaux*), has a cap whose color ranges from beige to chestnut, darkening with age to gray with violet; the swollen stem is white with gray. The insides, when cut, sometimes change color a little, to tan. The king bolete grows under oaks, chestnuts, beeches, spruce, and silver fir. When dried, it has the best flavor of any bolete.

B. aereus (in Italian *porcino nero,* in French *tête de nègre*) has no common English name. Its cap is brown or gray, darker than that of the king, and the stem is typically light brown. Although *aereus* are found under beeches, the best are said to grow under oaks. Scarcer than kings, they're often considered to have superior flavor.

In California, boletes have been examined more closely than they have in most other areas of the US, because the state is big, with so much conducive terrain and so many interested chefs and eaters. There the top five edible boletes are:

The spring king, *B. rex-veris* (formerly considered the same as European *pinophilus*), appears in the Sierras in late May or early June, at the end of morel season, growing under conifers, such as lodgepole pine. The cap, nearly white at first, turns pinkish tan, olive, and brown; the stems are white. The spring king is firmer than the king and tends to be less buggy, so some mushroomers prefer it.

The white king bolete, *Boletus barrowsii,* grows mainly in Arizona and New Mexico, under ponderosa pines; but the range extends into Colorado, under spruce and fir, and into southern California, under live oaks (it's found as far north as Lake Tahoe). Long thought to be a form of *edulis,* this bolete has an unusual white cap sitting on a white stem. According to the late Chuck Barrows, for whom the species is named, the white king bolete is the most delicious North American bolete. Others, less partisan, praise it but compare it with the spring king, which has a lesser flavor.

The king bolete of the West Coast, *Boletus edulis* var. *grandedulis,* looks like the European one, except that it can grow more than twice as large, the cap reaching nearly twenty inches (fifty centimeters) across. Near the coast, the king grows under Bishop and other pines and Douglas fir; inland it grows at higher elevations, under pines and firs. In fall the king can be particularly buggy, but some consider it to have the best flavor of all North American boletes, and it's universally regarded as the best when dried.

The butter bolete, *B. appendiculatus* (for now considered the same as European *B. appendiculatus*), has a firmer texture than *edulis*'s. The cap is pale yellowish when young, becoming brown or red-brown with age. When bruised or sliced, the pale yellow interior sometimes but not always slowly turns blue. Less common than *edulis,* the butter bolete appears in the high Sierras in May and June, under conifers, especially Ponderosa pine, but it's also found under hardwoods, including oaks. For flavor and texture, it's the favorite bolete of some California mushroomers.

The queen bolete, *B. regineus* (formerly considered the same as European *B. aereus*), is closely related to the king. It has a similar tan cap and dirty white stem, but the young queen bolete is covered with a white bloom, and the edge of the cap curls in over the edge of the pores. When *regineus* is cut, the interior darkens slightly. The queen bolete appears in fall on the coast and in the Sierras, and where *edulis* grows among pines, *regineus* grows in both deciduous and coniferous forests. Some California mushroomers, perhaps most, place the queen at the top in taste.

Boletes newly sprung from the earth are smaller, firmer, and less likely to have been nibbled on or bored into. The worms work their way up the stem and then into the cap, which is more often sound. Older boletes have usually been sampled by wild creatures, but they're bigger, and if they're not too old and the damage is mild, there's no reason to shun them.

A pure fresh taste comes from steaming whole boletes inside tight paper or foil with nothing more than salt, though the texture becomes very soft. Sautéing in oil or butter adds firmness and heightens the flavor. A large, oiled cap grilled over coals is similarly firm and even more delicious. The caps can also be stuffed and baked (filled, for instance, with a mixture of breadcrumbs, onion cooked in fat, grating cheese, parsley, and raw egg to hold it together, with butter or oil on top to ensure crunch). Boletes go easily with lots of other foods, adding flavor to pasta, risotto, polenta, potatoes. Dishes called *cacciatora* or *chasseur* are "hunter style," which can mean many different things, but often the first, and always the second, includes mushrooms.

HOW TO BUY AND KEEP FRESH BOLETES: Any fresh mushroom has a short life. Buy the freshest boletes you can find and the least nibbled on, meaning as a rule younger and smaller. If you can't firmly identify the species, which with boletes isn't necessarily easy, find a trustworthy seller. If you have to keep boletes for a day or two, then remove any slugs or insects, pare away the dirt-encrusted base of the stem, and put them in a paper bag in the refrigerator, which allows some of the moisture to evaporate rather than cause decay. Before use, carefully remove all other dirt with a brush or a damp cloth. Rinse mushrooms only if they're very dirty, because they absorb water, which dilutes flavor and makes sautéing difficult. You can dry thinly sliced boletes easily on the shelves of an electric dehydrator; in some places, they're still dried in the sun.

HOW TO BUY, STORE, AND USE DRIED BOLETES: Inside their clear plastic packages, lighter-colored dried boletes are more likely to be *B. edulis* and therefore more flavorful. But a lighter color also comes from commercial hot-air drying, which may be too fast for the complete change in aroma that occurs during drying. Old-fashioned slow drying, outdoors or indoors, produces a darker bolete that may have a stronger aroma. Maybe it's coincidence, but really flavorful dried boletes also seem to come in mostly whole pieces and to be free of tiny wormholes, although those boletes are more expensive (and some holes are acceptable). The best and cleanest dried boletes I've bought were in Italy, where there's generally a strong correlation between quality and price, and there you can buy a big package of them at a much lower price than you'd pay at home. They keep for months in a glass jar in the freezer. (At the small central market in Cannes, I once bought dried cèpes labeled "*Boletus edulis, pinophilus*" and "Qualité II." The seller advised me that they were untreated and should be stored in the freezer to prevent insect damage. I resisted the idea, and some weeks later, when I took the jar down from its shelf, insects had appeared and gone to work.) Depending on where you are, boletes, fresh and dried, also come from Eastern Europe and China, and it's not always clear what the species are.

A 25-gram packet of good dried Italian porcini, depending on how intense a flavor you want, serves three or four people in a sauce for pasta or in a risotto. Don't rinse the dried mushrooms unless they're very dirty. Pour boiling water over them and let them soak for at least half an hour. The texture of the rehydrated caps isn't bad, but the stems are stringy and I don't serve them. (I freeze them and then add them when I make stock.) The main point of dried boletes is the soaking liquid. Drain it through a kitchen cloth to remove grit, and add it to whatever you please.

COMPLEMENTS TO BOLETES: Boletes sautéed in olive oil or butter don't need anything more than salt and possibly pepper, but they're good topped with a little chopped raw garlic and parsley. With or without, they go with any meat. They're good, too, with the flavors of cooked onions, ham, and Parmigiano, though too much of either of the last two distracts. Cream is excellent in a bolete soup or sauce, as are meat juices or stock, a large spoonful or more of tomato, Madeira, the acidity and flavor of white wine, an almost imperceptible amount of sherry vinegar, or (sometimes also) a final squeeze of lemon juice. Asparagus provides a counterpoint to sautéed boletes, as do zucchini, spinach, and eggs.

NOTES ON WINE: Like so many other foods, boletes are best with a white or a light red wine free of oak, including Chardonnay from various parts of the world. Among reds, boletes go with good Burgundy, especially more earthy bottlings. They go with Pinot Noir from Oregon, traditionally made Nebbiolo from Piedmont and Rioja from Spain, and the Merlot-dominated Bordeaux of Saint-Émilion and Pomerol.

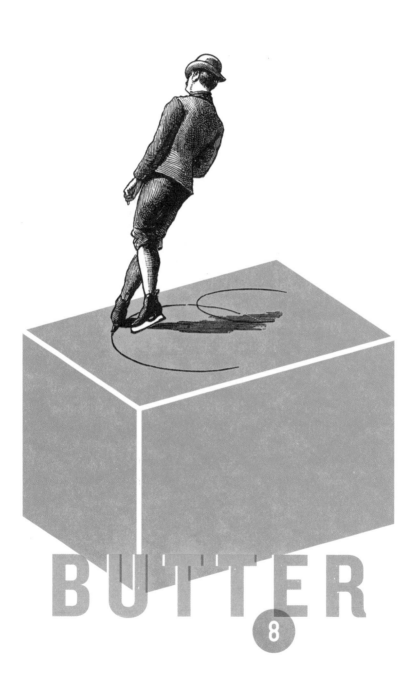

BUTTER

8

The best butter is exquisitely fresh, delicate in aroma, with a clear dairy taste. The most demanding French pâtissiers buy butter no more than a week old and use it within a week. Butter preserves dairy fat for a time because the readily spoiled watery part of cream has been eliminated. But fat absorbs whatever odors are around it, so butter is vulnerable, easily overwhelmed by off-flavors. From either the cream or the process, I've found unpleasant flavors of canned corn, sharp supermarket sour cream, and barnyard (probably from an unclean barn or what the cows ate). And the fat in butter gradually turns rancid. The only desirable ingredient, apart from cream and perhaps salt, is a culture to ripen the cream before it's churned and create a stronger dairy flavor. Raw cream gives the finest taste, though it takes experience to tell the difference: raw-cream butter is sweeter and faintly flowery. But with the prevailing regulations, you're unlikely to taste raw-cream butter in the US unless you buy cream directly from a farm and churn it yourself. Most butter is made from pasteurized cream, which has cooked, caramel flavors. And the butter in supermarkets often suffers from poor wrapping, old age, or both, so the quality of the cream and the methods used hardly matter. When you slice through a stick, you often see that the pale interior is surrounded by a halo of darker yellow fat, where the butter has dried out and gained a rancid taste. Butter's only defense, besides cold, is an impermeable wrapper, which it doesn't always have. On the tongue, butter is luscious because it melts at just below body temperature, between 90 and 96 degrees F (32 to 36 degrees C), depending on its precise mix of fats. As it melts, it should taste not just fresh but smooth, creamy, and light. The best process is minimal, involving nothing at all extraneous to butter. As Soyoung Scanlan, a California cheesemaker and butter-maker, once said to me, "Buttermaking is simple, so it can be very difficult."

The most flavorful butter of the year comes from cows (or goats, ewes, water buffalo) on spring pasture. A sign of the season is yellower butter. The deeper color comes from more carotene, which is hidden in the lush plants by the powerful green of chlorophyll. It happens that the fat from cows on pasture is also less saturated, which makes softer butter. The flavor can be affected by the particular soil and plants. Different breeds don't give different flavors to butter, but the most intense, eerie-looking yellow color comes from Jersey and Guernsey cows. (And because of the mix of fats they contain, their butter is a little harder at room temperature.) Mass-market butter typically contains added color so it looks the same year-round, and, at least in the US, coloring isn't required to be listed as an ingredient.

The best cream is perfectly clean and fresh, promptly separated from the milk. And no matter how good the cream, the flavor of butter is subtle by nature unless the cream is first ripened—soured, like crème fraîche—to give a slight tang and a more intensely buttery, rich dairy aroma, sometimes described as hazelnut. The acidity that gives the tang also helps to protect the butter against spoilage. The bacteria used to be part of the benign contamination of the barn, equipment, and creamery, but in today's clean dairy environment a culture must be added. Ripening, accomplished by various lactic bacteria, takes twelve hours or more at approximately room temperature. Otherwise, during the time before churning, the cream should be deeply chilled. Cultured butter—from ripened cream—is common in Europe, but in the US only unsalted butter is normally cultured, and because ripening takes time, most US producers of unsalted butter skip the ripening and simply add flavoring, which is a "starter distillate" made from cultured skim milk and containing diacetyl, the chief natural flavoring substance in butter. I'd like to criticize the taste from this shortcut, but actually it's good. It's often said that European "cultured" butter has more flavor than US brands, but when I've tasted them blind side by side, one sort wasn't markedly tarter or stronger in flavor than the other.

Butter is all too easy to make, as you know if you've ever whipped cream a few seconds too long and found it had turned grainy with fat. Hand-churning and the continuous machine process work on the same principle. Mechanical action breaks many of the globules of fat, which begin to stick together in grains, and those gradually form balls. As the fat comes together, it releases buttermilk, the watery portion of the cream, which is later poured off. (That's true buttermilk, as opposed to the cultured skim milk usually sold as buttermilk.) Homemade butter is kneaded in cold water using two hands or a paddle, and commercial dairies once did, and perhaps a few still do, "wash" their butter several times. That gets rid of the remaining traces of buttermilk, which would lead more quickly to spoilage, though too much washing makes the flavor flat. The new butter is further worked—not too much or it becomes greasy—to give it an even consistency and, in the case of homemade butter, to expel the drops of water that aren't mixed invisibly with the fat. (Where cream is an emulsion of fat in water, butter is an emulsion of water in fat.) From about 12 to 18 percent water remains in butter. A century ago, US butter contained more fat, sometimes much more, than it typically does today. Current technology allows a larger proportion of water to remain suspended, and butter can have the US federal minimum of 80 percent fat (the EU requires a more natural 82 percent). The rest is water and about 2 percent nonfat solids. When butter is "wetter"—larger droplets of water remain in emulsion—it's easier to perceive the flavor, which is of course a good thing.

Cold butter, when you cut it, should be firm and yet plastic. The firmness comes from the fat outside the globules. It crystallizes when the cream is cooled to 35 to 40 degrees F (2 to 4 degrees C) for four to twenty-four hours before churning, and it crystallizes further when the finished butter is cooled after churning. If more fat globules are broken, there's more fat available for crystallization; faster cooling to a lower temperature also makes harder, flakier butter. Winter butter is more brittle, harder to spread. Summer butter from cows on pasture is softer. But the texture can be made the same year-round by adjusting the crystallization of fat. (My own preference is for seasonal variation.) Between the extremes of waxy and soft lies the most exquisite texture.

Salt improves the flavor of merely satisfactory butter. It was originally added as a preservative. It dissolves in the butter's water, and if the brine that forms is strong enough, spoilage organisms can't work. Where once butter had 2 to 3 percent or even more salt, it now commonly contains

1 percent or a little more. The French generally prefer unsalted butter, but the butter from Brittany, on France's Atlantic coast, is piquant with salt, so much so that, if you aren't used to it, the saltiness can overshadow the rest of the taste. Breton salted butter can be fresh and superb, but in most parts of the world the best cream is reserved for unsalted butter.

"Dry" butter—sold at a premium, especially for pastry—is a little higher in fat, which makes it harder when cold and allows more distinct and flaky layers in pastry. But it's easier to produce a crisp, light texture with other fats—lard and Crisco-type shortening. They contain no water, melt at higher temperatures, and have other properties that keep the flour-water part of the dough better separated, whether tiny fragments in a sandy crust, thin pieces in a flaky crust, or the paper-thin layers of puff pastry. The industrial shortenings contain partially hydrogenated fat, which is less susceptible to oxidation and requires much less skill to produce a more tender, crisp, flaky crust. These fats can be so intensely fatty that they're hard to wash off your hands, even with hot water and detergent, and like lard they're greasy in the mouth. The industrial fats have no particular flavor, but home-rendered lard adds some porky flavor, which is good in savory pies. I like a lard crust (the crispest is made with leaf lard from around the kidneys), but to me, even if butter is trickier to work with, its flavor makes it far superior in pastry.

If you cook butter before using it, the color turns golden and then brown (classic French *beurre noisette* and *beurre noir*) and the taste becomes nutty. When you put butter into a hot pan, it foams as the water boils away and gets steadily hotter until it starts to brown and smoke at around 250 degrees F (120 degrees C), so if you fry in it, you risk a scorched taste. You have to clarify butter first: heating it, skimming off the foam, then decanting the clear fat and leaving behind the solids that would burn. Ghee, the brown, nutty clarified butter used in Indian cooking, is made from sour milk or ripened cream that is cooked until golden and then separated. Clarified butter and ghee smoke at around 400 degrees F (200 degrees C), roughly the same as lard and fresh olive oil.

Butter tastes best, however, when it isn't cooked to an oily state. Pieces whisked into a sauce, for instance, add the good qualities of butter almost without your being aware of it. There's no more flattering complement to other foods.

HOW TO BUY AND STORE BUTTER: You can find delicious butter even in North America, where little if any of the butter in stores is impeccably fresh and the variation in freshness can be extreme from brand to brand. Look for a wrapper that bars oxygen, light, and outside aroma—paper-lined foil or a special barrier film, which confusingly looks like paper. Choose, if you can find it, butter that contains only cream, culture, and, optionally, salt. Unless you know otherwise, the overwhelming likelihood is that unsalted butter will be fresher. Only if the butter tastes fresh and clean does it matter whether the cows were on pasture, the cream was raw, or the butter is otherwise special. If you have ready access to fresh butter, buy only as much as you will use in a week; raw-cream butter is especially delicate and vulnerable and should be eaten quickly. (When the fat globules are broken during churning, enzymes are released that cause rancidity; one advantage to pasteurization is that it destroys them.) Butter of any kind should have an even color throughout, and the taste should be clean and delicate. Keep butter cold and away from light and air. For longer storage, you can further seal the butter inside its wrapper with a layer of aluminum foil (avoid direct contact of butter with metal) and freeze it. But mostly, for immediate use, I discard the wrapper and put butter in the refrigerator in a glass dish with a glass cover, which is fine for a few days.

COMPLEMENTS TO BUTTER: Fats are chameleons, and butter allies itself with most foods, while they in turn complement butter. Two standouts are fresh bread and scrambled eggs. (Butter is brilliant in brioche, a form of bread that incorporates eggs and butter to maximum effect.) A different sort of combination is crisp raw radishes eaten French-style, with unsalted butter, coarse sea salt, and bread that's either fully dark or tan from flour containing a portion of bran. Lemon juice is a particular kind of complement to butter, in that a squeeze counters any heaviness.

NOTES ON WINE: The reflexive choice with buttery food, such as fish in a butter sauce, is a buttery-tasting Chardonnay, but don't opt for a very rich one. Other white wines that flatter butter include Condrieu, Loire Chenin Blanc, and the richest versions of Sancerre. When *beurre blanc*—the wonderful creamlike, not-quite-warm Loire Valley sauce, containing mostly butter—is served with a lean poached fish, one option is Coteaux du Layon (sweet Chenin Blanc), which has enough acidity to counter both the wine's sugar and the butter's richness. When *beurre blanc* is served with salmon, a better choice is Savennières (dry, mineral Chenin Blanc).

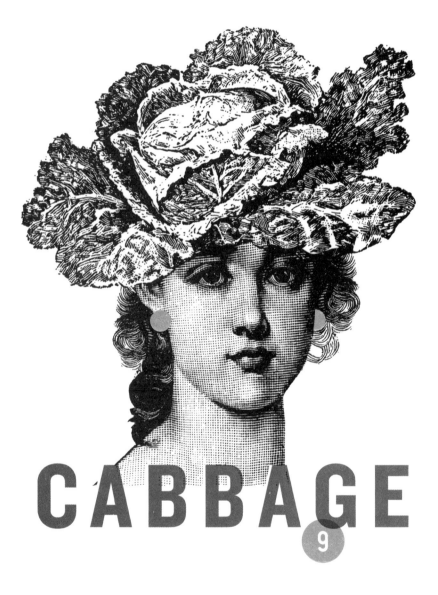

CABBAGE
9

9. CABBAGE

C abbage always tastes at least a little sweet and, when cooked, satisfyingly rich with its sulfurous edge. Easily grown to a large size and stored, cabbage is an old food of the poor, especially when cooked in flavorful soups that can form the heart of a meal. And yet cabbage belongs to haute cuisine, too, in soup, braised, or stuffed, just as in humbler cooking. Meaty stuffings of whatever kind turn cabbage into a substantial main course. Familiar green cabbage is *Brassica oleracea,* a species that also embraces broccoli, cauliflower, kale, Brussels sprouts, and Chinese kale (kai-lan). The broad cabbage family extends to further species and includes white turnips, mustard, and rocket (arugula). You may hardly be conscious of it, but raw cabbage has some of the same sweet pepperiness you find in rocket, garden cress, a new radish—all members of the big cabbage family. Less-evolved relatives, such as collards and kale, turn sweeter and less bitter after they're touched by frost, but the heading cabbages have been selected over centuries for sweetness. Cooked cabbage is savory but not far from the border with sweet. Cooked cabbage likes onions and garlic and has an affinity for chestnuts; red cabbage likes those as well as apples. Like other brassicas, cabbage echoes the rich, often faintly sweet taste of pork. Even better with cabbage is partridge, when the two are braised together in the great French dish *perdrix aux choux.* In a very different direction, the sugar in cabbage with an addition of salt allows the vegetable to ferment and achieve the tart zing of sauerkraut or kimchi (though the cabbage in the latter comes from a different species, *B. rapa*). In a mild climate, the cabbage season runs nearly year-round, starting with the small new heads of late spring and continuing through the large heads of summer, fall, and then, from the cellar, winter.

Familiar cabbage comes in hard heads—closed so tight that sunlight doesn't penetrate and the insides are nearly white—good keepers, but not necessarily the best in taste. The sweetest, most delicate, least sulfurous cabbage is savoy. Its crinkled, greener, thinner leaves form looser heads. We call it savoy because the type originated in the historical region of Savoy, once part of Italy and today belonging to France. Savoy cabbage is usually called *cavolo verza* in Italian, but also *cavolo di Savoia* and *cavolo di Milano,* the last for its popularity in that city's cooking. The famous Milanese cabbage dish is *casoeûla,* which includes braised pig's ears, tail, feet, rind, and ribs. Savoy comes in a number of varieties, of which the best US one, introduced in 1938, may be Chieftain.

Red cabbage doesn't taste very different from green. The many sweet-and-sour recipes for it are probably a reaction to the color. To keep the red from turning grayish-blue in cooking, which happens especially if you use hard water, cooks add something acidic, such as apples, wine, or vinegar, especially red-wine vinegar, which provides a trace of color of its own. The acidity reacts with the cabbage's pigments to create a strong, appealing red and, with the vegetable's sweetness, makes a sweet-and-sour effect.

As for cooking green cabbage, the cleanest, freshest flavor, the sweetest taste, and the brightest green come from a quick, hard boiling in plenty of water. I like full cooking to tenderness, but longer cooking comes with a sacrifice: the more you cook cabbage, the more you bring out the sulfur. Old French recipes call for changing the water and for cooking the vegetable almost to purée. However, one excellent old, minimalist cabbage dish, *chouée,* from the French province of Poitou, doesn't automatically call for overcooking. It's like some versions of Irish colcannon. The hot cabbage, cooked just until tender, is mashed to a purée, anywhere from rough to smooth, along with one part butter to perhaps eight of cooked cabbage and up to an equal amount of boiled potato. The butter gives *chouée* a surprisingly refined flavor.

Cabbage leaves are an inevitable wrapping in many countries for all sorts of foods, as in Russian *golubtsy,* Polish *gołąbki,* Hungarian *töltött káposzta,* German *Kohlrouladen,* and the sour-cabbage wrappings of southeastern Europe. In Italy, *involtini* or *cavoli ripieni* appear in variations in most regions, making it one of the rare national dishes, according to Slow Food's impeccable *Dizionario delle Cucine Regionali Italiane.* The leaves are typically filled with chopped beef or pork, egg, breadcrumbs, ewe's-milk cheese, and spices, then in winter baked in *ragù* and in summer in a simple tomato sauce. In France, *chou farci,* "stuffed cabbage," although most appreciated in the southwest, is also a national dish. It takes the form of individual leaves or hollowed-out whole heads, and the stuffing possibilities include sausage meat and chestnuts.

When you eat raw cabbage in salad, to make it more tender and avoid a watery dressing, mix the finely shredded raw head, green or red, with vinegar and salt, leave it for an hour, pour off the liquid, and season again with more vinegar or lemon juice, along with salt, olive oil, and a little finely chopped onion or whatever you choose (garlic, crushed cumin, almonds, sesame oil, cilantro). Even with the raw onion, which in most uses turns foul-smelling within an hour, the salad keeps for a day or two, while the cabbage becomes more peppery. Some people add mustard, but most heads have distinct pepper without it. When I don't use a vinaigrette, I prefer thick cream to mayonnaise. Besides raw cabbage salad, there's warm Alsatian semicooked cabbage salad: the shredded head is cooked in vinegar but retains a crunch, then it's seasoned and dressed with crisp sticks of bacon along with their rendered fat.

The best sauerkraut is made after the September-October harvest, when the heads are in peak condition and cool weather keeps the fermentation cool. The shredded cabbage is packed with salt, nothing else, in a crock or a barrel. The salt draws water from the vegetable to form a brine, and a stone-weighted plate or board placed on top ensures that the vegetable is immersed. Wild lactic bacteria then turn the vegetable's sugar into lactic acid and carbon dioxide. The salt discourages spoilage while it favors good bacteria (a series of different ones act as the acidity rises), and it captures some of the crunch of the raw cabbage. The fermentation may continue slowly for a very long time, but after about three weeks it's mostly done and the sauerkraut is ready to eat.

The raw sauerkraut, especially during the first months, tastes faintly to strongly prickly from carbon dioxide; it has a firm crunch and a bright, fresh tartness. The taste is refreshing and delicious as is. And, preserved by salt and acidity, sauerkraut keeps for months. What you gain from cooking it, generally with other ingredients, is rich melded flavors. As sauerkraut grows old, the flavor can veer off in a more rank direction, and then it's better rinsed and cooked. Similarly, sauerkraut cooked for any length of time smells and tastes more sulfurous. Most of the sauerkraut for sale, strangely, has been preserved twice, first by fermentation and then a second time by pasteurization, which replaces the raw taste and texture with a cooked one—the flavor is never very good. But certain stores sell delicious raw sauerkraut in refrigerated jars.

Fermented vegetables, not least those from the cabbage family, reach their highest level in the many varieties of kimchi. During the warm half of the year, Koreans traditionally make kimchi fresh and begin to eat it after a few days, consuming it within a month. In November, for winter, they typically prepare large amounts of what's called *kimjang* kimchi, which has more varied flavorings, and they eat it over the next months until warmer weather brings fresh vegetables again.

HOW TO BUY AND STORE CABBAGE AND SAUERKRAUT: Heads of regular cabbage, green or red, should be tight and feel hard and dense, heavy for their size, with no sign of mold or cracking (usually caused by swelling after too much rainfall). Freshly harvested cabbage is excellent from its first youth through maturity, and it stores well—under ideal conditions, for months. Even when the outer leaves look tired, the inside of a head usually remains in good condition. In contrast with regular cabbage, the ruffled heads of savoy, common from mid-fall through late winter, feel almost airy. More than regular cabbage, they should look as if they were still growing— where regular tight heads keep well, savoy starts to wilt within days. With any kind of cabbage, refrigeration and high humidity help to hold sweetness and flavor. The ideal storage temperature is precisely freezing, since cabbage freezes a degree below that.

Sauerkraut is best as soon as the fermentation is mostly complete. In cool climates, the season lasts from October through May—longer if the cabbage is stored and then fermented during the winter. Look for raw sauerkraut from a skilled organic producer, preferably a local one in the hope the sauerkraut will be fresher. Keep it refrigerated in a jar with a loose lid, so that carbon dioxide from any continuing fermentation can escape. If the sauerkraut tastes very salty or sharply acidic, then before you eat it raw, as is, drain it, rinse it, and drain again. And when you cook sauerkraut, according to its taste and yours, boil it in its own juice or else rinse it first and then cook it in a little fresh water; doneness depends on how firm or soft you like it. Drain and serve.

COMPLEMENTS TO CABBAGE AND SAUERKRAUT: The prime complement to cooked cabbage is butter. (You may immediately answer that butter goes with everything, but sweet butter has a particular affinity for the sweetness of cooked cabbage.) Alternatively, the savory, rich side of cabbage responds to goose or duck fat as well as to onions, garlic, and chestnuts. Red cabbage is good with any or all of them. It goes especially with game and fatty meats—duck, goose, pork, including any of them in the form of sausage. Cabbage of any sort—the whole family—goes with cured pork and cured beef (green cabbage is of course typical with corned beef). Cabbage also goes with tripe, and it forms a classic combination with partridge. Cabbage goes readily with potato, with shellfish (as in some Chinese *shumai* dumplings), and with egg in Japanese *okonomiyaki* (a sort of savory pancake). Sauerkraut is good cooked with a little chopped onion (first cooked gently in fat), white wine, sometimes juniper (for me, not caraway). And sauerkraut, with its salt and acidity, likes the same fats and fatty meats as other cabbage does, including the pork components of a *choucroute garnie.*

NOTES ON WINE: Cabbage, apart from sauerkraut, rarely dominates a dish enough to determine the choice of wine, but the sweetness of *chouée* (cabbage-butter-potato purée) suits barely sweet Chenin Blanc from the same region (the appellations include Anjou and the often finer Savennières), and Chenin goes with the white meats often served with cabbage.

Riesling is at least an equally good complement. Sauerkraut is hard on wine, but with the pork of *choucroute garnie,* the potential conflict is short-circuited by an aromatic Alsace Muscat or Gewürztraminer, in dry or nearly dry versions. (Muscat is often confined to use as an apéritif or dessert wine, but in Alsace it's an old option with three diverse foods: *choucroute garnie,* asparagus, and Munster cheese.)

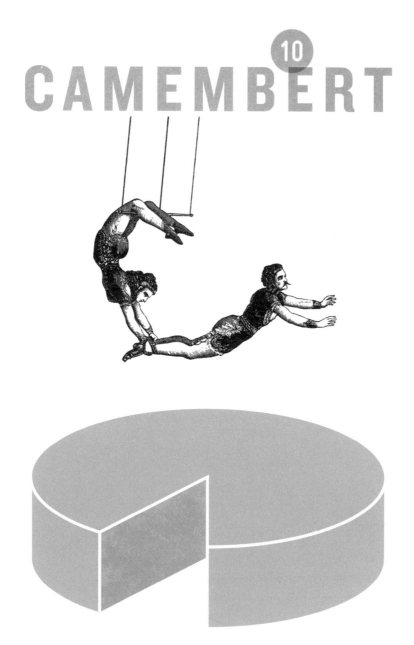

10. CAMEMBERT AND OTHER COW'S-MILK CHEESES THAT TURN CREAMY FROM THE OUTSIDE IN

Camembert can seem less a food that exists than one that lives in imagination, or perhaps memory. Of course, it *does* exist, and in very large quantities. One million Camemberts are said to be eaten each day in France. But can you find one with the taste evoked by the name? Wherever you live, ask your cheesemonger, "What's really good right now?" and the chances are almost zero that he or she will answer, "Camembert." When I called one of the more serious US retailers and tried to order one, the closest they could come was a ripe Coulommiers, which is a larger, thicker cheese from a different part of France. I turned to a cheese book by an important London seller with good access to French cheeses to see what she had to say, and she said nothing whatsoever about Camembert. She left it out. Twenty years ago, when Pierre Boisard published a widely noticed book, *Le Camembert, Mythe National,* he found only a single true artisan making the cheese; large-scale producers had taken over, the tail end of a long process. Today, like many cheeses, Camembert is covered with an all-white laboratory strain of *Penicillium candidum* mold. And where many French cheeses at their best are made from raw milk on farms, almost all Camembert is made from pasteurized milk, with an emphasis on control, safety, and durability. The most industrial Camembert has a thick plastic texture and a boring, invariable taste. The poet Léon-Paul Fargue famously compared Camembert with "the feet of God." But too often now His feet are very clean. And yet some producers do use raw milk, some large producers have a more handcrafted line, and even some pasteurized-milk

Camembert is made using relatively craftlike methods. It's possible to find a good, well-ripened cheese.

Camembert originated in the Pays d'Auge of Normandy. The often-told story is that it was invented in 1791 by Marie Harel in the village of Vimoutiers, four kilometers from the village of Camembert. A priest from Brie, a region just southeast of Paris, fleeing the Revolutionaries, is said to have given her the recipe, which was presumably for a very wide, thin disk of Brie. But there are earlier references to cheeses from Camembert, and the area had at least one additional cheese, Livarot, named for a village north of Vimoutiers and still widely appreciated. Possibly Harel was an innovator who followed the priest's recipe for Brie but put the cheese into the much smaller mold used for Livarot. Where the latter is a smelly washed-rind cheese, however, Brie has a *croûte fleurie,* a "flowering crust," or "bloomy rind" as we usually say in English. Not too far away, another stinky cheese, Pont l'Évêque, was made—Normandy may have been the land of stinky cheeses. We can't know for certain, because there are few early mentions of particular cheeses, and there is almost never any description. Still, what set the early Camembert apart and made it special may have been its combination of creaminess and bloomy rind.

National fame came to Camembert about 125 years ago when several things happened: the railroad from Normandy to Paris opened, yields of milk climbed, and the soft, vulnerable cheese was put into a lightweight wooden box with a colorful label—a marketing inspiration of around 1890. Sales and production surged. The cheese that became widely beloved was mass market from the start, and delicious, or it wouldn't have succeeded. The appeal in France and throughout the world was the creaminess coupled with a mild, earthy aroma. The small cheese, safe in its box, was also easy to ship, so there was less loss and perhaps a lower price.

In simple prosaic terms, cheese is milk that has been acidified, dehydrated, and salted—preserved. The quality of the cheese naturally depends heavily on the quality of the milk. If that's somewhat higher in protein and fat, for instance, the cheese has richer texture. Raw milk supplies essential wild microorganisms, picked up as benign contamination. Raw milk also gives better texture, and it carries more aromas from what the cows eat, including certain wild plants in their seasons. All else being equal, a raw-milk cheese is superior. These days, however, things on the farm are so clean that even raw milk contains only a limited number of wild organisms; almost all cheesemakers add a laboratory starter culture, or the milk would never become acidified and embark on its journey to become cheese. It's perfectly possible to make flavorful cheese with pasteurized milk, if it hasn't been heated too much. But cheese made with pasteurized milk takes longer to ripen and, unless the maker takes special care, ends up with a muted, generic flavor and a stodgy texture. A good raw-milk cheese conveys much more of the ensemble of local and regional influences, especially soil and climate, evoked by the French word *terroir.*

Each traditional cheese—Camembert, Roquefort, Cantal, Lancashire, Cheshire, Parmigiano-Reggiano, the little orangy Langres, the small, flat Pérail, the varied *pecorini* of southern Italy—has its own logic, its own idea of itself, a rightness that's not improved upon easily if at all. It reflects the place where it is made—especially the local environment, which determines the feed and milk and has a strong influence on the recipe, techniques, equipment, shape, and aging. While the quality of a cheese originates with the milk, the specific taste comes from human choices, down to the merest details.

As with other cheeses, to make Camembert the milk is warmed and rennet is added. Originally, the rennet for cow's-milk cheeses always came from, and sometimes still does, the fourth, or true, stomach of a calf. The rennet's enzymes turn the milk into a gel—curd. That's transferred to molds pierced with holes, so that as the watery whey slowly separates, it will run out and leave an increasingly solid cheese. After a few days it's substantial enough to be unmolded. It's salted, and every day or two it's turned, so it dries evenly. Then it goes into a cool, humid *cave* to ripen.

The essence of this *affinage*—ripening—is the breakdown of part of the protein and fat; the first softens the cheese, and the second gives flavor. (Drier cheeses take longer to soften, and during that time more flavor develops. Hard cheeses such as Gruyère and Parmigiano, which are very large and pressed in their molds to make the curd quite dry, evolve much more slowly, never softening. They're brushed to reduce surface mold and to encourage a hard rind that will protect the cheese during its slow evolution.) Camembert, being moist, small, and somewhat thin, is ripened very quickly from the outside in by varied microflora, especially penicillia, that need air and multiply on the surface.

Raw-milk Camembert for sale in France is aged three to four weeks, but for the US market, raw-milk cheeses of any kind must be aged for at least sixty days, which alters the evolution and the taste. (In any case, these days no raw-milk Camembert is being sold in the US.) The taste of any cheese depends heavily on the ripening. A cheese needs the right time at the right temperature and humidity to produce maximum flavor for its type. Natural cellar temperatures produce better flavor and do it faster than chilled aging does, but a producer can add special laboratory cultures to the milk so that Camembert excels only after eight weeks, time that's spent mostly in the cold. (After nine or ten days, most Camembert is wrapped and refrigerated. The close covering suppresses the surface mold, while the cold slows ripening, favoring the changes accomplished by enzymes. Much of the ripening occurs in distribution—that's the plan from the start.) Only with care does a cheese develop all its potential, which is why a Camembert from a top Paris cheesemonger may stand out; the *affinage* took place in the cellar beneath the shop.

Some people say that Camembert became less interesting early in the twentieth century, when the wild mold on the surface of the cheese began to be replaced by a different laboratory one. Camembert had been ripened by wild *Penicillium album,* which turns the surface of the cheese at first white, then gray or blue-gray. Now the cheese began to be seeded with *P. candidum,* which is always very white. The clean look probably added to Camembert's appeal and success. The two molds produce different enzymes and flavors, but a cheesemaker who has used both tells me that the flavor from *album* isn't obviously better. There are so many diverse commercial strains of *candidum,* however, that it's hard to generalize. Into the second half of the twentieth century, the color of Camembert, like that of Brie, was described as orangy or orangy yellow, probably because the mold would wear off in places and the skin would show. A more orange skin comes from the same organism that's associated with stinky cheese and occurs only with the right conditions, including high enough humidity, temperature, pH, and oxygen. Now the white layer is often so thick that it doesn't wear off.

One problem with Camembert is that the Norman producers lost legal control of the name in a ruling by the court of appeals in Orléans in 1926, just the period when the French appellation system was being set up. The cheese was already too widely produced, too popular and well-known. Camembert is made all over France and the world (not least in the United States, but the more large-scale versions lack interest, and although North American farm cheesemakers produce many outstanding cheeses, their Camembert-style efforts are almost invariably without character, not very different from industrial ones). Only a tiny amount of all Camembert is "Camembert de Normandie," one of approximately four dozen French cheeses protected by an Appellation d'Origine Contrôlée (AOC), or nowadays the European Union's Appellation d'Origine Protégée (AOP). An appellation supports but doesn't ensure the best quality. The Normandy rules insist on raw milk and require the molds to be filled with a ladle, so the curd is little broken, giving a moister texture. More recently, the rules mandate cows of the brown-and-white, often brindled, Normande breed. You may think of real Camembert as coming from a particular small area, but the list of ancient Norman villages permitted to make the cheese is so long as to seem satirical. And the ladling has long been done by machine, for better or worse. Beyond that, the white surface mold must come from *P. candidum*—the original wild *P. album* is out. The official description calls for a layer of "white felting," though it allows for possible spots of "red."

France has many other creamy, surface-ripened cheeses from cow's milk, though few are quite like Camembert. Some people would place the little rounds of cow's-milk Saint-Félicien and Saint-Marcellin in the same category; they also ripen quickly and turn creamy, but they can run. The obvious cousins are just two: Brie, especially Brie de Meaux, and Coulommiers.

BRIE DE MEAUX (AOP) Along with Brie de Melun and the half-dozen other Bries, Brie de Meaux originated in the region of Brie in the

Île-de-France, the old province that embraces Paris. Today the Brie de Meaux appellation covers an enormous area, lately proposed to include a dozen French departments. The milk must be raw, and the molds must be filled by hand with a special perforated shovel in just one or two passes, for maximum moisture. A wheel of Brie de Meaux is much wider and yet thinner than one of Camembert—almost fifteen inches by just one inch (thirty-six by two and a half centimeters). With its proportionately greater surface area, Brie would ripen more quickly than Camembert, but its greater acidity slows and prevents that. After about four weeks it's only a quarter ripe; full ripeness takes six to eight weeks. Even before Camembert reached Paris, creamy Bries were popular there. It probably goes without saying that Brie de Meaux has nothing in common with US supermarket "Brie," which is the epitome of a plastic-textured industrial cheese. The present rules for Brie de Meaux call for "a subtle aroma of cream, butter, and hazelnuts." The cheese has been called elegant.

COULOMMIERS (NO APPELLATION) Named for the Brie market town, this is a form of Brie, no matter the small size—often just five inches (thirteen centimeters) wide. Coulommiers is still sometimes called Brie de Coulommiers or Brie *petit moule,* "small mold." Part of the appeal of Coulommiers has always been that, compared with the large pancake of Brie, the small cheese, like a Camembert, is less vulnerable in shipping. Most Coulommiers is now made from pasteurized milk, and often it's made by producers of other kinds of Brie. No rules govern the making, but a very good one comes from raw milk, the molds for it are filled with a ladle, and after about a month its texture has become very creamy. (It sometimes used to be made with added cream.) I've had rich-flavored, lusciously creamy ones, with odors of fresh white mushroom plus a slight garlickiness, recalling Camembert but less intense.

Most Camembert—sad fate for an icon—has been taken far into the realm of control, divorced from nature. And yet, with cheese, *nature is the point*—its variety from season to season, from farm to farm, even from one cheese to another ripening side by side on the same shelf. If I were to describe the ideal Camembert: It's soft but holds its shape; it doesn't flow when cut. Its rind is thin and supple, like a skin, and its color is white (or perhaps blue-gray), though in places where the surface mold has been rubbed off it shows a distinct orange skin. Inside, the color is creamy and so is the texture, which tends toward buttery and even silky. The scent is of cultivated white mushrooms and something that might be garlic. There's just the right balance of salt. The taste is rich, slightly peppery, with a nutty, fruity, fungal earthiness, which is to say a very mild stink. If you have a little luck, or know where to look for this Camembert, you can find it.

HOW TO BUY CAMEMBERT: Turn if you can to a skilled cheesemonger who may have done the ripening or, if there's no wonderful Camembert, will guide you to something similar. Buying a Camembert is an act of faith. A seller won't normally sacrifice one for tasting, and you may not even be allowed to touch the cheese in its wrapper to judge its softness. If you're able to feel it, look for a degree of softness that suggests the cheese is fully creamy without flowing. A dip in the center implies too much softness, and then the flavor may not be the fullest and most characteristic. Often you can buy just a half cheese, and then, if one is already cut, you can at least see the texture. (Make sure the half cheese is as ripe as you want it, because no cheese ripens well after it's cut.) In Europe, look for raw-milk Camembert de Normandie, though others, including pasteurized-milk versions, can be good. The best season for any cheese is the best season for milk in its part of the world, usually spring. But in most dairy regions, good cheeses are produced from late spring through fall, when the animals are outdoors eating living plants. And if the maker is skilled, even a winter cheese from cows eating mostly hay can be excellent. Seek a Camembert whose surface isn't entirely covered with a heavy white felt but shows signs of orangy yellow skin.

HOW TO KEEP CAMEMBERT BRIEFLY AND, IF NEEDED, RIPEN IT A LITTLE: When you get the cheese home, unwrap it and smell it. There should be no mustiness, no strong ammonia; even a cheese wrapper with tiny perforations can hold in too much. Usually, though, an excess will disappear as the cheese breathes.

If the cheese is already ripe and you plan to keep it longer than half a day, and your house is warm, with no cool pantry or cellar, then surround the cheese somewhat loosely with its wrapper and refrigerate it. A cheese can survive for a time under refrigeration—imported cheeses have crossed the ocean to North America in a "reefer" and been kept chilled at least until they reach the retailer. But cold suppresses the life in a cheese, and the longer the cold lasts, the harder it is for the cheese to recover, so consume it promptly. Be certain to take it out a few hours beforehand: unwrap it and let it breathe as it warms to cool room temperature.

If the cheese seems firm and you think it would benefit from further ripening, and you have a spot at around 55 to 60 degrees F (13 to 16 degrees C), then unwrap the cheese, set it on a plate, give it a fine spray of water (or fling drops with your fingers), cover it with an inverted bowl, and place it in that cool spot. At least once a day, lift the bowl (allowing in fresh air), turn the cheese over, and add more moisture—there should be enough that it will condense on the inside of the bowl. Judge the evolution of the cheese by touch. How soft it becomes depends on how moist it was to begin with. It might need two or three days or more—but better underripe than over-ripe. Many people prefer Camembert while there is still a thin, contrasting white chalky core.

Some cheese lovers believe all rind is only a container for the cheese inside, and some rinds have a taste that obviously detracts. The mold on a Camembert is often so thick and chewy, from having been ripened too warm for too long, that it has developed a slight crunch. I taste, and if I'm lucky enough to have a cheese with a thin, tender, mild rind, I eat it.

COMPLEMENTS TO CAMEMBERT: Camembert needs only bread, and nothing is better than a fresh baguette.

NOTES ON WINE: Each cheese has its successes with wine, sometimes big ones, but contrary to what has so often been said, cheese and wine aren't automatic partners. And a mixed platter at the end of a meal makes wine selection difficult if not impossible. Because cheese generally goes better with white wine, the usual progression from white to red doesn't work, and a sommelier often suggests switching to a sweet white wine, at least to go with firm and blue cheeses. If at the end of a meal I offer several diverse cheeses, I don't worry about the wine. Those who want can sip a little of whatever dry red is on the table.

To turn specifically to Camembert, it's one of the more difficult cheeses with wine. It strips red wine of all pleasure, turning it harsh and metallic. The usual tactic when you don't know what wine to drink with a cheese is to try a traditionally made white from the same region, which tends to work. Normandy, however, makes cider instead of wine, and in my experience, neither Norman sparkling cider nor perry (cider made from pears) forms a magical combination with the cheese. The wine that sommeliers generally suggest as the best solution for Camembert is good Champagne. But to me, as with the cider, in most cases the flavors simply coexist, though sometimes the drinks bring out a bitterness in a cheese. Occasionally there's a small synergy, such as an intensified mushroom flavor on both sides. The one sure success with Camembert is water, which is an excellent drink with any cheese.

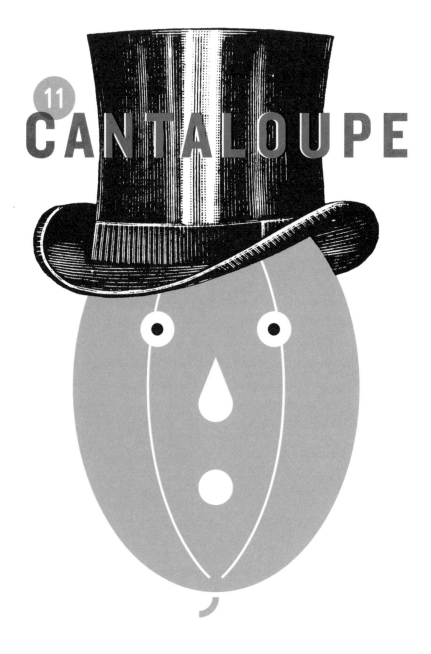

11
CANTALOUPE

II. CANTALOUPE

The melon, *Cucumis melo,* came into being in Africa from unknown wild parents and arrived perhaps three thousand years ago in the hot, dry valleys of Persia and adjacent lands. Melons cross readily, and the family grew large as kinds and varieties were developed. They're smooth or netted, round or long, wrinkled, bulbously warted, ribbed, striped, and blotched. The many delicious sorts testify to the high value always placed on melons. The species, called melon or muskmelon, includes cantaloupe, Persian, honeydew, canary, and casaba melons. (Watermelons belong to their own species.) Somehow, the name "cantaloupe" moved from one melon to another when it crossed the Atlantic. North Americans consider any netted melon with orange flesh to be a cantaloupe, while the true cantaloupe, called by that name in Europe and distinguished botanically as *cantaloupensis,* is different and not commonly grown in the United States. It has a smooth skin, usually green and yellow, with shallow or deep ribs; it's often smaller than other melons. The first cantaloupe is supposed to have reached Europe in the sixteenth century, brought by missionaries from Armenia to the pope's castle at Cantalupo, near Rome, giving the name. For my purposes, the cantaloupe embraces the European kind as well as the netted muskmelons. At their perfumed peak, even as they pass full ripeness and the aromas become partly cloying, cantaloupes are a concentration of summer.

Compared with most other edible garden plants, varieties of melon are more sensitive to conditions in the region where they're grown. Although different ones ripen at different times, melons are all most delicious in periods of greatest heat. Certain varieties grow in the north and in a hot year can excel. When I've grown melons in the cool place where I live, they've ripened only during the last of the hot weather in the first week of

September; for every ten melons I grew, not the first or the last but only the two that ripened in the middle had an extraordinary perfume. The crop barely had the time and heat it needed to ripen, and melons that ripen in mid-season, for their variety, tend to be most typical and flavorful.

Two things are especially important to melon flavor: variety and ripeness. The essential book for anyone who loves to eat melons (not necessarily grow them, despite the title) is Amy Goldman's *Melons for the Passionate Grower,* the outcome of thirty years of melon growing. She has a powerful appreciation for the most delicious old varieties rather than modern hybrids that come and go. The best true, smooth-skinned cantaloupe varieties, she says, tend to be French, including Petit Gris de Rennes, Prescott Fond Blanc, and the relatively small Charentais (now more than one variety and constituting most of the melons grown in France). Some excellent true cantaloupes do come from elsewhere, such as the green-fleshed Ha'Ogen from Israel, which perhaps originated in Hungary.

The netted muskmelons and Persian melons, orange- or green-fleshed, are classified as *reticulatus.* In addition to the Persian melon proper, they include the excellent Jenny Lind, Anne Arundel, Banana (long and narrow), Delicious 51 (for colder climates), Eden's Gem, Emerald Gem, Fordhook Gem, Golden Gopher (part honeydew), Green Nutmeg and its offspring Rocky Ford, and Montreal Market and its offspring Oka.

(Certain ripe melons, also called winter melons, don't smell at all until they're opened. They require a long growing season and include the smooth honeydew, the canary, cavaillon from the South of France, crenshaw from California, and casaba from Turkey. The ones called Christmas, Santa Claus, or Piel de Sapo, Spanish for "toad skin," will keep in the cold until Christmas.)

As they ripen, melons move from a crunch to, like most great fruits, a melting texture but one especially filled with juice. Some varieties are more floral, some more musky. Some split when very ripe. Like almost every fruit, melons ripen first at the blossom end, which remains the sweetest, most aromatic part. (Even the blossom end of an avocado ripens faster and tastes better than its stem end.) If you taste and compare, the difference in a melon is dramatic. Always divide melons lengthwise, and if you compare the taste of different ones, make certain you don't measure a blossom end against a stem end.

Little that you can do to a truly ripe melon will improve the taste. But you can change the form with a blender or food processor and turn it into an excellent sorbet or ice or, adding a good portion of citrus juice, into a dessert soup. The pastry chef Shuna Lydon strains the stringy material mixed with the seeds scraped from the interior and adds that juice, too, for its concentrated flavor, when she makes a frozen dessert, soup, fool, or gazpacho. Some people enjoy melons with black pepper, and in Hungary they're eaten with paprika. Melons fit with the mixed fruits of a *macédoine*. In the heat of summer, there are good arguments both for eating melon with a deep, refreshing chill and for eating it warm and fully aromatic from the garden.

HOW TO SELECT A DELICIOUS CANTALOUPE: The first step is to find a great variety, most likely at a farm stand or farmers' market, picked at or close to maximum ripeness. But melons in a pile can look like so many blank faces, and the challenge is to know which are really ripe. In the garden, generally the closer a cantaloupe or any muskmelon is to perfect ripeness, the more easily it slips from the stem with pressure from your finger. A home gardener can wait for "full slip," when a slight crack shows all around the stem where it meets the fruit, and when you push the stem away, it leaves a smooth surface. If you're buying a cantaloupe or any muskmelon and see that the stem is attached and was cut with a blade, then it was probably harvested early. To be fair, growers can't afford the labor it takes to pass through the rows daily checking each fruit, and if they did pick only fully ripe, soft melons, they might lose many of them to bruising. Besides, the slip test doesn't work with every variety. More reliable indicators are that the blossom end yields a little to pressure, the aroma is distinct, and the color has changed from green to more yellow or brown. Beware that honeydew, crenshaw, and casaba are nonslip. With them, look for yellower color, which is more obvious in the spot where the fruit touched the ground. A melon that's picked only partly ripe will gain in juice off the vine but not in aroma or sugar. If ripe melons are in danger of going by before you can eat them, then refrigerate them.

COMPLEMENTS TO CANTALOUPE: Thin slices of raw dry-cured ham set off a perfect melon, and lemon or lime juice flatters a melon short on acidity and flavor, but I don't find that much else helps. A skilled pâtissier can present stimulating herb and spice complements in an elaborate plated dessert, but perhaps none of the individual ones on their own make a lasting combination with melon. See also the notes on wine just below.

NOTES ON WINE: Many people believe that a perfect melon is improved by filling its hollow with sweet wine—vintage Port, Banyuls (including *rancio* versions), Muscat de Beaumes-de-Venise, excellent Italian Moscato, sweet Champagne.

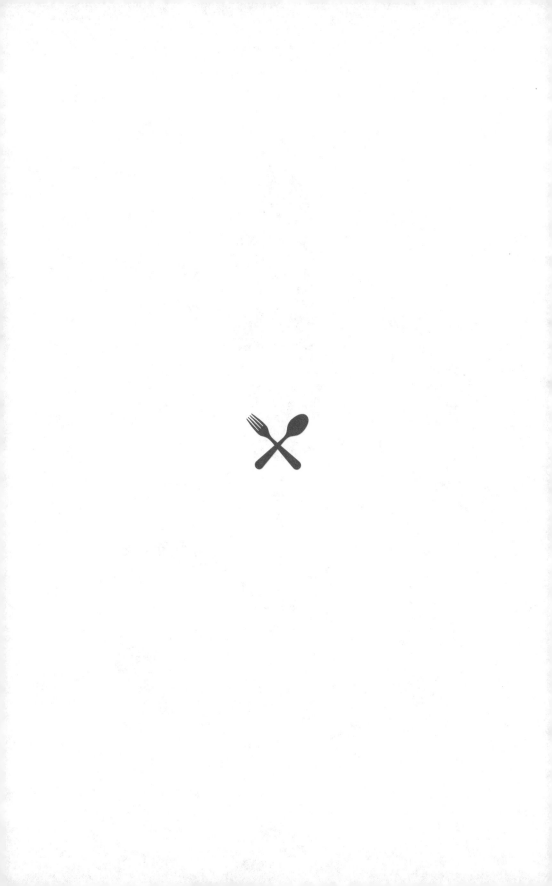

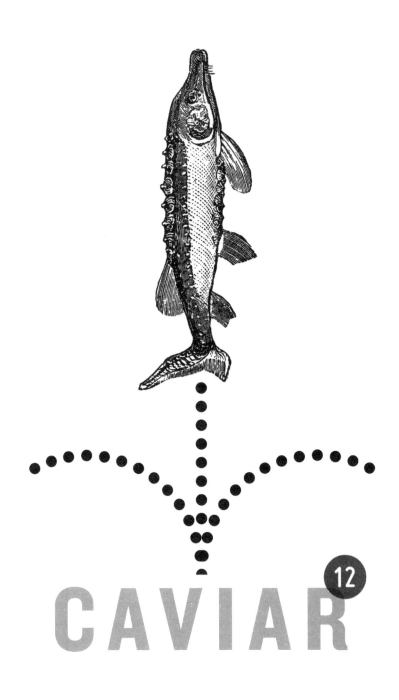

CAVIAR 12

Really good caviar, the only kind worth eating, tastes fresh—only slightly salty, not fishy at all. Each small, shiny, moist, perishable egg is covered with a frail membrane that, when the eggs are exceptionally firm and pressed with the tongue against the palate, gives a pop, or close to it. Texture is important. Caviar is served on ice to firm it and make the taste more delicate. Salt preserves the eggs and enhances their flavor, but it shouldn't be a large part of the taste. The eggs are certainly, however, somewhat fatty—rich. Caviar hasn't often risen to the ideal. A dealer once said to me, "The ultimate buyer has a low level of knowledge in this business." Until a few decades ago, most caviar was Russian, taken from wild sturgeon caught as they swam up the Volga River and other tributaries of the Caspian Sea. That caviar, once abundant and inexpensive, has retreated into folklore. The fish were diminished by dams and pollution, and after the collapse of the Soviet Union they were poached nearly to extinction. Imports from the Caspian and Black seas have been banned altogether at times, although more recently, notably for Iran, the Convention on International Trade in Endangered Species has allowed extremely limited quotas. Somewhat ironically, now that wild caviar has nearly disappeared, we've entered the era of more consistently well prepared and much fresher caviar from farmed fish. The sturgeon are raised in a number of countries, and some caviar is certified organic and appears sustainable. Even before the decline of wild caviar, good US caviar from farmed sturgeon tasted better than much of the wild did, at least partly because domestic caviar suffers less and stays fresher during its shorter journey to the domestic consumer. Sturgeon farmers have learned to produce caviar of high quality, and the average caviar for sale may be better than ever, although the taste of the wild, perhaps more intense, remains the point of reference. Meanwhile the price has been steadily rising, making any caviar more and more a luxury. The taste remains special, an important part of the big picture of taste.

The word "caviar" is often used loosely. Strictly it comes only from sturgeon and no other fish. The salted eggs of paddlefish (spoonbill), whitefish, or salmon may perhaps taste harmless, but they can be crude and fishy and leave you wishing you hadn't tried them. The three main kinds of real caviar are called by the Russian names for the sturgeon that produce them: sevruga, osetra, and beluga.

Sevruga comes from the starry sturgeon, *Acipenser stellatus,* the smallest of the caviar species, which commonly grows three to four feet long. The eggs, too, are the smallest, light gray to black in color, and in texture they're the most fragile. Yet the taste is strongest. Sevruga caviar is the least prized, least expensive of the three kinds.

Osetra comes especially from the Russian sturgeon, *A. gueldenstaedti,* and the Persian sturgeon, *A. persicus,* which may be the same species. Both are middle in size and produce middle-size eggs, light yellow to brown-black in color. Caviar from the yellower eggs has long been sold as "golden osetra." Osetra eggs are the firmest of the three kinds, and compared with the famous beluga, the caviar is stronger in flavor, commonly described as "nutty" and sometimes as "iodine."

Beluga, which has always been the most expensive and prestigious caviar, comes from the beluga sturgeon, *Huso huso,* the largest European freshwater fish, capable of growing twenty feet long. Beluga eggs, too, are the largest. The caviar is light gray to nearly black, the lighter color (coming from older fish) being more prized. The texture is buttery, and the taste is elegant. Whether or not beluga is truly best is a matter of taste; some in the trade have always preferred osetra.

Besides those species, caviar from the Siberian sturgeon, *A. baerii,* which is now farmed in the US and elsewhere, is sometimes called osetra. But certain experts consider that this caviar belongs to its own category and even is closer to sevruga—creamy and nutty. It can be excellent. Another sturgeon, the sterlet, *A. ruthenus,* produces a golden, highly prized caviar, a little of which still comes at a high price from Iran.

One more kind of caviar these days is very important and often compared with osetra: caviar from the white sturgeon, *A. transmontanus,* which is native to the Pacific Coast of North America. The wild population is still relatively strong, but the caviar comes from farmed fish, and in North America it's the kind you're most likely to find. The flavor can be complex, subtle, and extremely delicious.

When the eggs are taken from the sturgeon to make caviar, they're immediately passed by hand through a sieve, without crushing them, rinsed in salt water, and then mixed with salt. The final concentration of salt, determined by a caviar master, is typically 3.5 to 4 percent. Caviar with this amount is called *malossol,* Russian for "lightly salted"—today almost the only kind. At first, the salt is somewhat prominent and there's less character. The ideal is to hold the caviar for roughly three months before sale while the taste matures, but in practice the time is often a month or less, especially during periods of high demand.

Caviar was once much saltier than it is today, and there still survive saltier, drier forms of roe, whose origins go back millennia. *Avgotaraho,* to use the Greek word, or *bottarga,* to use the more familiar Italian one, is a whole preserved roe sac of, especially, gray mullet, which always used to be cured with enough salt to last without refrigeration. As it dries, the individual eggs are lost in the mass. Best of the type, however, is the modern, less dry and salty, carefully executed *avgotaraho* made by the Greek firm Trikalinos. This does require refrigeration. Eaten in thin slices, it has a slightly soft, waxy texture, and the flavor, implausibly and very satisfyingly, combines fishiness with the antifishy, ultrafresh flavor of a straight-from-the-ocean raw oyster. With its long aftertaste, it's one of the world's great foods.

The taste of caviar, besides reflecting species and execution, is influenced by differences among individual fish and by the precise maturity at which the eggs are taken. Caviar from farmed fish additionally reflects the cleanliness of the water and naturally the feed, primarily fish meal, which shouldn't be too fatty. Each egg is firm and distinct; the taste is fresh and oceanic, lingering.

HOW TO BUY AND STORE CAVIAR: Buy caviar only from a source with an outstanding reputation. The most important criterion is freshness—a nonfishy taste. Without that, nothing else matters. Some caviar is pasteurized, which preserves it better than just salt and cold, but the heat of pasteurization changes the taste. Raw caviar, kept continuously cold and sealed from air in its unopened container, remains relatively fresh for up to a year. Once purchased, a container will last in a home refrigerator, unopened, for several weeks. After it has been opened and the caviar has been exposed to air, eat it within three or four days. Serve it very cold in a dish set on ice. If you can, avoid contact with metal (plastic is better)—the traditional spoons are made of mother-of-pearl. Look for firm eggs that "pop" in the mouth, a mild, balanced saltiness, and a clean flavor like that of the freshest raw fish.

COMPLEMENTS TO CAVIAR: Most of the old accompaniments—chopped hard-cooked egg, capers, lemon wedges, chopped raw onion—are flavorful if not aggressive and were intended to hide defects. They also hide strengths. You don't need anything at all, but delicious caviar is set off by buckwheat blinis, whole-wheat bread, slices of steamed waxy potato, and perhaps crème fraîche.

NOTES ON WINE: Champagne is a common first thought with caviar, but for most people who love either one, Champagne isn't the ideal choice. Caviar needs a very cold drink with very little flavor, and caviar lovers have limited enthusiasm for any option other than vodka. (I've also heard a preference for deeply chilled, very light-flavored beer.) The danger with any kind of wine is that it will bring out a metallic fishiness in the caviar. If you'd really prefer wine, then the important thing is to avoid a negative taste. Choose a dry, nonfruity, somewhat acidic wine, such as a dry Riesling or Sancerre. If you have to have Champagne, then choose a young, crisp one without much character—deeply chilled.

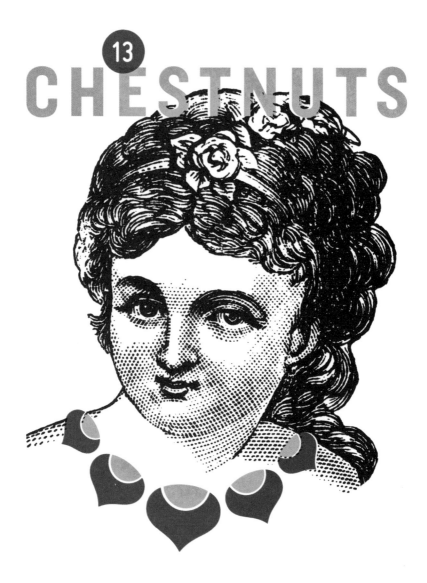

13
CHESTNUTS

H ot chestnuts, with their delicate, luxurious aroma of honey, straddle the line between savory and sweet. Only fresh chestnuts in the weeks after the harvest carry such clear flavor. Toward the end of September, the remarkably hostile, spiked green husk splits open to reveal, typically, two to four ripe nuts inside their brown shells. By Christmas, the quality is already in decline. The old way to keep chestnuts through the year is to dry them, which takes away much of the flavor. The nuts become as hard as the hardest wood, because where other nuts are filled with oil, chestnuts store energy for a future plant as starch. And they differ from other nuts because they're eaten only cooked (though they're harmless raw). If you mash the cooked chestnuts into purée, their soft starchiness requires lubrication with fat or liquid or both—milk, cream, butter, chicken stock, which are all impeccable complements.

In the West, we eat the European chestnut, *Castanea sativa.* (The Chinese eat the sweet Chinese chestnut, *C. mollissima;* the Japanese eat the sweet Japanese chestnut, *C. crenata.* Americans used to eat the American chestnut, *C. dentata,* until it was almost entirely eliminated by blight in the twentieth century; a resistant version has been bred at last, based on a small percentage of Chinese, and it's possible that chestnuts will once again take their place in eastern North American forests.) The European chestnut probably originated in the Transcaucasus and from there spread to Asia Minor and Europe, growing among hills and low mountains. The trees shun limey soils in favor of acidic ones; they like heat in summer, followed by rain before harvest.

In English, we have the single word "chestnut," but Italian and French have the general words *castagna* and *châtaigne* and the specific ones *marrone* and *marron,* to describe a superior variety of chestnut, generally containing just one seed. Chestnuts from other sorts of trees have two or three seeds folded together within the same shell. *Marroni* and *marrons* are often bigger, and they're what you need if you want whole chestnuts. Modern hybrids, which have been created especially in France, bear bigger, more beautiful *marrons.* Better flavor, though, comes from older varieties, without regard to size.

In Europe, the main producer is Italy, with the largest number of chestnuts coming from the hills of Campania. The many Italian kinds are tied to particular places: the *castagna Cuneo, di Montella, del Monte Amiata,* the *marrone di Castel del Rio, di Combai, di Roccadaspide, di San Zeno—* more than forty in all. The one with the greatest reputation, and possibly the best, is the small, delicate *marrone del Mugello,* from the area of the Mugello in Tuscany, northeast of Florence. The variety is best appreciated roasted in the oven. One fall I visited Palazzuolo sul Senio, a town so deep in the Mugello that the dialect spoken is not Tuscan but Romagnolo, that of the adjoining region. At a hillside *agriturismo* with an old, out-of-use, stone *seccatoio* for drying chestnuts, I ate *marroni* with *porcini* mushrooms, a combination of the season.

The starch and flavor make chestnuts good partners with meat and, particularly, with different forms of cabbage. Old European recipes are mostly savory, not sweet, if only because so many of them come from the countryside, where sugar used to be a luxury. In various regions, chestnuts were important sustenance for the poor. Especially when a meager crop made wheat a luxury, dried chestnuts were ground and baked into bread. In Italy, the chestnut tree is *l'albero del pane,* "the bread tree," partly a symbol of poverty. Chestnut polenta is older than maize polenta. Chestnut flour mixed with wheat flour made and sometimes still makes certain kinds of pasta and gnocchi. Mixed with grated cheese and nutmeg, mashed chestnuts sometimes fill *tortelli,* which are served with butter and more cheese. Whole chestnuts are sometimes cooked as a *ragoût,* which in France might mean simmered in water or white wine with onions, garlic, smoked bacon, a clove, a branch of fennel, and several branches of parsley.

All the charms of chestnuts are evident in a smooth soup, thinned with milk and chicken stock and often flavored with leeks and celery. The outstanding addition to the soup is butter-fried croûtons—so underappreciated and so little used, so mistakenly out of fashion. (I don't make them as often as I should.) Cooked to golden at the last minute and thrown on top, their effect isn't heavy but toasty and crunchy, a textural counterpoint. *Soupe aux marrons* from the region of Bourbonnais in central France takes a different tack: onions, carrots, turnips, and celery are cooked with a mere fat handful of chestnuts, and all goes through a sieve; added last are crème fraîche and chervil. One of the best ways to eat chestnuts is as a thick purée, like a more interesting form of mashed potato, especially good with turkey, goose, or wild boar. For a perfect consistency, pass the purée, like a smooth soup, through a fine-mesh sieve.

Chestnuts have long been cooked in sugar syrup to make *marrons glacés,* whose roots go back to the 1500s, and yet the famous sweet is always in my experience starch-textured and dry, tasting only of sugar and added vanilla—awful. The main problem is surely the long cooking, which drives off the innate flavor. Canned chestnuts and canned chestnut purée are useless for the same reason. (Yet I'm told that, exceptionally, a *confiseur* makes *marrons glacés* very well, and they are superb with Pedro Ximénez sherry.)

The famous rustic Tuscan dessert *castagnaccio* is hardly sweet at all. The batter of chestnut flour and water commonly contains pine nuts and a selection of other ingredients—raisins, walnuts, sometimes rosemary, fennel seed, orange peel, all topped with olive oil. The batter is baked in a thin layer, giving a cracked surface and a puddinglike consistency, solid enough to cut. The rosemary-chestnut flavor is fascinating, but *castagnaccio* evokes ambivalence in me and some others. For flavor, it helps to grind the chestnut flour fresh.

Most chestnut desserts exploit the fresh nuts. The classic French Mont Blanc, known in Italy as Montebianco, addresses the potential dryness by covering sweetened chestnut purée with whipped cream—the name comes from the snowy effect of the cream on top of the mountainous pile of chestnut. Nesselrode pudding in its haute cuisine form combines chestnut purée with custard and whipped cream, candied cherries, orange peel, and raisins (the fruits being previously soaked in sweet Málaga wine); the whole is flavored with maraschino liqueur. Chestnut purée is sometimes lightened with beaten egg whites, like a soufflé, baked in a mold, and then served with a custard sauce.

HOW TO BUY CHESTNUTS: By Christmas, some chestnuts in a batch may have begun to mold, and there's no way to know until you open them. Within a variety, bigger nuts may be better, and yet the small Italian variety *marrone del Mugello* may be the best of all. Unfortunately, unless you're in the right place in Italy and can buy a special variety like that, you have to trust the seller and hope for the best. Alternatively, cooked chestnuts sold vacuum-sealed in plastic can hold good flavor (they're available that way in Europe, and maybe we'll see more of them in the US). For cooking and eating plain, the quantity you need depends on how much your audience loves them and how delicious the particular chestnuts are. A pound, roasted, might satisfy four after a light meal and twice as many after a big one. To keep the chestnuts hot, bring them to the table in a covered cast-iron pot, if that's what you cooked them in, or if you roasted them over a fire, put them in a warm bowl with a cover.

HOW TO KEEP, PEEL, AND COOK CHESTNUTS: Keep fresh chestnuts chilled, to slow the loss of moisture and discourage mold. Before you cook them, so they don't explode in the heat, cut an × through the shell on the rounded side.

Merely to peel them for another preparation, put them into boiling water for eight minutes, and then remove the pot from the flame. Take out a few nuts at a time, wait a minute until you can stand to touch them, then peel off the shell and the papery inner skin, which is so unpleasantly astringent that it ruins the taste. (The skin comes easily from freshly harvested nuts, but as the weeks pass it clings and peeling can be slow and frustrating.) If the skin holds annoyingly tight, loosen it with the point of a small knife. As the nuts begin to cool, the skins stick more; return the nuts to the hot water to reheat. As you peel, discard any that show mold or worm damage or don't have a reassuring chestnut smell—when in doubt, taste.

Finish the cooking according to the dish, adding the peeled chestnuts, for instance, to a simmering braise or *ragoût*. To make a purée, simmer the peeled nuts in milk until they are completely tender, usually about twenty minutes. (Peel a pound, or 500 grams, of chestnuts as above, and cook them in milk until they fall apart when pressed with a fork, drain while saving the milk, and push them through a fine sieve; add ½ cup, or 100 grams, butter and ½ cup, or 100 milliliters, heavy cream or crème fraîche; thin further as needed with the milk from cooking.) Be careful not to overcook chestnuts or hold soup or purée on a hot burner for too long: the delicious flavor goes off into the air.

To fully cook the scored chestnuts inside their shells, you can boil them, which may take twenty minutes or more; open and taste to know whether they're ready. If the chestnuts are quite fresh, you can roast them in the oven at 400 degrees F (200 degrees C), which may take up to an hour, as the shells open outward from the cuts—again, taste to know when they're done. I've never roasted chestnuts over a fire, but as with other hearth cooking, you need a fire that has settled from active flames to glowing coals, and preferably a pan made just for roasting chestnuts, with holes and a long handle. The range of advice is to roast them for twenty-five to forty-five minutes, frequently turning or shaking the nuts.

COMPLEMENTS TO CHESTNUTS: They go with the flavors of leeks, celery, parsley, a fennel branch or fennel seed, chicken broth or stock, milk or cream. They make a happy combination with cabbage (regular green heads, Brussels sprouts, sweet-and-sour red cabbage). They're often put with boletes, and the two do go together but no more than that. Chestnuts are sometimes said to go with a range of meats: chestnut purée with beef isn't bad, but there's little or no conversation; the chestnut flavor is mildly at odds with pork, good with wild boar, and very happy with turkey and goose. Beyond these, which I've confirmed recently, the French gastronome Édouard de Pomiane recommended chestnuts with the delectably odorous sausage *andouillette de Troyes,* which makes sense. Besides, the purée is often put with pheasant, partridge, and guinea fowl, as well as veal, lamb, and mutton.

In desserts, the best complement is vanilla. (Or not, if you accept the minimalist argument that closely related flavors are competition and it's better to use diverse and contrasting ones.) Chestnut honey is often proposed with chestnuts, but it treads on the chestnuts' own delicate honey flavor. (Cinnamon, another common recommendation, inevitably takes over—I rarely use it with anything.) Chocolate respects chestnuts, though the flavors don't interact. As flavoring, very good in both sweet and savory dishes are the intentionally oxidized wines—Marsala, Madeira, sweet sherry.

NOTES ON WINE: Whole chestnuts in a savory dish, unless it's a soup or stew, badly need a moistening wine. With turkey or goose with chestnuts, a red Bordeaux, aged without oak, goes well. With a purée with wild boar, turn to one of the reds that usually goes with that meat, such as one of the gamier examples of Syrah or an old traditional Rioja. With roasted chestnuts, drinking the brand-new white wine from the same harvest is more traditional than it is delicious. Instead choose a more fully formed wine from the previous year, such as a fresh, light Beaujolais, which at its best has its own quality of sweetness. Much less expected and excellent with roasted chestnuts is a very sweet (Sélection de Grains Nobles) Gewürztraminer from Alsace.

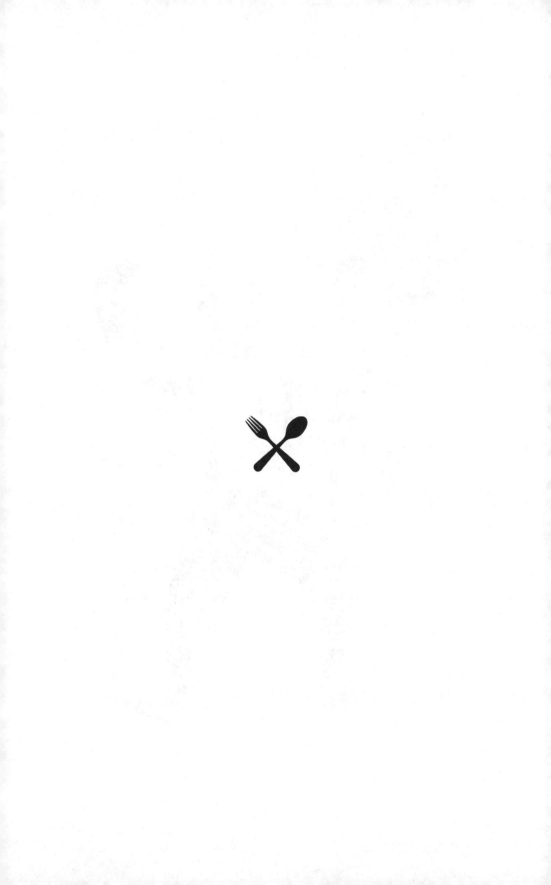

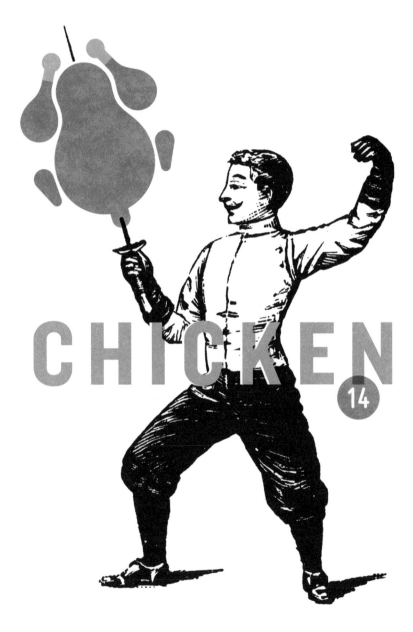

CHICKEN

14

Chefs have always placed a high value on chicken, and as commonplace as chicken has become, they still do. For centuries in the West, and perhaps the entire world, more recipes have existed for chicken than for any other meat. It doesn't hurt that, more than most foods, a roast chicken is likely to succeed with wine. Yet the occasional illustration that appears in an old text shows a comparatively scrawny bird with a meager breast, very unlike the current industrial model. Still today, chickens of old breeds have smaller breasts and longer legs than mass-market ones. Neither a *fermier* bird bought in France nor an Amish one bought in Manhattan is plush, but, like the birds in the old pictures, they have real flavor. When you bite into the meat, it's tender while offering some gratifying resistance. The farm chickens I've cooked in France are drier than almost any North American bird and yet more succulent. Nearly all chickens in North America are industrial, fast-growing and high-yielding. They descend from the old Cornish and White Rock breeds, though they've been so much crossed and selected that the concept of breed hardly applies. They're white-feathered, so that any feathers left behind are less obvious. The flavor of these intensively farmed chickens is weak, diluted, even somewhat unclean. The white meat seems to me spongy. (The way these chickens are raised, both the special strains for meat and the separate ones for eggs, is about as inhumane as the intensive methods used to produce pork.) Delicious chicken naturally comes from a higher tier of bird, allowed outdoors during the day so it can exercise and eat what it finds—grass and other plants, insects and worms.

Chefs sometimes cook *poussins,* very small, young chickens, and present them as a special meat, though they have little to offer. Industrial chickens that reach "fryer" size in six or seven weeks, such as those used in fast food, aren't much better. A chicken of any kind doesn't have real flavor until it's nine weeks old. Heirloom breeds take about fourteen weeks to reach fryer size, and they eat a lot more feed during that time, but in return their meat tastes much more delicious.

The chicken best known for flavor, as well as its blue feet, is the French Poulet de Bresse, a selection of Gauloise. For now, Bresse stock is all but unavailable in the United States. But there are plenty of good breeds, old-fashioned dual-purpose ones, meaning they produce both eggs and meat. Some of the more interesting breeds raised in North America are Buckeye, Blue Andalusian, Columbian Wyandotte, Dark Cornish, Black-Breasted Red Game, Cochin, Plymouth Rock, and New Hampshire Red. It's important to get good examples; some of the farmers who keep particular breeds and sell chicks select and maintain quality much more carefully than others.

It's not just the breed and the way the birds are raised that count. Everything matters, not least the slaughter. It's important that the birds stay calm and feel no surge of fear and adnenaline. After they're killed, to keep the meat from becoming tough, it should be first kept for about ten hours at 50 degrees F (10 degrees C). Air chilling is good, because otherwise the meat is chilled in water, which it absorbs, and the water isn't necessarily clean. Nonetheless, to loosen the feathers for plucking, the carcass is put briefly in hot water. Dry-plucking is probably better, but it has to be done by hand. The chicken should then wait for two days, for more tenderness and flavor.

Famously, roasting a chicken presents a puzzle. The legs, to be tender, must reach at least 160 degrees F (70 degrees C), and yet the breast starts to dry if it rises much higher than 150 degrees F (65 degrees C). At those temperatures, there will and should be a few reddish juices at the bone. To achieve the dual temperatures in a single bird, many tactics have been tried, including trussing and not trussing; covering the breast with slices of pork fat; chilling just the breast with an ice pack beforehand while the rest of the bird warms up; stuffing just the breast under the skin, which works well; and cooking the bird upside down on a rack. You need a rack that raises the bird higher than the sides of the roasting pan, but whatever part is down will cook more slowly, because the bottom of the roasting pan reflects heat away. If you skip the rack and place the chicken directly in the pan, it partly sautés in the fat, which isn't roasting, though that may not matter. To have the pleasure of the crisp, deep-golden skin, you dry, oil, and salt it before cooking. Humidity from the bird quickly softens the crispness unless the skin is served right away.

Rather than struggle to achieve perfect light and dark meat in traditional roast chicken, I accept some difference, but to be sure that the legs don't cook more slowly than the breast, I nearly always cut down the backbone, open and flatten out the bird, and "roast" it that way. That's called spatchcocked in English and *à la crapaudine* ("toad style") in French. In Italy, *pollo al mattone* is cut open and flattened, weighted under a brick (*mattone*), and grilled slowly. *Pollo alla diavola* is opened flat like a book and grilled, sometimes with hot pepper (the "devil" in the name is variously attributed to either the pepper or the fire). A flattened chicken, like a whole roast chicken, needs a fifteen-minute rest, and then the breast slices beautifully.

Chicken is also one of the "boiled" meats in Italian *bollito misto,* served with sauces that are really condiments. *Poule au pot* is a whole chicken cooked in broth with vegetables, parallel to the treatment of beef in a pot-au-feu. Italian chicken dishes called *alla cacciatora* involve the cut-up bird and have some regional consistency but no fixed meaning: the most common addition may be tomato, but instead there might be white wine, onions, and pancetta; hot pepper, garlic, and rosemary; or capers, anchovy, and lemon; sometimes there are bolete mushrooms. In place of liquid, the impression of moisture can come from fat. Assuming a tender but flavorful chicken, the point of fried chicken is the contrast in textures—the luscious effect of the crisp batter, partly impregnated with fat, and the usually juicy meat, protected by that batter.

Lately I've been roasting chickens, but over time I've been much more of a sauté cook and a braise cook. You take the chicken breasts out before the legs, or you add them last, or you cook just legs or breasts and avoid the problem of disparate cooking times altogether. For a sauté, normally of an entire cut-up chicken, you color the pieces in fat and continue cooking in a covered pan until done; then you deglaze the pan with liquid (wine, tomato, vinegar, cream, broth) to make a sauce and then add sautéed mushrooms, vegetables, or whatever you like, the flavors remaining much more separate than they are in a typical braise. *Poulet au vinaigre* is an originally home-style sauté that stresses vinegar; the recipe I've used tempers it with tomatoes and cream. The original idea behind coq au vin, a sauté that becomes a braise, is that a tough old rooster cooked long enough will finally become tender (if dry) while it gives flavor to the sauce, but that tough old bird has long since given way to a young chicken. Apart from the meat, the recipe is like that for bœuf bourguignon.

One of the great flavor combinations is *poularde aux morilles et au vin jaune,* from the Jura Mountains of France; it combines the region's *vin jaune* ("yellow wine") with cream and morels—the sauce is excellent even without the morels. *Vin jaune,* which increases the chickeny-ness, is aged *sousvoile,* "under a veil," something like sherry, but it has its own particular set of *rancio* flavors (always compared with rancid walnuts, as well as fresh ones and caramel; then, depending on the bottle, there are butter, toast, dried fruit, curry, and more). Other more affordable, traditional Jura whites serve almost as well.

Chicken livers are as mild as any. Blond ones, sold separately in France, are better—fattier and milder. One dish that especially focuses on them is *gâteau de foies de volaille,* the rich chicken-liver flan of Lyon, unmolded and surrounded with tomato sauce. Generally, chicken livers are sautéed with enough heat to color the outside while leaving the inside rare, and then a quick pan sauce is made, such as with Madeira and cream. The sautéed livers can be turned into an excellent mousse with shallots, whipped cream, salt and pepper, and a little Cognac.

I'm almost never without stock, for soup and risotto, to make pan sauces, to enrich pasta sauces. I make stock after we've roasted a chicken (with a houseful, we often roast two chickens at once), maybe every two weeks.

HOW TO BUY CHICKEN: For a tastier bird, choose a fresh-killed chicken raised humanely outdoors (during the snowless months). If you can find it, choose a bird from a more old-fashioned breed, less plump but more flavorful. I like a chicken so fresh that it smells of almost nothing more than clean air. (There *is* a subtle odor, and you can smell the differences among very fresh chicken, duck, and goose.) An "air-chilled" bird is drier, and the skin will color and crisp faster. There should be plenty of neck skin left to cover the openings at either end. For my purposes, the liver, heart, gizzard, and neck should all be present, if only so the cook can fry the liver as a reward and add the rest to stock.

Cook a fresh chicken on the day you buy it, or else marinate or salt it (you boost flavor if you salt the chicken a day or two in advance, using a little more salt than you might normally), keeping the chicken very cold until an hour or two before you cook it. Often a small farm sells only frozen chickens, and it's no sin to buy a frozen bird, especially a local one, although there's some sacrifice of juice and freshness. (The USDA, defying common sense, allows a chicken to be called "fresh" as long as it hasn't been frozen below 26 degrees F, or –3.3 degrees C.)

COMPLEMENTS TO CHICKEN: Of the many things that go with chicken, a few stand out. *Vin jaune* and similarly made white wines from the Jura in France intensify the chicken taste in combination with cream and, if you have them, morels. Chicken benefits from the flavor and acidity of red and white wine, vinegar, verjuice, and lemon juice and zest. Chicken likes ham and bacon (smoked or otherwise), garlic, onion, rosemary, tarragon with cream, sage (not "rubbed"), thyme, dried-herb mixtures, fresh fines herbes (chervil, parsley, chives, tarragon), mustard, and the combination of saffron and tomato. Excellent with chicken are cooked greens, green beans, fried or grilled zucchini (from the Costata Romanesco variety), mushrooms of all kinds, and potatoes, especially fried brown and crisp. An excellent traditional garnish for roast chicken is watercress.

NOTES ON WINE: A simple roast chicken is a gift to many wines—young and old, dry and sweet, white, pink, and all but the stronger reds. With fairly plain roast or grilled chicken, I like to show off, for example, a flavorful Riesling, whether from Alsace, Austria, or Germany. A red wine might be a lighter Burgundy or a Pinot Noir from Sancerre, Alsace, the Jura, or Oregon. The path is more open to a red if the chicken is more deeply browned in cooking and flavored with a little ham or bacon, or accompanied by *lardons* and sautéed mushrooms. Generally, the wine that goes with chicken is determined by what's in the dish. With *poule au pot,* perhaps a medium white Burgundy; with *vin jaune,* cream, and morels, then *vin jaune* or a related Jura white; with *poulet au vinaigre,* a Chinon or Bourgueil; with Madeira, mushrooms, and cream, a Pinot Noir; with a saffron and tomato sauce, a dry rosé; with fried onions, an aromatic Friuli white; with fried zucchini, a plain light white; with cold roast chicken, Champagne. Those aren't rules, just possibilities.

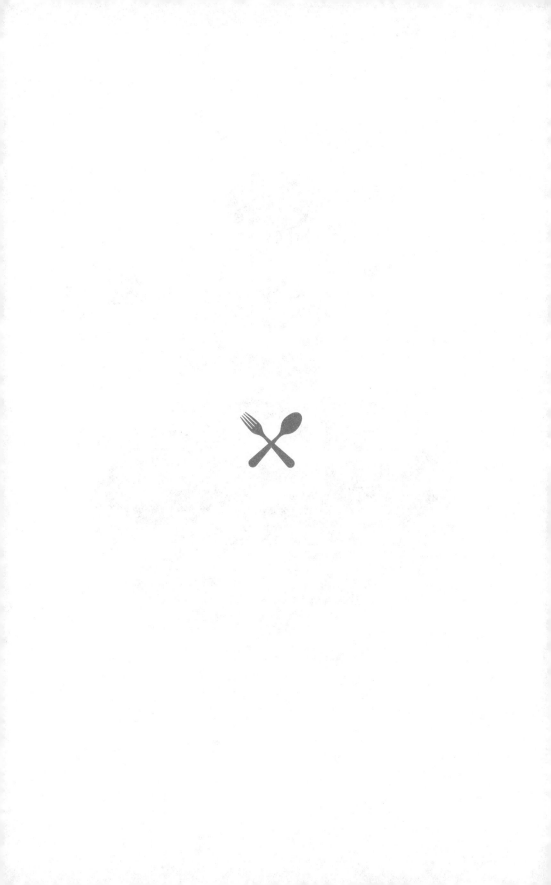

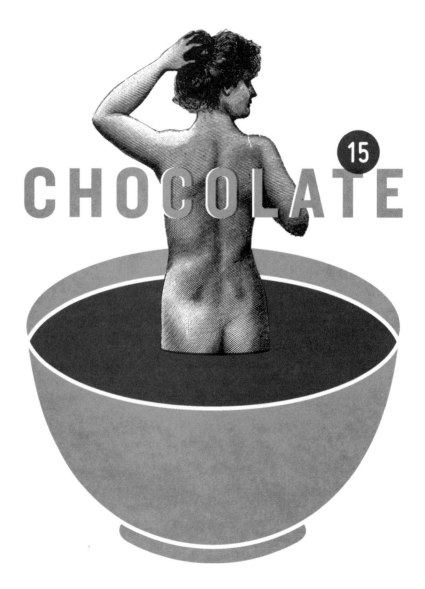

CHOCOLATE 15

15. CHOCOLATE, DARK

The best chocolate tastes strongly of ripe fruit and even flowers, and of roasting flavors; it has a pleasing acidity and a firm bitterness. (As a package, the taste of chocolate is very much like that of good coffee.) Darker chocolate tips the balance from sweetness toward aromatic intensity—it's more fun. By darker, I mean in the range of 65 to 75 percent chocolate; the number is usually indicated on good bars. The rest is almost entirely sugar plus, as a rule, a tiny amount of vanilla to underline the fruit. A few people like 100 percent chocolate—zero sugar. But sugar provides relief, and without it chocolate's bitterness and astringency are so powerful that it's hard to make out aromas. A higher percentage of chocolate tends to taste stronger, though that's not automatic. The percentage represents the combined dark aromatic portion plus cocoa butter, whose ratio can be adjusted by the maker. Chocolate with too much cocoa butter has notably reduced aroma and, in its place, the unpleasant fatty texture typical of Belgian chocolate. Yet a certain amount of cocoa butter is essential. Together with sugar, it gives chocolate its characteristic snap when you break a bar or bite into it. And like regular butter, cocoa butter melts at slightly below body temperature, which is why chocolate melts in your mouth. Velvety texture is a large part of what makes chocolate so gratifyingly sensual.

Mass-market chocolate doesn't have fruit flavor. And milk chocolate hardly counts as chocolate at all; it's dominated by the potent caramel flavors of cooked milk, added in powdered or condensed form. White chocolate to me is just a disagreeable form of fat, made mostly of cocoa butter, with a flavor that depends entirely on what's added: sugar, milk solids (including butterfat), and vanilla—often cloying artificial vanilla.

The world center of chocolate culture, of transforming beans into chocolate and chocolate into candies, has long been France and, for candy, especially Paris. At least for now, it still is. Top-quality chocolate is also made in other countries, including Italy, Switzerland, and more recently the United States and some of the cacao-growing countries, including Venezuela and Ecuador. ("Cacao" refers to the tree and the beans before processing; after that the word is "cocoa.") Most good chocolate, though, still comes from a few major European manufacturers: Valrhona and Michel Cluizel in France, Lindt in Switzerland and elsewhere, and Cacao Barry, originally French but today part of the global giant Barry Callebaut, whose headquarters are in Switzerland. Other good brands are smaller in scale, even minuscule, and lately new ones are steadily appearing. Now in the US, as an alternative to the big names and occasionally far surpassing them in fruit flavor, there's a wave of tiny, sometimes one- or two-person chocolate makers, including Amano, Dandelion, Patric, Ritual, Rogue, and Taza. They buy top-quality beans, often at the source, and push hard to preserve all their fine flavors in the finished bar.

Good chocolate used to be made by blending beans from complementary sources, for consistency and complexity. Today producers seek to identify superior beans at the source—90 percent of cacao is still grown on farms of just five to a dozen acres (two to five hectares). Most of the best bars are labeled by provenance now, and a few bear the name of an individual farm. Besides Ecuador and Venezuela (where the famous place-name is Chuao), you find bars from Bolivia, Colombia, Congo, Costa Rica, Cuba, Dominican Republic, Haiti, Madagascar, Mexico, Peru, Vietnam, the islands of Java in the Pacific and Trinidad in the Caribbean. Africa produces mostly bulk cacao, but there are exceptions; Ghana, for instance, has a reputation for grading and higher quality. (Some African beans have a rubber taste from being dried over fires.)

Very recently, new genetic work has overturned our understanding of cacao trees, which always used to be divided into three kinds. Criollo ("native"), with white seeds, was best and scarcest, vulnerable to insects and disease, and found mainly in Central America, where it has been cultivated for three thousand years. Forastero ("foreign"), with violet seeds, was robust and high-yielding, supplying the mass market with beans anywhere from devoid of interest to richly chocolatey. In the middle was Trinitario, a hybrid originally from Trinidad. It was well-known that among the three types there were many varieties and intentional and natural crosses, with seeds in a range of color from white to violet. Now the name Trinitario is no longer considered useful. We know there are a dozen or more genetic groups, each with its geographic locations: Criollo forms one group, and all the rest are Forastero, with perhaps a few more to be identified.

In theory the skin of Criollo beans is white, but there's only a loose correlation between color and flavor. Criollo is less bitter and astringent than Forastero and has more acidity and more delicate fruit. A few special Criollo bars are labeled Porcelana, which is named for the translucence of the white skin covering the pod and comes from certain trees in Venezuela. And even Porcelana further subdivides. It has flavors of nuts, such as macadamia. At least a couple of US microroasters make bars using beans from particular stands of wild trees.

The cacao fruits—the pods that hold the beans—resemble elongated melons, and, weirdly, they're attached directly to the tree trunks and main branches. The ripe pods, according to the tree, can be anywhere from green to yellow, orange, or red. To determine whether a fruit is ripe, you tap and listen to hear whether the bean mass has pulled away from the pod a little. The ripe pods are cut from the trees and hacked open, and the seeds are pulled out by hand, along with the surrounding sweet mucilage. Together they undergo a triple fermentation that gives a large part of chocolate's flavor. Wild yeast act on the sugars in the mucilage to create an alcoholic fermentation; a first group of bacteria consumes sugars and citric acid to make lactic acid; then other bacteria turn the alcohol into the acetic acid of vinegar. The vinegar and high temperatures kill the seeds, leading to further complicated changes, particularly as enzymes form flavor precursors. Times, temperatures, equipment, even stirring—all influence flavor. A lot is happening, and a lot remains unknown. A fermentation can go awry and produce funky flavor and too much vinegar. More fruit flavor may result from a longer, cooler fermentation, but Criollo benefits from a shorter one than most beans. Afterward, drying the beans slowly with only the sun's heat preserves more fruit.

Roasting increases the cocoa-y flavor and adds those of grilling, dried fruit, and freshly baked bread—strong flavors that easily hide those of fruit and flowers. Just as a lighter roast of coffee beans preserves more fruit in a cup of coffee, so a lighter roast of cocoa beans preserves more fruit in chocolate. Roasting also accomplishes one smaller thing. When I visited the Valrhona factory in Tain l'Hermitage, France, I was surprised to find the courtyard filled not with aromas of either fruit or roasting but instead with a strong smell of vinegar. Roasting drives off some of the acetic acid from the fermentation, though not that much—a little vinegar produces a strong odor. The roasted beans are reddish-brown, a color that carries over into the finished chocolate.

Vanilla is the flavor most complementary to chocolate, combined with it in South America long before the first Europeans arrived. Some of today's purists, however, argue that vanilla only interferes with the innate flavors of good beans. They compare added vanilla with the oak flavor, from barrels or chips, found in so much current wine. But the overwhelming quantity of chocolate contains vanilla, and then the ideal, not necessarily the practice, is to grind whole vanilla beans with the cocoa. Often manufacturers also add a tiny quantity of lecithin, a substance widely found in nature, which has beneficial effects on texture and perhaps on flavor.

Steel rollers, or very exceptionally stones, grind the beans to a powder that is sifted and reground until it's fine enough to convey full aroma and provide smooth texture. The powder, which might contain 50 to 55 percent cocoa butter (the range is from 46 to as high as 65 percent), is then mixed, and the heat of mixing melts the fat and creates a watery paste. Big operations press the paste to expel the cocoa butter, and then reassemble the two components in the proportions they want. Almost any good large-scale manufacturer adds cocoa butter in a higher ratio than the natural one. (It's probably needless to say that purists don't do that.) The extra fat comes from selling off some of the cocoa powder as just powder (and keeping the butter from it) or from buying in extra cocoa butter from a manufacturer that sells powder. The reassembled paste is mixed thoroughly with sugar and ground again.

The chocolate is then mixed in another way: it's conched in specially designed machines, the nineteenth-century original of which was shell-shaped, giving the name. The machine repeatedly works the soft mass, transforming it through heat, movement, and exposure to air. Experts disagree about all that happens during conching. But it clearly turns the paste of fat and dry material into a smoother, more fluid, more homogeneous suspension, achieving that creamy smoothness you feel as good chocolate melts in your mouth. It also breaks up and moves the minute flavor compounds between particles in such a way that they come out in your mouth at different rates, creating a layered effect. And conching allows certain off-flavors to evaporate. ("I come home smelling terrible on the days I conch," a US microroaster said to me.) It costs time and money to conch, so low-end bars are conched for no more than a few hours. A high-end bar might be conched for up to three days.

Yet the exposure to air during conching removes some desirable aromas, and lately in the US some small-scale producers take the antediluvian position that any conching at all is a mistake, because it takes more than it gives. The small company Taza, in Massachusetts, for one, follows the Mexican model and doesn't conch at all, and for the same reason—concern that more manipulation takes more flavor—it doesn't fully grind either the cocoa or the sugar, leaving detectable fine sugar granules in the bars. Unconched chocolate, even when the sugar is ground smooth, is less refined in texture, and its flavor is more rustic, wild, and more often full of fruit. Next to Taza, the widely available Lindt "Excellence," which I've enjoyed on its own, appears dull, muddy, and off-flavored, and Valrhona's Guanaja, while free of defects and outstanding, shows mainly deep, nutty flavors, falling short on high notes and fruit. Taza is more vivid and intense than either one, full of the flavors of small red fruits, though perhaps not as focused.

It's not that conching is a mistake. It gives a more settled flavor and a more gratifying texture. And you need a delicious smoothness for coating fine chocolates. The highly knowledgeable small-batch maker Colin Gasko of Rogue Chocolatier, in Massachusetts, stresses that conching is easily oversimplified to longer or shorter, yes or no, while in truth the results depend on potent variables, such as temperature and different ways of using different machines. His own chocolate shows a distinct conched effect, although his times are short, from twenty-four to as few as six hours. And his bars can have very strong fruit. As a taster, it's hard to know what comes from the beans and what comes from technique. The best bars from both approaches are exciting to taste, though I strongly prefer the traditional velvety texture.

Before chocolate is molded into bars, it's tempered: carefully heated to 115 to 120 degrees F (46 to 49 degrees C) to melt it completely and then cooled to 82 to 84 degrees F (28 to 29 degrees C) and raised again to 88 to 90 degrees F (31 to 32 degrees C). The effect is to give the fat a more stable crystalline structure, shown in a cleaner snap, a brighter shine, and a greater resistance to the defect called "bloom." That's the harmless powdery white surface composed of either sugar or fat (and caused by, in the case of fat, too-warm storage and, in the case of sugar, either too-cool storage or too much humidity). Each time chocolate is melted to use for coating or molding, it must be retempered.

Some people find a big advantage to chocolate that's just been made—less than a week old, when there's a bright edge of flavor. And yet inside its foil wrapper a bar of chocolate remains delicious for months. A few people even like the effects of age, up to perhaps six months. Changes occur quickly during the first two or three weeks as flavors meld, and more and more slowly after that. As in wine, flavors come and go before they diminish altogether.

Then there is the high craft of the chocolatier, at least as practiced by certain celebrated craftsmen, mainly in Paris, such as Michel Chaudun and Pierre Hermé. The first thing any chocolatier must do is decide what kind of chocolate to buy, since almost none roasts beans and makes chocolate from scratch. Instead, they buy from one of the big manufacturers, and for most the choice is determined less by taste than by a combination of price, the technical qualities of the chocolate, and the technical support provided by the manufacturer.

The craft of a chocolatier is both repetitious and exacting. A large part of the skill and pride lies in hand-dipping chocolates, with the center balanced on the tines of a special fork, to create a thin coating with a sharp snap. A dipped chocolate shouldn't, for instance, have a "foot," a border around the bottom where the chocolate settled before it set. Yet to achieve any economy of scale, you need an enrobing machine, which can be adjusted to shake off much of the melted chocolate and avoid a foot. Part of the logic of the chocolate coating is that it allows a soft center to be eaten at room temperature. A classic chocolate truffle, for instance, is always coated; a naked one, merely dusted with cocoa powder, must be chilled, or it will be too soft to pick up.

Modern chocolates are smaller, more bite-sized, and more thinly coated than any chocolates used to be. The thin coating gives a larger proportion of interior, but there should be enough chocolate to provide a balance in taste and texture. Some modern chocolates have too-thin coatings, and, besides, a thicker one holds its flavor longer. Molding can be done well, too, but as a rule it gives a much heavier, more irregular coating, and generally it's a shortcut.

One of the most satisfying of all forms of chocolate—more delicate than a truffle—is the *palet d'or,* a "golden disk" that is a little more than an inch in diameter by about a quarter-inch thick. The upper surface, which was the bottom when it was dipped and set down to harden, is flecked with gold foil, a visual charm that neither adds to nor takes away from the taste. The fascination of the *palet d'or* is its double form of chocolate: the firm, intense, dark outer chocolate in a thicker or thinner layer, according to the views of the chocolatier, around a soft center of ganache, which is chocolate mixed with nothing more than fresh cream or crème fraîche and sometimes a little butter. The soft crunch of the bitter exterior contrasts with the smooth, yielding, often slightly sweeter interior.

Some chocolatiers only repeat familiar flavors, but for others an important part of the job is to seek fresh, sometimes highly innovative flavor combinations, and the list of possibilities is endless. Ganache is a good medium for other flavors, but it's easily made, not a test of skill. Other interiors play on other textures: jelly, nougat, fondant, caramel, *praliné,* candied fruit, and, exceptionally, liquid. Often overlooked is crunch. I sometimes wonder why chocolatiers haven't pursued new gastronomic technologies in the way some high-end chefs have, putting familiar tastes into previously unimagined textural forms. Why aren't there novel inside-out chocolates with, say, nonsticky fruit coatings over chocolate insides that are liquid, foamy, gaseous, even somehow gently exploding? Two-compartment fillings that mix and form some unexpected third element? Sweetness lends itself to fantasy.

HOW TO BUY CHOCOLATE: You can't tell much of anything before you open a bar or box and bite in, so choose a chocolate maker you know is good, or knowingly take a risk on an unfamiliar one. Some big manufacturers produce both high- and low-level bars, and the difference isn't necessarily reflected in the price. Usually, however, the major manufacturers' bars labeled with a geographic origin are good to excellent. And often a label usefully states the percentage of chocolate, 65 to 75 percent giving a balance with wide appeal. Once you've opened a bar, signs of high quality are a bright shine, a dark reddish-brown color, and a good snap. In your mouth, look for a smooth texture and marked fruit flavor. Any small off-flavors should be offset by a superabundance of good ones.

HOW TO STORE CHOCOLATE: Keep both chocolate and chocolates protected in the package they come in; set them in a place free of dampness and strong odors and at a slightly cool temperature (if possible, 60 to 65 degrees F, or 16 to 18 degrees C). A bar, even inside its tight foil wrapping, gradually loses flavor as time passes, so don't ignore it for weeks. (And if you melt chocolate for cooking, don't heat it too much or too long, or the aromatic high notes will give way to a peanutty taste.) Dipped and molded chocolates taste best as soon as the chocolate has set and hold good flavor for only about ten days.

COMPLEMENTS TO CHOCOLATE: Chocolate's strong acidity, tannin, and nutty, roasted flavors stand up well in an enormous range of combinations. It's tempting to say that everything goes with chocolate. Yet being so strong, chocolate merely coexists with a lot of those other things. One item that goes beautifully with chocolate is vanilla, already present in conventional chocolate in a calibrated amount. Cream and butter are complementary in both flavor and texture, and they do well in quantity, like some other additions—caramel, toasted nuts, coconut, candied orange peel. Certain things require restraint—rose, coffee, cinnamon (the last is classic, though not my favorite). More complements by category: *strong alcoholic drinks,* such as rum and fruit eaux-de-vie; *browned, roasted, nutty items,* including sesame, balsamic vinegar, and rum with raisins; *fruits* of very many kinds; *floral items,* such as violet and orchid but also muscat; *herbs and spices,* such as Earl Grey tea, cardamom, basil, and mint. Newish ideas are lychee, passion fruit, saffron, Thai basil, Szechuan pepper, powerful kinds of honey, green tea in pistachio paste, and a reduction of sweet vinegar. (Distinctly bad combinations with chocolate, in my experience, are licorice, maple, blue cheese, and rosemary.) A common successful addition is hot chile pepper, though it's less a taste complement than an intellectual one that recalls the pre-Columbian origins of chocolate. And then there are complements, such as tomatoes and prunes, that work particularly in savory dishes.

NOTES ON WINE: Chocolate destroys most wines. Some people insist on drinking dry red wine with it, and in that case there's more chance for success when the wine is made from very ripe grapes that give extra alcohol and leave some residual sugar, as in Recioto della Valpolicella and certain California Zinfandels. (With a savory sauce merely flavored with bitter chocolate, such as Mexican-inspired moles with various meats, choose a rich red that also has a savory side, which might be a Côtes du Rhône or, better, a Rhône Syrah.) With chocolate in dessert, to give any wine a better chance, the chocolate shouldn't be too sweet (no less than about 70 percent chocolate), and to overcome the chocolate's strength, astringency, and sweetness, the wine must be powerful. It needs concentrated flavors carried by sugar or high alcohol or both. Very-high-alcohol options include Armagnac, good marc or grappa, the plum eaux-de-vie mirabelle and quetsch, and single-malt Scotch.

But no drink goes better with chocolate than Banyuls, the intentionally oxidized, fortified, and often sweet wine from the Mediterranean French coast beside Spain. Modern versions, labeled "Rimage," have a somewhat lighter, fresher set of flavors that are less adapted to chocolate.

Better in every way is the traditional oxidized, deep-flavored, mahogany-colored Banyuls (there's also white and even rosé) from, above all, Domaine du Mas Blanc but also Domaine de la Rectorie, Domaine la Tour Vieille, and the cooperative L'Étoile.

Closely related to Banyuls and similarly successful with chocolate is wine from the nearby appellation of Maury, where again the traditional style is better. Affordable and outstanding with chocolate is Mas Amiel's Cuvée Spéciale Maury, with its *rancio* flavors (see "Walnuts"). In the same region, the much larger appellation of Rivesaltes produces some similar wine, but a good traditional bottling is harder to find. All these wines are sweet, though from a label it's hard to know just how sweet. All you have to go on is the imperfect relationship of sugar to alcohol: bottles of Banyuls at 16 percent are sweeter as a rule, and better with chocolate, and those at 18 or 19 percent are drier. Serve the sweeter wines at 60 degrees F (16 degrees C) in winter and a few degrees cooler in summer. Once these wines are opened, you don't have to consume them right away; a recorked bottle can last for a month in the refrigerator.

Still in the oxidized realm are Pedro Ximénez sherry and aged tawny Port. (Vintage Port is on almost everyone's list, not so much on mine.) Also outstanding with chocolate are certain bottlings of Madeira, though it's hard to predict which ones before you taste. Like Banyuls, Madeira has oxidized flavors—dried fruits, walnut, almond, caramel, coffee, chocolate itself, sometimes *rancio*—similar to but not quite the same as those in the chocolate.

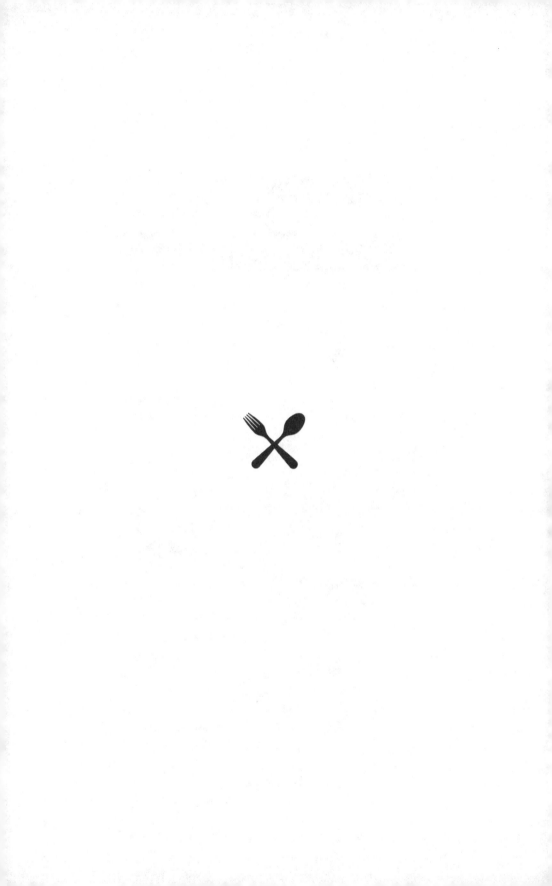

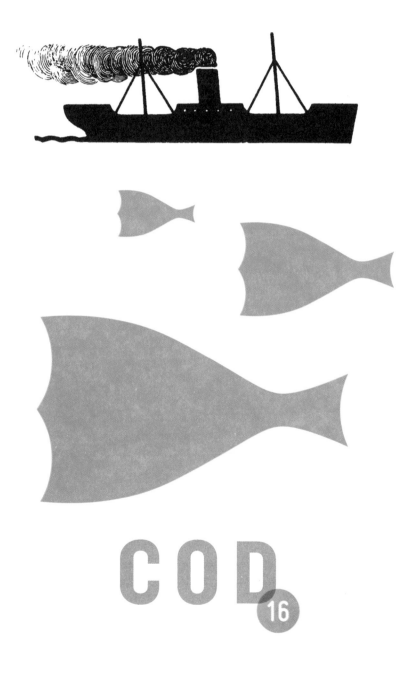

COD
16

Cod once filled the North Atlantic Ocean, particularly on the American side, and for centuries it was one of the most important fish. The fresh fish is lean and meaty, easy to separate from the bones, neither delicate nor coarse. (To compare it with two of its relatives, it's finer than haddock and much finer than pollack, which is fibrous. Some fish with the name, such as black cod, or sablefish, and lingcod, aren't part of the family at all.) Cod had enormous value above all because it lends itself to salting and drying. Overfishing has reduced the stock of Atlantic cod to a fraction of what it was, though limits have been imposed that may someday allow the depleted Georges Bank and Gulf of Maine, the main US cod fishing grounds, to rebound. The Atlantic cod, *Gadus morhua,* lives in deep, cold waters from Cape Hatteras north to Ungava Bay and Hudson Bay, by Greenland and around Iceland and throughout northern Europe all the way to the Barents Sea. The fish can reach a length of four or five feet (130 centimeters) and a weight of 50 to 75 pounds (25 to 35 kilos), exceptionally much more, but the average today is much less. Cod is one of the groundfish, living near the ocean floor and feeding on other fish and seafood, even lobsters. The Pacific cod, *Gadus macrocephalus,* always less abundant in nature, lives in a vast arc from the coast of California northward and across the Aleutian Islands. Pacific and Atlantic cod are close in taste.

The word "scrod," referring to young cod, sometimes appears on menus, but today small fish are the norm. The fresh fish, being lean, is often fried or cooked in liquid, or broiled or baked very simply. It's one of the fish that can make chowder, which in New England homes is centered on salt pork, potatoes, and long cooking in milk—nothing like the typical gluey restaurant chowder. Cod is one of the main fish sold as fish and chips. The French *cabillaud* means fresh, not necessarily young, cod; *morue* is normally salt cod. In cod-fishing ports, the most highly regarded part of the cod is the cheeks; also popular are tongues, sounds (air bladders), and throat muscles.

Besides being eaten fresh, cod is salted and partly dried to make salt cod and fully air-dried, without salt, to make stockfish. The latter are whole fish, opened flat and dried; they become rigid, like wood. Originally, the fish was salted onboard ship and then dried outdoors on land. Fresh and salt cod are related in taste, though salt cod can be very tender by comparison, and in cooking sometimes, as in the Veneto, the two are treated as interchangeable. Salt cod tends to evoke a definite like or dislike. I feel a strong aversion to any fishiness in fresh fish, but salt cod, like cured anchovy, has a different, desirable fishiness that isn't spoilage but richness. (I've eaten stockfish, but I've never sought it out to cook it myself.) Salt cod is made especially in Canada, Iceland, and Norway. And with the decline of cod, you may see some other fish sold as salt cod. Both salt cod and stockfish require soaking, but stockfish, being completely dehydrated, requires more soaking. Salt cod was traded and consumed throughout Western Europe, partly because it could be eaten on fast days. It became a fish of the Mediterranean table, common food, not something special. With rare exceptions, salt cod is soaked before it's cooked to remove some of the salt and return it closer to the state of fresh fish. Until a few decades ago, salt cod was still eaten in inland parts of New England, often breaded and fried as fishballs. Overcooked salt cod, especially if it was very salty to begin with, is dry, fibrous, and tough. But good, carefully cooked salt cod has a consistency not so far from that of the fresh fish.

When you buy it, the best salt cod has some of the lustrous appearance of fresh fish. The world center for appreciation is Catalonia, in northeast Spain, where you see it displayed in central stalls of La Boqueria, the main market in Barcelona. The whole fish is salted, but it's sold in different cuts: belly is darker and inferior, used only in flaked preparations; the best parts, thick and white, come from the part of the loin toward the tail.

In Catalonia, it's said there's a *bacallà* (salt cod) dish for every day in the year. It's mostly fried, sometimes baked. It loves garlic and olive oil; it goes with tomato and olives. The famous dish of the city of Tarragona in Catalonia is *peix amb romesco,* a mixture of fried fish in a hot *romesco* sauce (garlic, parsley, toasted almonds, and Romesco peppers) that can also be applied to *bacallà.* (This *romesco* is very different from the creamy cold sauce for grilled onions.) In Catalonia, *bacallà* is cooked *amb panses i pinyons:* floured, fried, and cooked with fried onions, a paste of pine nuts, a little water, raisins, and more pine nuts. It's also baked with lightly browned garlic and fresh tomatoes in the oven, then finished with finely chopped raw garlic and parsley. It's cooked with artichokes, or with honey, to make an exotic taste. In modern Spanish cuisine, salt cod is sometimes served raw, as if it were sashimi or carpaccio, such as in salad with oranges, raw onions, and olives.

In Italy, *baccalà alla vicentina,* the famous dish of the Veneto, is finely flaked and cooked in onion, garlic, parsley, anchovies, milk, grated cheese, and olive oil, never stirred, and served with polenta. *Baccalà alla livornese* is floured and fried with tomato. Tuscan *baccalà con i porri* is with leeks and tomato. *Baccalà mantecato,* from the Veneto, is beaten with olive oil with a wooden spoon to a creamy consistency and served on crostini. *Baccalà* is also cooked in milk in layers with potatoes, onion, a bay leaf, a little oregano, at the end some hot pepper, chopped raw garlic and parsley, and finally, optionally, served with olives (which added earlier would stain the dish) and hard-cooked egg—a recipe given by Patience Gray. Salt cod can be deep fried as croquettes. Sauces for salt cod often include anchovy.

In Provence, salt cod is at the center of a *grand aïoli,* and there are many more Provençal dishes. To make *brandade,* which is associated with the city of Nîmes, the cooked salt cod, together with mashed raw garlic, is beaten with olive oil to make an emulsion like mayonnaise; it's thinned with a little hot milk and finished with a touch of lemon juice. The result, which looks a lot like mashed potato (and looks and tastes like *baccalà mantecato*), is eaten with toasted bread. Salt cod can be flaked and added to eggs *à la tripe,* which are hard-cooked in béchamel, with butter-fried croûtons on top. Salt cod goes into dishes *à la provençal,* meaning various cooked-tomato concoctions. One of the best is salt cod fried and cooked *en raïto,* in a sauce of olive oil, onion, tomato, bay leaf, red wine, garlic, parsley, and at the end chopped capers.

HOW TO BUY FRESH AND SALT COD: The season for fresh cod is year-round, and the most important thing is always freshness. (Cod frozen immediately on shipboard is much better than questionable "fresh" fish.) Fresh-caught cod comes from day boats, of which in the northeastern US, under current limits, there are few. The best method for catching the fish, for quality and the environment, is hook-and-line (there's commercial gear for the purpose). Least good is trawling, which damages the bottom habitat and picks up other species along with cod. Various better and worse methods are used in the healthy cod fishery in the seas off Iceland, Norway, and Russia. (It's incomprehensible that the burden of making complex environmental choices about fish is placed on each consumer, rather than any professional or governmental organization.) From Alaska, avoid cod caught by trawling. Keep fresh cod, like other fresh fish, on ice, and cook it on the day you buy it. Salt cod is scarce in North America; try to find a fishmonger who cares about it. One good brand is Bacalao Giraldo, from Basque Spain, which has a centuries-old tradition of salting cod. Keep salt cod well wrapped in the refrigerator.

HOW TO PREPARE SALT COD: The time required for soaking varies according to the saltiness and thickness of the piece—anywhere from twelve to thirty-six hours—and it helps to change the water as many as half a dozen times. The goal is to remove salt and introduce moisture, but the more salt that is lost, the more flavor goes with it, and you need a balance. The difficulty is telling how much soaking is enough. Good salt cod swells to more or less its fresh condition; it feels like a firmer version of the fresh fish. For moist texture, cook salt cod gently, starting it in cold water and merely poaching it—boiling dries it out. The time might be from seven or eight minutes to ten or twenty, depending on the amount of soaking and the thickness. (For *brandade* or *mantecato* slight underpoaching avoids dryness.) Probed with the point of a knife, the fish should be tender but shouldn't fall readily into flakes. For some dishes, salt cod remains whole;

for others you take out the bones, which flakes the fish, but generally keep the pieces as large as you can. Remove the skin.

COMPLEMENTS TO FRESH AND SALT COD: Fresh cod, like other fish, goes with a range of flavors, including lemon, parsley, butter, potatoes, capers, onions. It goes with spinach and a generous range of vegetables, including bell peppers and steamed or boiled potatoes. It goes with milk in chowder. Salt cod and stockfish go easily with a huge variety of other flavors. They're especially complemented by garlic, olive oil, spinach, chard, artichokes, fennel, olives, aioli, and all the fixings of the *grand aïoli* (which includes tomato in season, green beans, boiled potatoes . . .), onions, milk, parsley, black pepper, saffron, tomatoes, wine, raisins, and pine nuts.

NOTES ON WINE: Fresh cod isn't especially picky about wine. It's often matched with white Burgundy. I like simple baked cod with Muscadet; a full-flavored dish goes with, for instance, a dry Alsace Pinot Gris or Pinot Blanc. When in doubt, follow the old, sometimes-mocked rule, and avoid red wine with fish. Simple breaded and fried balls of salt cod, like fish and chips and other fried foods, go with Champagne. Salt cod, such as in *brandade* or as part of a *grand aïoli,* goes first of all with dry rosé, not too strong, and with a southern French white. It goes with a white Hermitage. With salt cod in a flavorful sauce, or with salt pork or bacon, a light fruity red can work. Salt cod goes with Fino and Manzanilla sherry.

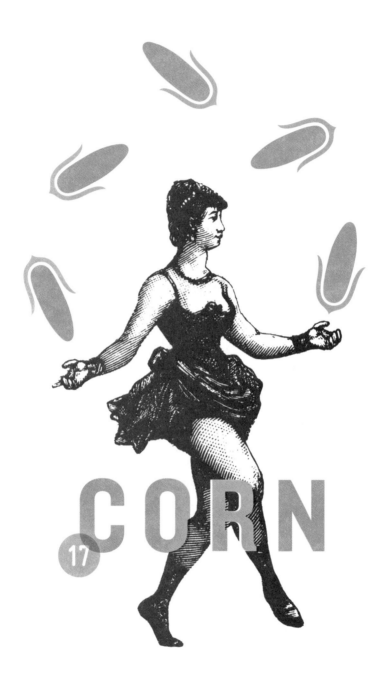

CORN

17

F or really great sweet corn, it used to be that, just as the old advice had it, you had to put the pot of water on to boil and then go out to the garden to pick the ears. The sugar in the old varieties began to turn to starch immediately. Few people grow those varieties anymore. Now we have vastly sweeter genetic categories—sugary supersweets, sugary enhanced, fully modified, single-gene replacements, multiple-gene replacements, and "triplesweet," which combines supersweet with sugar-enhanced. The extra sugar used to taste very strange to me, though I've become slightly used to it. Still, compared with the old sweet corn, the new kinds don't fit as comfortably on a plate of savory food. Occasionally in August I see a stand with a sign for one of the old varieties—usually Silver Queen, but there were and are others, such as Country Gentleman and Golden Bantam. They're more flavorful—they taste more like corn. Sweet corn is delicious boiled, on and off the cob, mainly with butter, and generous salt and pepper pulls it back toward the savory. Even the old kinds to me don't have enough flavor to stand up to grilling or, more romantically, to cooking inside their husks buried in the coals of a fire. But I've loved a totally modern vegan soup that a chef made from the sap pressed from the raw kernels, subtly flavored with saffron and half a dozen other ingredients.

Dried corn, ground into meal, isn't more delicious, but it's more complicated and interesting. It makes grits, mush, and polenta—all names for humble, delicious corn porridge. Grits in the US South are traditionally eaten at breakfast and supper rather than at dinner, in the sense of the old-fashioned midday meal, which was the biggest of the day. And they're eaten, not with milk or cream and sugar, like a breakfast of New England mush, but with butter and salt and pepper, or alongside eggs, fried chicken, fried fish, sausage, country bacon, or country ham. In Italy, where polenta used to be eaten at any meal, it similarly goes with all kinds of savory foods. Often, like pasta, it receives a sauce. Sometimes it's sliced and then fried or grilled very slowly over a cool fire. Whatever the method, butter and grating cheese are commonly stirred in first—both Italians and American Southerners like cheese with their ground corn. Fine cornmeal also makes corn bread, raised once always by yeast and now by baking soda and powder. It makes tender spoon bread, pancakes, and cookies.

Of course most cornmeal is mass-produced and refined, in Italy as in the US. It's one even color, yellow or white, and deprived of the flavorful germ. It doesn't taste like much at all. Delicious meal comes from a flavorful milling variety. It must ripen fully in the field (or your porridge will taste like split peas), and, once dried, the whole kernels must be freshly ground. In the kitchen, the porridge must cook slowly and long; at a point between one and two hours, a much stronger corn flavor appears, akin to the corniness of fresh sweet corn from one of the old varieties.

Coarser, more shattered cornmeal retains more flavor; old-fashioned polenta and old-fashioned Southern grits are about equally coarse. The word "polenta," to be clear, refers to the cooked dish, not the raw meal, and it's made more in the north of Italy than in the south. I've visited Italian mills that use stones and grind only flavorful old *ottofile,* "eight-row," varieties, eight-row corn being the original kind. (Modern corn has as many as fourteen and even sixteen rows of kernels.) In Italy, low-tech polenta was the food of the poor, and now it's the food of the affluent. You find it in certain high-end restaurants at its delicious best: organic, *ottofile,* coarsely stone-ground, whole and fresh, perfectly cooked. The fresher the cornmeal, the better the taste. When you cook the freshest meal in a covered pot and lift the lid, you smell a floral perfume.

The millers who care most about grits grind theirs on stones, although there's no clear advantage beyond the pleasant link with the past. Milling can be done well or badly with stones or steel rollers; in either case, it's important that the meal remain cool. Grinding exposes the germ's oil, source of much of the flavor. The only way to slow the oil from turning rancid is to keep the meal cold or frozen or in some way protected from oxygen.

The old North American regional varieties haven't evolved that much since they were received from Native Americans. Most American cornmeal today is, like the meal for some Italian polenta, ground from softer types of corn. Southern grits are typically milled from dent corn, whose kernels have hard sides and a central column of floury starch; as the ears dry, the ends of the kernels become dented. Certain old varieties of dent, often saved in farming families and never given formal names, make especially flavorful grits. It's perhaps less a question of one variety being better than another than of planting the right one in the right spot, the place to which it's best adapted. The old way to dry corn, still practiced here and there, was to let it stand in the field until fall. That way, the ears can't help but be fully ripe, and there's no risk the grain will be damaged by mechanical drying.

Cornmeal, once an important food in New England, continues to be eaten here a little, as corn bread, jonnycakes, and mush. The traditional New England corn comes from the very hard varieties called flint, full of protein and varying in color from white to yellow to red. Rhode Island White Cap was *the* corn in southern New England. Its Maine and Vermont relatives were each saved from extinction by a single family. The Vermont corn, called Roy's Calais Flint, has perhaps the best flavor of any flint, not so much of corn as of subtle bran and malt. A large handful of other old flints are grown around the country; some people especially like Amish Butter popcorn or Sea Island White from South Carolina. The American flints became the European ones, and there are "unimproved" Italian varieties with all the old virtues. Only this year did I learn just how good flint corn can be. I cooked some excellent flint meal that a farmer had sent me, the last of which had been sitting for a month in the freezer, and it still held a strong floral quality along with its delicious grain flavor. Meal like that gives a completely different sense of corn flavor.

The precision-minded, deeply informed South Carolina miller Glenn Roberts, of Anson Mills, is a fervent believer in the value of heirloom grains. He chills the dried corn to minus 10 degrees F (minus 23 degrees C), grinds it on stones, chills it again afterward, and ships the meal the same day. During the grinding, delicate, short-lived flavors, even of violets, fill the mill, and for Roberts they're the real point. Both milling and packing are done in an atmosphere of CO_2. Without it, he says, "the top mill flavors are gone within seventy-two hours." Corn was commonly ground at home once a week, or more often.

Most Southern grits are white, but there has always been some yellow corn in the South, as well as mixed colors, including red. In taste, the white and yellow belong to slightly different categories, both of them good. Yellow grits are stronger; the corn flavor leads, followed by, to borrow Roberts' description, citrus and mineral flavors. He considers white grits to have more aroma of flowers and limestone, with corn flavor coming afterward.

Then there is hominy. The word comes from Algonquian and in its broadest sense means "hulled corn." In the South, the hull that coats each kernel was typically loosened by soaking the kernels in water mixed with lye from wood ash (the same can be done with mineral lime); then the hulls could be rubbed off and rinsed away. The treatment gives a distinct nutritional benefit. Many consumers believe that any hominy for sale today is made that way, but the old procedure, associated with poverty, went into such decline that some years ago when I looked for lye hominy for sale in the South, I found none at all. When I did taste hominy like that and made it myself, which is easily done, I was surprised to discover that the lime simplifies and heightens the floral perfume of fresh corn. The aroma is an essential component of corn, but I like it better as an indicator of freshness than as the central part of flavor. And when hominy is cooked in soups and stews, it becomes a balanced part of the whole.

The common Mexican word for hominy is *nixtamal,* which is ground wet to make *masa* ("dough") for tortillas and tamales. The dough, too, should be fresh. *Masa harina,* flour ground from dried *nixtamal,* doesn't have much flavor. One more form of corn is prized in Mexico: the pearly gray fungus, producing bizarrely swollen kernels, called in Mexico *huitlacoche* and known in English as corn smut. It has a good, mild fungal flavor and can be used in as varied ways as mushrooms.

HOW TO BUY AND STORE FRESH SWEET CORN AND CORNMEAL: Buy sweet corn only from a farm stand or farmers' market. Even very sweet modern varieties of sweet corn taste better when the ears were picked an hour ago rather than eight hours or two days ago. And if you come across an old-fashioned variety of sweet corn, it's best that it was picked an hour ago at most. With any variety, look at the base of the ear where it was torn from the stalk to see how dry it looks; as time passes it also shrinks. To determine ripeness, you can look at the silk, which should be brown and not too dry, but it doesn't tell much. The only way to be sure of ripeness, although some stands discourage it, is to pull back the husk just enough to see the tip of each ear, which should be mostly but not quite completely filled out. (You may see a worm, proof that the farmer's methods weren't toxic.) When you take the cooked ears from the boiling water, wrap them in a towel to absorb water and keep them hot. When I slice the kernels from the cob, I hold the ear upright on a board and use a regular dull table knife so as not to include any of the tough part of the cob.

For flavorful fresh cornmeal, buy directly from a conscientious mill, aiming to get meal ground no more than a week before. There aren't many such mills, but a few in the southern US will ship. Sometimes there's a choice of fine or coarse meal (I suspect most people would prefer coarse). A good mill chooses its dried corn carefully from a ripe, flavorful old variety. Use the meal within a week if you can, a few weeks at most; keep it in a tightly sealed glass jar in the refrigerator or freezer.

HOW TO COOK GRITS, MUSH, AND POLENTA: There's one detail to consider in preparing old-style whole-ground corn. Before cooking, some Southerners take the trouble to "wash" their grits to remove the loose dark hull, which does take longer to cook and never becomes as soft as the rest. (Sifted out and cooked separately, the bits of hull have a rich odor and taste of bran.) To wash raw grits, stir them with a lot of cold water, skim off the floating dark flecks, then stir and skim again.

The usual ratio of water to meal, by weight, is about 5½ to 1, which is about 1 cup meal to about 3½ cups cold water (150 grams meal to 825 milliliters water) with from one-half to one teaspoon salt. (Rather than water, some Southerners prefer the richness of milk.) *In the traditional method,* to avoid lumps, you slowly sift the meal from one hand into the boiling water while stirring continuously with the other hand. *In one modern method,* also to avoid lumps, you stir the grits all at once into the cold water and then raise the temperature to a boil while stirring. With either method, once the pot begins to bubble, you adjust the heat so the grits barely bubble, stirring frequently at first and occasionally after that, and you can even transfer the pot to a low oven. *In a second modern method,* you cook the grits in a double boiler, which ensures slow cooking and eliminates the need for vigilant stirring. With any method, you add more water as needed. Polenta, like grits, should be cooked very slowly for one to two hours, until a stronger, sweeter taste of corn appears. In northern Italy, the preferred consistency varies from one area to another. To my taste, grits and polenta should be neither runny nor stiff; they should flow just a little on the plate.

COMPLEMENTS TO CORN: Sweet corn goes especially well with butter, cream, bell pepper, chile pepper, onion, salt and black pepper, and a gentle flavor of thyme. It goes with lobster and other seafood. Grits-mush-polenta are as easygoing as wheat bread, a good counterpoint to strong-flavored foods, such as *ragùs,* braised meats in rich sauces, and grilled sausages. They're good with butter and grating cheese stirred in, with varied other cheeses, cooked onions, boletes, shrimp, and white truffles.

NOTES ON WINE: Sweet corn is too sweet for wine. With grits or polenta, the wine is determined by whatever is served with it.

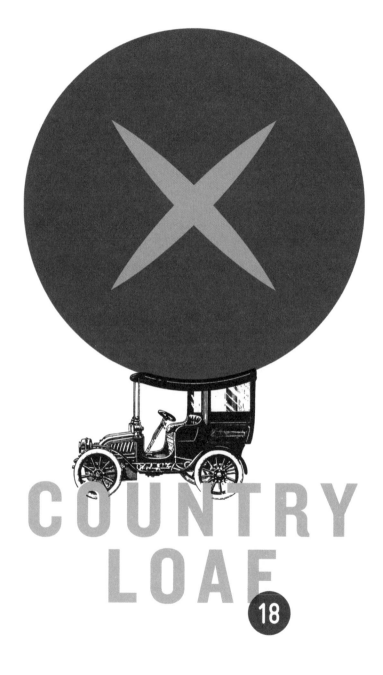

COUNTRY
LOAE 18

18. THE "COUNTRY" LOAF— BIG BREAD

The "country" loaf is the timeless, traditional household bread of much of Europe. It's big and typically round, a primordial, efficient shape. The French *boulanger* is a maker of *boules,* "balls," although for more than two centuries the big loaf has also been, less often, oblong, long, or ring-shaped. Today, it usually weighs two kilos or less, but I've seen five-kilo loaves, and some loaves used to weigh more than that. To call the big loaf *pain de campagne,* "country bread," is misleading. It was and is city bread, too—universal bread, going under many names. (In France, the name *pain de campagne* has been so overused in recent years that, to have the same connotation of rustic authenticity, the partly synonymous *pain au levain,* "sourdough bread," has taken its place.) The flour for "country" bread may be all white, or it may be tan from a proportion of wheat or rye bran or both. At the last minute before baking, slashes are often cut in the top of the raw dough, but the traditional loaf doesn't swell much in the oven, so the cuts hardly open. The just-baked crust is crisp and good but not typically delicate or flaky.

A famous version of the bread is the light brown sourdough baked by the Poilâne family in Paris, a type that was once common all over France and in other European countries. A few diverse Italian forms of the big loaf are the bran-coated *pane di Genzano* of Lazio, the pale unsalted bread of Tuscany, and the yellowy, hemispherical *pane di Altamura* from Puglia (although that's made of durum flour and may belong in its own category).

The big country loaf at its best is outstanding, full of flavor from good wheat, a complete fermentation, and a dark, nutty crust. The logic of the loaf proceeds from its large size and round shape, a combination that gives the least crust in proportion to interior. By no coincidence, the insides are substantial, a little dense. The big fundamental loaf is meant to keep: the point is the long-lasting, full flavor within.

Most farm families, living far from the nearest village and baker, used to bake their own bread once a week or every two weeks, or less often. In Mediterranean Italy, which we associate so much today with pasta, the foundation of daily meals not long ago was bread. Bread was and is delicious, inexpensive, portable, ready to eat. The loaves were big because there were many mouths to feed, because with big loaves you can fit more bread in the oven, and because, once baked, a bigger loaf dries out more slowly, which was important with infrequent baking. Not just the size helped the bread to keep, but also the somewhat compact texture. That came from a slightly dry dough, from using flour other than white (when that was the case), often from a sourdough leavening (whose acidity tightened the dough), and from forceful shaping (which pressed out more of the bubbles from fermentation).

In France, the greatest country for wheat bread, the very image of bread today is the baguette. But until the 1930s, when the baguette first became widely popular, and even after that, "French bread" to the French meant a big sourdough loaf, variously called a *miche, tourte, boulot, gros pain,* or simply *pain.* In 1922, Édouard de Pomiane, a doctor and leading gastronome, wrote in *Bien Manger pour Bien Vivre* ("Eat Well to Live Well"): "*Pain boulot* is the very type of *pain français;* it is globular, the eyes are very large, the crust is hard." There were and are other shapes and many regional breads, but if there is one timeless everyday French bread, it is the *gros pain*—the "big loaf." By contrast, the skinny baguette is archetypal city bread, different in nearly every way.

You can list their opposed qualities in a chart:

"COUNTRY" LOAF	BAGUETTE
big	small
round	long and narrow
white or tan flour	white flour
frequently sourdough	always commercial yeast
dark to very dark crust	golden-brown crust
narrow slashes or none	wide slashes filled with crust
crust usually thick and tough	crust thin and crisp
slightly dense insides	bubbled and open insides
durable flavor	short-lived flavor
for keeping	for eating fresh

Still, both kinds of bread require no more than four ingredients: flour, water, yeast or sourdough, and salt. Never sugar, never fat. And like the baguette, most big loaves have been creamy white for a long time, wherever people could get and afford white flour. Flour means "flower," the flower of ground wheat—the finest, whitest part.

A relatively small amount of bran is enough to hide the subtle flavors from the white core of the wheat berry. The more bran there is, the denser and stronger-flavored the bread. Bran provides its own excellent flavor, and after the fresh-baked flavor is lost, the bran flavor compensates. But flour with a lot of bran can make bread bitter, just like whole-grain flour whose oil has gone rancid. With sourdough, darker flour with more bran allows the acidity to rise higher, though when all goes well, the acidity doesn't stand out amid the greater flavor of the darker flour. And bran makes sourdough, compared with dough containing commercial yeast, ferment more quickly. Most of all, however, the bran particles interrupt the gluten fibers, giving a denser, heavier loaf that stays moist longer. Bran also absorbs more water than white flour, and that along with the extra acidity helps the bread to keep. Because the big loaf is intended for keeping, you might argue that by definition it must contain at least some darker flour or perhaps be entirely whole-grain.

In rye, too, the strongest flavor comes from the bran, whose flavor can be particularly delicious. In much of the West, the archetypal mixed-grain bread was roughly half wheat, half rye. The late chef Charles Barrier, of Tours, who was born in 1916, once told me that during his childhood not just wheat and rye but sometimes barley, sometimes oats, were all sown together in the same field, as they always had been, as a form of insurance. If one grain fared poorly in the weather that year, the others might do better. (Once ground, he said, the flour was sifted to remove almost all the bran.) The French word for the mixed grains is *méteil,* and the bread was *pain de méteil.* The nearly forgotten English word for both the grains and the bread is "maslin," which like the French comes from the Latin for "mixed." A little rye flour is occasionally still combined with the white flour for a country loaf, heightening flavor and improving keeping without giving a clear rye taste or a soft, compact rye texture.

At the mill, either steel rollers or traditional stones can grind well or badly. A small difference between the two is that a roller mill flattens the bran and leaves it in flakes, which keeps the dough from rising quite as much; while stone-grinding shears and tears the wheat berries, which puts more of the germ and its oil into the flour, and includes more of the aleurone layer, just beneath the bran, with its protein and other nutrients that help feed the yeast. For a tan country loaf, it's better not to mix whole-wheat flour with white but instead to use a French-style type 80 or type 110 flour, which contains some fine-ground bran along with part of the germ. (These flours lie between type 45, the whitest kind, used for pastry, and type 150, whole wheat.)

Where the taste of white bread comes especially from the skill of the baker, the taste of darker bread depends more on the variety of wheat or other grain—its genetics—plus fresh grinding. For flavor, the fresher the better, at least for rye. (I admit that in very fresh whole-wheat flour I find a taste like cinnamon that for me is out of place in bread.) The assertive taste of bran can be delicious, but even the best whole-wheat bread tastes simpler than the best white bread, because the bran flavors overwhelm everything else.

As to water and salt, bakers today add more water to their dough, sometimes much more, than they once did, so that country loaves have become more open and light. A wetter dough stretches more easily during fermentation, producing a more open texture that traps more aroma, which means more flavor in the fresh bread. Salt, at about 2 percent of the flour by weight, strengthens the dough (which was important in the past when the flour was commonly lower in protein and in some years very weak). In addition, salt enriches flavor by slowing the fermentation, helps to darken the crust, prolongs freshness, and, according to almost everyone outside Tuscany and some nearby parts of central Italy, bread without salt tastes flat.

A sourdough leavening, timeless for the big loaf, contains yeasts and acid-producing bacteria. Different combinations of the two came into being in different places, some cultures producing noticeably different flavors from others. And the more often a culture receives fresh additions of flour and water, the sweeter and livelier it is and the sweeter and lighter the bread is. More water and a warmer temperature favor milder lactic acid, while less water and a colder temperature favor sharper acetic acid (the acid in vinegar), as you can readily taste in the baked loaf. The more sour the dough is, the tougher the bread, including the crust. Too much sourness easily dominates the delicious *bread* flavors. (Ironically, as an expert baker I know argues, the French legal definition of *pain au levain* now requires too-acid bread.) When the starter is sweet and the fermentation is lively, sourness may become apparent only the next day, after the fresh-baked flavors have begun to disperse.

For centuries in beer-drinking places, the big loaf was raised by adding foam skimmed from fermenting ale. The foam is filled with *Saccharomyces cerevisiae,* the same species as in today's commercial baker's yeast. (In Italy, baker's yeast is still called "beer yeast.") For flavor, it's better that the amount of commercial yeast be small, so that the fermentation doesn't go too fast. From initial mixing to the moment the loaves enter the oven, a full commercial-yeast fermentation takes around five hours, where sourdough requires around seven. Commercial-yeast bread tastes sweeter and lighter than sourdough, but neither one is better than the other. There's no best kind of bread—a baguette, a country loaf, various flatbreads, rye are all forms of excellence.

Inside the oven, the transformations of the country loaf are like those of other kinds of bread. But where the baguette is baked at 480 to 500 degrees F (250 to 260 degrees C), so the crust will brown before the inside dries out, the big country loaf is usually baked 25 to 45 degrees cooler, so the crust doesn't form too early, imprisoning the loaf before it has finished expanding. The crust of the traditional big loaf contributes important flavor, and it tends to be darker and thicker in rural France than in the city. Some bakers can tease a lot of darkness out of the crust, particularly sourdough, without burning it.

I've met people in the French countryside who don't like the fresh taste. They wait several days before eating a new loaf. I suspect the reason is that often in the past bread dough wasn't fully fermented, and perhaps sometimes still isn't, and in that case the bread tastes unpleasantly raw at first. But today most people want fresh-baked flavor—I do. And there are more and more good bakeries, so it's easier to buy fresh bread as often as we want.

As the days pass, any sort of loaf becomes steadily firmer, more crumbly, and less enjoyable to eat by itself. But "stale" may not be the best word to describe an older big loaf, if you consider that most country bread never used to be eaten fresh and maybe still isn't. Instead of stale, I often say "older" bread. Italians say *pane raffermo,* "firm bread." The French say *pain rassis,* which has sometimes meant "firm," though today it means "stale." Older bread just needs something to go with it, generally something to moisten it while adding delicious flavor.

Above all, traditionally, a slice is placed in a bowl and hot soup is poured over it. Fresh bread raised with commercial yeast all but dissolves in the liquid; slightly old sourdough holds much more substance and is far better. And these days most people would probably prefer it toasted. Tuscans moisten older bread with water and then add cut-up tomatoes, among other things, to make *panzanella,* a salad commonly described as a "cold soup." Jacques Médecin, a longtime mayor of Nice (who was accused of corruption and fled to Uruguay), wrote in his excellent cookbook, *La Cuisine du Comté de Nice,* that the city's *pan bagnat,* "bathed bread," was also originally a salad, made with hard bread "reduced with a hammer or a pestle to pieces the size of a mouthful"—even shatteringly dry bread never used to be thrown out. The pieces of bread were combined with the rest of the ingredients of a *salade niçoise* an hour before serving, so it could drink up the olive oil and tomato juices. These days, *pan bagnat* is a salady sandwich made with fresh bread, still assembled an hour before eating, and containing, according to purists: tomato, thinly sliced small green peppers, small onions, young fava beans, black olives, and either anchovy or tuna with plenty of olive oil, basil, and of course salt and pepper. The original ingredients, far more variable, were dominated by whatever was in season.

HOW TO BUY A COUNTRY LOAF: You can't tell a lot about the quality of a big loaf before you bite in, but you can tell something.

Shape, size, weight, and keeping. There should be no sign of a pan or a mold. The bread should have been baked directly on the hearth, so crisp crust formed all around. On the bottom, you may see the outline of bricks or oven tiles. A big loaf is often much wider than it is tall, but a cross-section should show no corners, the bottom curving smoothly upward. Rather than a taut sphere, which indicates less flavor and often lighter weight, a big loaf should appear slightly relaxed. Any slashes in the top may have scarcely opened; it's better that they open at least a little. If you're in a position to smell, then with sourdough the sourness should be no more than a trace among rich fresh-baked odors. A large sourdough loaf often tastes better than a small one, because a large one springs more in the oven. For best keeping, choose a round loaf that weighs at least a couple of pounds, feels slightly heavy for its size, and contains some darker wheat or rye flour.

Crust color and texture. Fresh, golden-brown crust is delicious, but in a country loaf, especially sourdough, more flavor comes from a darker crust, almost to the point of being burnt. But the insides shouldn't have dried out in the oven. In the opposite direction, with very moist dough and light-colored crust, if the loaf didn't dry enough in the oven, its crust quickly softens. Some versions look as shiny and crackled as a baguette, and they tend to be more swollen and lighter. But typically the crust of a big loaf, especially sourdough, is dull, slightly rough, and irregular. For more visual appeal, a big loaf is often given a light flour coating, more than is needed to prevent sticking as the dough rises in its basket. But too much flour reduces browning, and the powder tastes no better on the top of bread than it does eaten straight from the sack.

Insides. A flavorful white loaf isn't truly white inside but always cream-colored, and it's slightly better for flavor and texture that a darker loaf be made with finely ground flour than show visible flecks of bran. Even a somewhat dense big loaf is filled with countless irregular holes, some of which should be rather large, although not as large as those of a good baguette—too many large holes cause even a big loaf to dry out quickly and lose flavor. If the dough was well cared for and the fermentation complete, the holes are filled with delicious aroma.

HOW TO STORE A COUNTRY LOAF: Keep fresh bread at room temperature—chilling turns any just-baked bread instantly stale—and for best flavor, slice it no more than ten minutes before it will be eaten. Where a well-fermented big loaf raised with factory yeast holds its fresh flavor for a day or at most two, a sourdough one will taste fresh for a day or so beyond that. And a big round loaf remains useful for two weeks and more, although in dry weather the loaf may lose moisture too fast and in humid weather may develop mold. Accordingly, leave it exposed, protect it beneath a cloth, or put it inside a paper or plastic bag, and as needed refrigerate it to discourage mold. Many bakers consider either plastic or chilling to be heresy, saying flavor and texture are altered. But with older bread they seem to me harmless.

COMPLEMENTS TO A COUNTRY LOAF: Compared with white commercial-yeast country bread, sourdough and darker country loaves go better with stronger-flavored foods. But there's no rule, and the complements to any good country loaf are nearly infinite. It's excellent with meat terrines and fresh cheeses and with dry-cured meats and strong cheeses. Bread is a wonderful way to eat soup and sauce. Olive oil, especially newly pressed, is shown off by toasted country bread, preferably grilled over coals. Traditional Italian bruschetta is simply a hot toasted slice (optionally, the abrasive surface is rubbed with a clove of garlic) with olive oil poured generously over, the warmth exalting the smell. You can add salt, especially if the bread is unsalted.

Bread, olive oil, and tomato have a particular affinity for one another, and not just in the form of pizza. Browned crumbs of any good white bread, with oil, go impeccably on a tomato gratin. (Layer thin slices of ripe tomato with salt, grindings of black pepper, a trace of finely crumbled Greek sage or oregano, and paper-thin slices of garlic, ending with tomato; top with white crumbs, and pour a thin stream of olive oil all over.) The best stuffed tomatoes are also topped with white bread and oil, so that the bread is in effect fried in the oven. (Remove the seeds and ribs from the fruits, salt the insides, and drain them upside down; fill them with a mix of coarse crumbs or tiny cubes, salt, black pepper, sautéed onion, the chopped tomato ribs, chopped parsley, and olive oil; pour more oil on top, and bake in a hot oven.) Slightly more complicated than bruschetta is *pa amb tomàquet,* "bread with tomato," one of the great foods—omnipresent in its home of Catalonia, where it's eaten at any time of day. Cut a thick slice from a big country loaf that's at least a few hours and up to a day old. Optionally and possibly less traditionally, toast the slice lightly and rub it with garlic. Then cut a fully ripe tomato in half and rub it on *both* sides of the bread, discarding the skins. Add a sprinkling of salt, and irrigate the whole with olive oil. The only way to eat *pa amb tomàquet* neatly, if that matters, is with a knife and fork.

NOTES ON WINE: Although darker loaves are less adaptable than lighter ones, any wheat bread makes food go more easily with wine.

19 BLUE CRAB

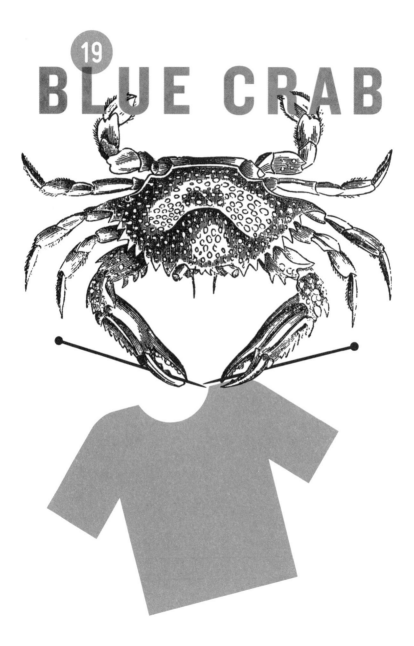

19. CRAB, BLUE

The blue crab, *Callinectes sapidus,* whose Latin name means "beautiful swimmer" plus "delicious," may be the best of the world's crabs. I admit I'm prejudiced, because it's the kind I know best. There are of course other wonderful crabs, such as, in North America, the Dungeness, found from Alaska to Mexico; the Florida stone crab, which lives from the Carolinas to the Gulf of Texas; and the sweet, delicate Maine crab (more properly the Atlantic rock crab; chefs call it "peekytoe"), which inhabits the cooler waters north of Cape Cod, the arm that sends the warm Gulf Stream out into the Atlantic. To offer just one more example, the shore crab in the Venetian lagoon makes the city's *moleche,* its softshell crabs. Blue crabs are common along the Atlantic Coast from Cape Cod to Florida, in the Caribbean, and as far west as Texas; they live in South America all the way to northern Argentina and have been introduced into parts of Europe as well as Japan. But the blue crab thrives especially in the Chesapeake Bay of Maryland and Virginia, with its vast, rich, shallow waters and great marshes, and that's the region where the blue crab is most appreciated. (The bay's shallowness and the huge area that feeds it and makes it rich—tributaries flow in from six states—combine to make the bay vulnerable to pollution. There are steady efforts to protect the bay, and the crabs continue to thrive.) The shells of the crabs are blue, but cooking turns them red. Around the Chesapeake Bay, blue crabs are eaten steamed, boiled, fried whole as softshells, made into soup and gumbo, deviled, fried in cakes, and dressed with mayonnaise as salad.

At crab houses near the water, customers sit down to mounds of steamed crabs on paper-covered tables, breaking open the claws with wooden mallets and eating the crabs plain, washed down with pitchers of ice tea and cold beer. The most serious eaters dissect the crabs with a stony intensity. Unlike some crabs, whose meat is almost all in the claws, the best meat of the blue crab is in the body. At a certain point, after you've lifted the top shell, you break the body in half, so the two big, prized, tender pieces of backfin meat come out. Blue crab is delicate and doesn't benefit from being dipped in butter like lobster. (Too often the crabs are flavored with Old Bay seasoning, a product that dates from around the Second World War and tastes of celery salt and baking spice. A little fresh celery is an old flavoring for crab, but the seed and spice flavors of Old Bay have no precedent in earlier Maryland cooking and don't complement any seafood.) Female blue crabs caught in winter and spring are likely to contain tasty orange roe. Most flavorful is the mustard-colored fat, called the "mustard," tomalley, or liver (scientifically, it's the hepatopancreas). It's safe to eat as long as the crabs were taken from water free of chemical pollutants.

Crab cakes are emblematic of mid-Atlantic cooking. A great one contains little but crabmeat—"lump," ideally, for the most delectable texture—mixed gently, to keep the pieces whole, with soft white breadcrumbs. There shouldn't be enough bread to taste, only enough to hold the cake together. (And so what if it falls apart a little?) You flavor the mixture as you like, with maybe a little fine dice of cooked bell pepper, maybe some chopped parsley, possibly some cooked onion, and probably a little hot red pepper. The old regional variety is the Fish pepper, just undergoing a revival. Hot pepper is one of the important African contributions to the cooking of the South.

Crab lends itself to soup and gumbo, and if you pick the meat yourself, you extract maximum flavor by making a broth of the shells and using that as the foundation of whatever you make. Charleston's she-crab soup uses female crabs full of roe. The point of reference is the recipe of William Deas, an African-American chef, in the 1930 cookbook *Two Hundred Years of Charleston Cooking;* he calls for she-crabs, milk, cream, onion, sherry, and Worcestershire sauce.

As it grows, a blue crab big enough to catch legally sheds its shell as many as half a dozen times a season. (The smallest, youngest crabs shed every few days.) Crabs identified as "peelers" are put into shedding floats, which sit on the water or next to it with water pumped through continuously. The crabs are checked frequently through the day and night so they can be removed soon after they shed. When a crab first breaks out of the shell, it's extremely soft and utterly exposed. Immediately it begins to form a new shell, drawing calcium from the salt water. Just-shed softshells, sometimes called "velvets," are so completely tender and weak that if they're shipped, they die. For eating, they're ideal, but to make them strong enough for the trip, they're left in salt water for about four hours while they form a slightly crunchy new shell. After six hours, they're "papershells," not as pleasant to eat but still considered soft. After eight to ten hours, the shells are definitely too crunchy to eat. Softshells lend themselves to preparations with all sorts of flavors, but they're probably best simply floured and fried in butter or olive oil and served with lemon, or finished by adding to the pan a little white wine and parsley.

HOW TO BUY BLUE CRAB: Along the mid-Atlantic coast where there's a strong crab fishery, you can buy freshly cooked and picked crabmeat. Freshness is key. The meat should be no more than a day old, to my taste, though longer is usual. To steam or boil crabs yourself, buy lively, just-captured ones. If you decide to pick your own crabmeat, know that it takes twenty or more crabs to make a pound of picked meat. Remove it in as large pieces and flakes as you can. Save the flavorful mustard, if the crabs come from unpolluted water. The season in the Chesapeake starts in March or April and ends in November or December. The meatiest, tastiest crabs of the year are caught in September and October, after their final molt and before they hibernate.

Blue crabs are sold by size in half-inch increments, measured tip to tip across the width of the shell. There are no official names, but you might find anything from "small" (four and a half to five inches) to "jumbo" (six to six and a half inches) and larger. Softshells have their own set of unofficial names, from "medium" through "hotel," "prime," "jumbo," and "whales." Picked meat with the largest pieces may be called "colossal," "jumbo lump," "lump," or "backfin," descending to "flake," "regular," the ironically named "special," the redder, stringy but flavorful "claw," and the intact claws of "cocktail claw."

With softshells, the more tender, the better. They should be tender enough to eat in their entirety without making you pause to consider the crunch. (In the worst case, you can always discard the top shell, the hardest part.) For freshness, the ideal is to eat the softshell on the day it sheds. (I once talked with a man tending floats of peelers, and he actually laughed at the idea of eating softshell crab in a restaurant.) But softshells kept at around 45 degrees F (7 degrees C) remain alive and good to eat for perhaps four days. Softshells frozen immediately can have a very fresh taste.

COMPLEMENTS TO BLUE CRAB: Butter is excellent for sautéeing crabcakes and making sauces (not for dipping, because the crab's subtle flavor is lost in so much butter). Blue crab also likes sweet corn, tomato, bell pepper, avocado, lemon and lime juice, and lettuce (for its texture and fresh flavor with a crab salad). Blue crab goes with onion, salt pork, hot red pepper, curry, and other spice. The merest suggestion of mace or nutmeg underlines the dairy taste of cream in soup.

NOTES ON WINE: With blue crab, drink a medium-weight white wine, such as one of the better *cru* Chablis, a white Burgundy (Mâcon, Pouilly-Fuissé, Saint-Véran, Mercurey), or another Chardonnay from elsewhere, without oak. Also good are a lighter, dry Chenin Blanc, a dry Riesling, or a light white Pessac-Léognan; Condrieu goes with crab in a cream sauce. When crab, like other food, is prepared with strong Asian spices, the common wine recommendation is Gewurztraminer, but I'm skeptical because the wine makes complicated sets of strong flavors and the crab may be left out of the conversation. Some people are fond of sake with crab, and the popular choice is light (in color) beer; I opt for pilsener or wheat.

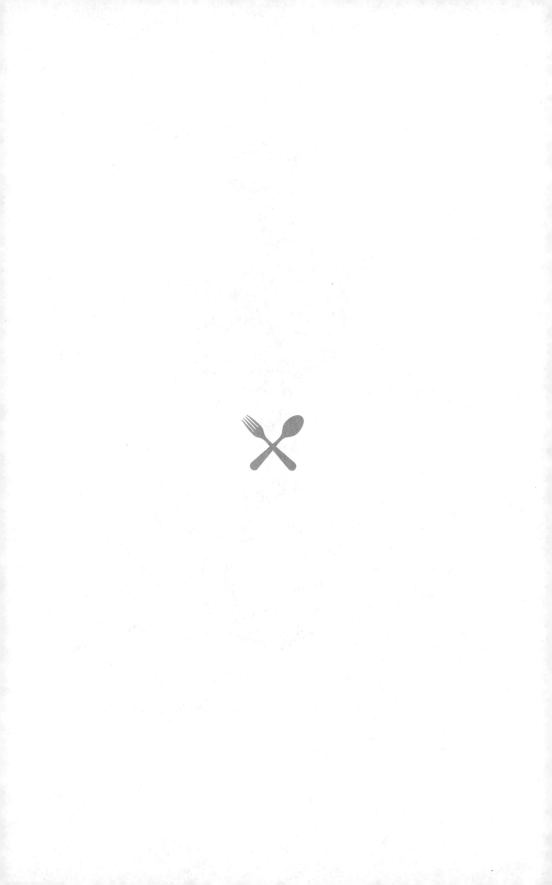

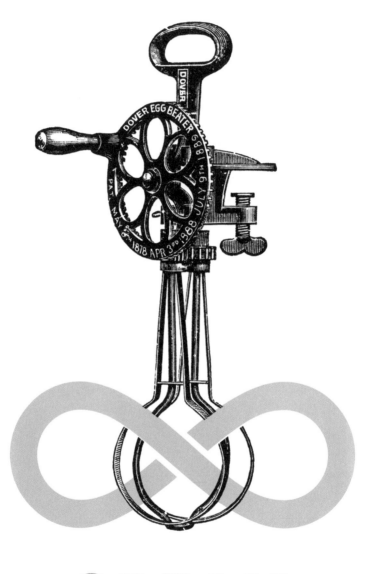

CREAM

20

20. CREAM

One of the most flattering of all foods to other foods is thick, rich cream, with its suave dairy taste and paradoxical lightness. Cream can be sweet or sour, and pourable, spoonable, or whipped. It tastes heavy if you eat too much of it or if you cook it until its fat turns to oil. Otherwise, the fat in cream is what makes it taste light—in soups, sauces, quiche, dessert custards, pastry cream, panna cotta, and ice cream. And cream is delicious even when it isn't light, as when it's combined with potatoes in a *gratin dauphinois*. The most flavorful cream comes from cows grazing on deep-rooted, permanent pasture at that moment in spring when wildflowers are in bloom. The new growth gives the cream an especially yellow color, which also reflects breed. (At the bright extreme is cream from Jerseys and Guernseys, selected in the Channel Islands long ago for the strong color of their milk, which is also high in fat and other solids.) Perfectly clean, fresh *raw* cream, like raw milk, tastes sweeter, milder, subtly floral. Pasteurized cream, having been cooked to preserve it temporarily and make it safe, has instead a somewhat caramel and custard flavor. Today almost all US cream isn't just pasteurized, it's ultrapasteurized or entirely sterilized through ultrahigh-temperature processing. Most of this UHT cream is heated instantly by adding steam, which then evaporates, taking with it some of the aroma. Afterward all UHT and other conventional cream is homogenized to prevent skim milk from gathering in the bottom of the container. The texture of UHT cream has been so damaged that it must be homogenized at higher than usual pressures to break the fat globules still smaller—homogenization works by breaking up the fat so it can't gather and rise. After that, additives are required, or the cream will be almost impossible to whip. (The dispersed fat from the broken globules prevents the cream from foaming well, the same way that a bit of yolk or other fat makes it harder to beat egg whites successfully.) As usual with the raw materials of cooking, the less processing, the better. Happily, here and there around the US you can find excellent, minimally handled, delicious local cream.

Pasture is the best feed (for the health of the animals and the quality of the milk), followed by hay, the immemorial option in winter when pasture isn't available. On industrial farms, however, cows rarely if ever go outdoors. Sometimes they're brought some fresh-cut grass, but more often they receive a mix of hay, grain, and other feed, especially silage. The last consists of various plants that have been chopped and fermented to preserve them, which can give barnyardy off-flavors to the milk. Other flavor problems come from feeding cows turnips, from wild onions that show up in a field, or from a barn rank with manure, since milk readily absorbs the aromas around it.

The oldest, gentlest way to separate cream from milk is to wait for the fat to slowly rise. You leave the milk overnight in a shallow pan at around 50 degrees F (10 degrees C) and in the morning skim off the cream. The fast method is to put the milk through a mechanical separator, a form of centrifuge, whose exaggerated gravity flings the heavier, more watery portion of milk to the periphery, sending skim milk out one pipe and cream out another. A poorly functioning separator breaks so many globules that loose granules of fat rise and fill the top of a bottle of cream with an undesirable buttery "cream plug." When you taste cold cream that hasn't been homogenized, and you bring your teeth together, you can feel the sticky globules pressed between them.

The more fat, the thicker the cream and the more flavor it has, the rest being mostly water. US "whipping cream" is at least 30 percent fat, "heavy cream" is at least 36 percent, and double cream in some countries can be up to 48 percent. Clotted cream, associated with Cornwall and Devonshire and closely related to Near Eastern *kaymak,* is thoroughly cooked. The process is nearly the same today as when Richard Warner described it in *A Tour through Cornwall, in the Autumn of 1808:* The cream is "submitted to a heat that produces boiling as nearly as possible. Here it continues until it be thoroughly scalded, when it is taken off, returned to the dairy, and in about ten or twelve hours a thick crust of cream rises to the surface of the vessel, which is the excellent article in question." The result is a mix of thick and thin textures, too thick to pour, with a nutty flavor and around 60 percent fat.

A few practical points about cooking and use: When you add cream (or béchamel sauce) to cooked spinach, the dairy protein eliminates the vegetable's tannic astringency; it's the same thing that happens when you add milk to tea. You can add cream to nearly any sauce, although if the cream isn't quite rich enough, it can make the sauce runny; you have to boil down the cream first or boil the sauce afterward. Heavy cream won't break when you boil it by itself, and you can add it to many soups and sauces and boil them without their breaking (curdling). But if you add heavy cream to a thin, acidic liquid, such as a mussel soup containing white wine, and you boil it, it will break. You can avoid the whole topic by using rich ripened cream as a sauce by itself without any cooking. When you whip cream, the colder the cream and equipment, the faster and lighter the result and the less risk there is of a grainy texture. It's not the number of strokes that hastens the process but how fast the wires of the whisk pass through the cream. The added air increases the volume by 50 percent or more.

Before refrigeration, raw cream kept in a cool spot would remain sweet for perhaps a couple of days in summer and twice that in winter, before you could taste the sourness. (That good sourness is very different from the repulsive decay of pasteurized cream or milk.) Under refrigeration, raw cream remains sweet for perhaps a week. The souring, or ripening, creates US sour cream (12 to 18 percent fat), inspired by Central and Eastern European–style sour cream, and it makes French-style crème fraîche (30 to 40 percent fat). Lactic bacteria, present in the dairies and kitchens of the past, turn the milk's sugar into lactic acid, and the acidity causes the cream to thicken.

You can easily ripen sweet cream at home, except that you can't easily get the right live culture, which isn't likely to inhabit your kitchen in significant amounts. The common recommendation to add a little store-bought cultured buttermilk gives a strong buttermilk flavor never otherwise found in cream, and adding yogurt with a live culture gives a yogurt flavor. Commercial crème fraîche with a live culture, however, if you can find it, is just right. (Crème fraîche, although ripened, is oddly called "fresh" in French, something that appears to coincide with the widespread use of pasteurization. Before that, probably most cream was a little fermented. Sweet cream in French today is distinguished as *crème fleurette.*) Cream ripened on the farm can be more than half fat. The thickness of ripened cream comes not only from high fat but also from the particular culture, which can make the cream even more luscious.

The *very* best cream comes from milk taken straight from the cow and put into a bowl or other container for the cream to rise—never trucked, pumped, put through a separator, or pasteurized. Kept cool but not cold, the cream thickens slightly over the succeeding days, taking a week or longer to turn distinctly sour. Randolph Hodgson of Neal's Yard Dairy, in London, who eats such cream at the company's farm in Herefordshire, says, "Obviously this is an idealistic state of affairs these days, although probably quite normal fifty years ago and more." Milk and cream that have undergone "mechanical battering of any kind" and changes in temperature, he says, won't withstand the old treatment.

HOW TO BUY AND KEEP CREAM: The fresher the cream, the better (unless you have the more or less unobtainable perfect cream described just above). If you can't find wholesome raw cream with a clean dairy taste, then look for gently pasteurized (not UHT) cream without additives. Even ripe cream should have a fresh immediacy, along with a clean but not acidy tang that doesn't hide the dairy flavor. Kept in the refrigerator, cream loses a little purity each day, slowly gaining a hint of rancidity and perhaps picking up off-flavors. Even so, the refrigerator is the best place to keep it. Consume it, if you can, within a couple of days. Cream that hasn't been homogenized will continue slowly to separate, and the bit of watery liquid that gathers in the bottom of the container isn't a defect but a sign of honesty. To mix it back in, shake the container gently once or twice or turn it upside down. A glass bottle is appealing, but an opaque carton protects against the oxidized flavors caused by light.

COMPLEMENTS TO CREAM: Cream, sweet or ripe, complements an almost limitless number of other foods, and in turn they make cream more delicious—leeks, potatoes, spinach, sorrel, beets (in borscht with sour cream), saffron, eggs, and all kinds of meats and fish served with cream sauces. Dairy flavor occasionally benefits from the merest hint of nutmeg (it's easy to add too much, much better to add none at all) and from European bay leaf (which has a nutmeg component along with its more aggressive, almost resinous side). The greatest complement to cream may be the little-known French wine *vin jaune* in combination with morels or chicken or both. Other intentionally oxidized wines, such as Madeira, also go with cream. In sweet contexts, most flattering is vanilla, followed by rose, caramel, and coffee (a very little nutmeg is good here, too, now and then). Cream also goes with all sorts of fresh and cooked fruits, and it goes with dessert wines used as flavorings.

NOTES ON WINE: Cream in a savory dish is echoed by an elegant Chardonnay with a buttery flavor (meaning most white Burgundies but not Chablis or other mineral wines), including sparkling wine made from Chardonnay grapes. Other white wines that speak to cream are Condrieu from the Rhone Valley, Pinot Gris from either Alsace or northern Italy, Chenin Blanc from Anjou and Touraine, well-made Cour-Cheverny (containing the little-known Romorantin grape) from just east of Touraine, and traditional *sous voile* Jura whites. Dry Riesling complements cream sauces when there is some extra element in the dish, such as saffron or curry, to tie things together. And cream in dessert is complemented by the whole range of sweet white wines.

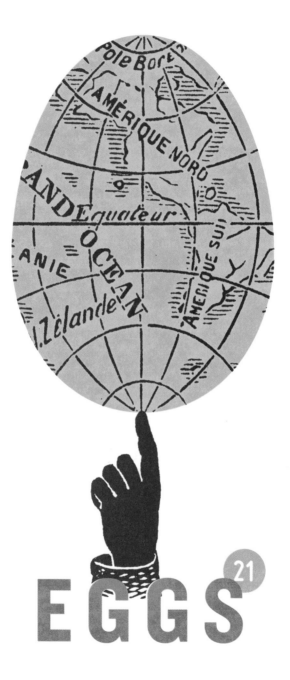

EGGS ²¹

21. EGGS

The wonder of eggs is their combination of richness and diverse texture. Eggs are architecture. They're delicate, velvety, airy, flowing, firm, crisp. Egg batters, hardly different one from another, make crêpes, clafoutis, and Yorkshire pudding and almost explode to make popovers. A stiff egg dough swells up into hollow, crunchy cream puffs. Eggs combined with yeast inflate brioche. Eggs form the strands of egg-drop soup. The yolks thicken and enrich sauces. The fat is in the yolks, while the whites give most of the structure. Either yolks, whole eggs, or both make custard that in the oven becomes delicate crème caramel (protected by a water bath) or quiche (protected by a crust). Hard-cooked eggs pressed through a sieve make a mimosa to go on leeks vinaigrette. The flowing yolk of a poached egg enriches the dressing of a frisée salad. Whites whisked into foam give volume to meltingly light soufflés and to cakes; whites whisked with sugar become soft or crisp meringue. Whole eggs whisked with sugar form airy "ribbons" that lighten cakes; whisked with sugar and wine over hot water, they become zabaione (sabayon). To all these things, eggs bring mild but definite flavor.

Chicken eggs have a rich, chameleon quality that allows them to fit nearly anywhere. Their flavor and especially aroma become strong only when eggs are overcooked, which releases sulfur. Counterintuitively, that comes not from the yolks but from the whites. Ultramild and almost sweet are the small, speckled eggs of quail, a byproduct of raising the birds for meat. Duck and goose eggs are subtly more animal-tasting, faintly gamier, with something of the flavor of the meat of each bird. Not to get into wild bird eggs—so many different ones were eaten in the past. Within the shell of a duck or goose egg, the yolk takes up considerably more space, leaving less white. Neither has all the architectural qualities of a chicken egg.

Flavor is influenced mainly by what the birds eat. The flavor is stronger when the hens live outdoors, eating plants, insects, and worms. Green plants, like the corn that's the usual base of the diet, contain carotene, which makes a more orange yolk. When you crack open a just-laid egg from an outdoor hen, its bright yolk and robustness set it far apart from flaccid industrial eggs. Fresh outdoor eggs make firmer, lighter baked goods, so you may need fewer eggs, or you may have to add some liquid to them to make a tender omelette. Breed is at most a minor influence on taste, though it's surely better that the hens belong to an old-fashioned, less productive meat-and-egg breed rather than a specialized egg-laying industrial one.

Simple boiled eggs are delicious, from very soft- to fully hard-cooked. Each small step along the way yields different texture and flavor. Precise cooks say soft- and hard-*cooked,* not -boiled, because a full boil easily leads to overcooking. Safest is to start the eggs in cold water, bring them just to a boil, take them from the heat, let them sit for twelve minutes (for fully hard), and promptly put them in cold water to avoid a grayish yolk. Some science-conscious high-end chefs have focused on the tenderest soft-cooked egg, cooked in water at precisely 147 degrees F (64 degrees C) or a little less, according to the chef, for thirty to sixty minutes or sometimes longer, the variables giving slightly different results in texture and taste. The white, still partly translucent, is almost but not quite fully set, and the yolk has thickened but still flows.

Not quite as gentle as that is regular poaching, meaning the egg is cooked in water that barely shows a bubble. Don't add vinegar to it on the old theory that it will keep the egg neater—the main effect is to flavor the egg. Instead, for neatness, use a very fresh egg, break it onto a perforated spoon, let the thin part of the raw white drain away, and then slip the egg into the water. The most intense poached-egg dish must be *œufs en meurette,* whose red wine is strong enough to stain them mahogany.

Eggs scrambled in the French way as *œufs brouillés*—cooked slowly and gently with steady stirring and a lot of butter—are a form of custard, containing a minimum of tender curds and still slightly flowing. They're a medium for asparagus, morels, truffles, smoked fish.

An omelette is as essential as any egg dish, though it rarely if ever appears today on the menu of an ambitious restaurant, as if it weren't a serious thing to offer. The old savory fillings for omelettes are a catalog of sure companions for eggs: cheese, mushrooms, ham, fines herbes, asparagus, tomato and shrimp, roe, sorrel, onions, kidneys, chicken livers, spinach. A French omelette uses a lot of butter and remains partly liquid at the center. A really good one requires skill, and the ideal is not quite agreed upon. The classic, for delicacy, is entirely pale. A homier version shows golden spots, exchanging a little toughness for more flavor. (I go with flavor.) The omelette is very quickly cooked, in less than a minute, even fifteen seconds. Stirring with a fork makes mingled layers of butter and raw and cooked egg. It's possible to achieve that by shaking the pan over high heat with practiced motions, tossing the cooked bottom onto the still-liquid top. To finish, the omelette is slid against one side of the pan, and the edges are folded in to make, classically, a neatly pointed torpedo. An omelette rises a little in cooking, much more so in the case of an Italian frittata or a Spanish *tortilla,* which holds a relaxed position beyond the fringe of the French idea. Where a French omelette is small, quickly cooked, still partly wet, and for pleasure must be eaten immediately, a frittata or *tortilla* is typically large, cooked slowly and fully, the additions mixed evenly throughout, and often it's eaten later.

Eggs allow you to leaven baked goods without yeast or chemical powders, although plain eggs make firmer cakes than powders do. American waffles or pancakes are fairly tender and light when they're raised with only the eggs beaten into the batter (I often make them that way). Before breaking cold eggs, put them into a bowl of warm water, because a warm egg inflates more. And of course separating eggs and whisking the whites into foam multiplies the leavening effect. I whisk whites in the wide copper bowl I once carried home from Dehillerin, the serious cook's equipment shop in Paris. Copper gives a more sensual experience and creates a more durable foam, but you need a big bowl, and high prices have made all copperware a luxury. As you whisk, a minuscule amount of copper bonds with the whites to strengthen the foam and keep it from turning grainy and weak as you fold it into whatever you're making. In theory, adding a little cream of tartar to the whites accomplishes the same thing, though when I do it, I'm never quite convinced. And in fact you can make a reasonably good foam in a regular bowl, adding nothing at all to the whites, if you're careful not to overbeat or later overmix them, though the foam doesn't have quite the same volume and isn't durable.

Flans and other forms of baked custard sometimes contain flour to ensure that they won't release watery liquid if they overcook. But delicate, light custard contains no starch, and it's cooked as gently as any form of egg, often covered and in a water bath, only enough to set it—with experience you can tell from a slight jostle that the center has gelled. Overcooked custard is shot through with small bubbles; pushed far enough, it becomes rubbery. Custard is often made richer with an additional yolk for each whole egg (one of each per cup of milk or cream). All custard, including crème caramel, with the caramel made dark enough that the bitterness offsets the sweet, should be smooth and elegant.

HOW TO BUY AND STORE EGGS: Buy the freshest eggs you can, from justlaid to no more than a week old if possible, and keep them refrigerated. An older egg shows its age by the larger air space at the wide end. (The lower an egg floats in water, the fresher it is.) Older eggs, broken onto a plate, are flatter and seem runnier—the yolk *is* runnier, because more water has seeped into it from the white. It's best to protect eggs from absorbing aromas, but I leave them in the carton, which is usually just cardboard. For flavor, strength, and goodness, buy eggs from small, preferably organic farms, whose hens spend the day on pasture, at least during the warm months. I've never come across large-scale production that competes in quality. Kinder treatment usually coincides with better taste, and some eggs are certified humane, though small farms can rarely afford certification. Shell color—white, brown, or blue—reflects the breed and has nothing to do with quality, albeit blue eggs are normally Araucana and come from good small farms. All else being equal, eggs from older, less-productive breeds are better. For flavor and strength, use eggs promptly (except that, for easy peeling, eggs must be at least a week old), but they'll keep in the cold for two weeks or much longer.

COMPLEMENTS TO EGGS: They're wide open to other flavors, from onions to lobster to ham to fruit. Butter is an ideal complement in brioche. Eggs go with fines herbes (parsley, chervil, tarragon, and chives) as well as dill, with bacon and other cured meats, with Gruyère and Parmigiano, with mushrooms (especially morels) and truffles. Hard-cooked eggs go with tomato and greens in salad (the best greens for the purpose may be mixed spinach, sorrel, and rocket, better known as arugula). In a spinach salad, hard-cooked eggs go with anchovies and olive oil–lemon juice dressing. Hard-cooked eggs have a homey deliciousness when they're buried in the white sauce of a cauliflower gratin. In a frittata, they go with combinations such as fried zucchini and grating cheese, sautéed potatoes and green bell peppers, and tomato and cooked onion. Eggs go with milk or cream and vanilla in custard, which in turn goes with fruit, such as pears or peaches in a custard tart. (I mean common *Vanilla planifolia.* The exotic floral perfume of the somewhat rare Tahitian vanilla, *Vanilla tahitensis,* makes it much less useful, though it complements tropical fruits.)

NOTES ON WINE: Plain eggs aren't flattered by wine, and red wine with its tannin is impossible. But a flavorful accompaniment—the more of it, the better—opens the possibilities to diverse wines. Egg dishes with cream and cheese go with Chardonnay or Pinot Blanc, for instance, and eggs with strong-flavored, especially meaty additions go with light reds.

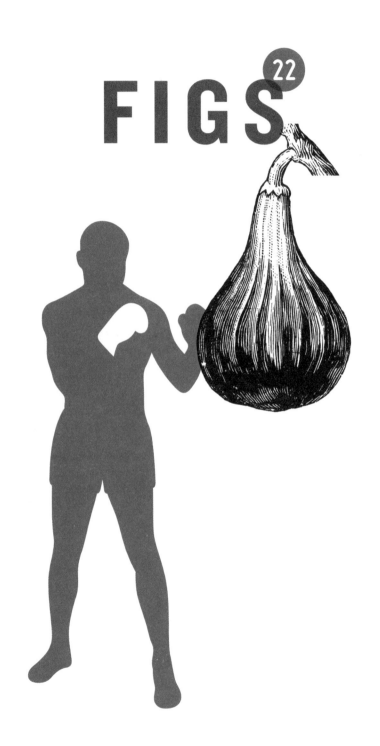

F igs like heat. As they grow, they stand alert on the branch, sometimes
upright, and when they ripen in August, the stem withers and they
hang. Some varieties show their ripeness by a drop of nectar that appears at the open eye where the petals were attached. The color, according
to the variety, is green, violet, bronze, brown, dark-purplish, or mixed. The
skin and flesh are giving, almost animallike. Ripeness is essential, yet a ripe
fig is so vulnerable and the time between ripeness and decay is so short that
a ripe fig can't be shipped. It lasts only hours. To enjoy figs in an ideal state,
you have to be in the warm places where they thrive. Some of the best grow
in Turkey. A friend from Istanbul says, "It's a huge thing; every well-to-do
family, even in Istanbul, had fig trees. They would teach you where to pick,
how to peel, how to eat them." David Karp, the fruit connoisseur and
writer who haunts Los Angeles farmers' markets, has said, "The fig lover
develops almost a mystical rapport with his fruit, alert to the many external
hints—striated or stretch-marked skin, a touch of sunburn, and a drop of
honey at the bottom"—revealing perfect ripeness. Figs have little acidity,
which underlines their warm-climate sensuality. The flavor, so often compared with honey and berries, to me can also have a nutty note; it's hard to
pin down. Many varieties dry admirably, something once always started in
the sun and then finished in a bread oven (to eliminate possible insects).
The best dried figs are very sweet and viscous inside, not yet crystallized,
with a deep caramel taste. The seeds, so tender and insignificant in the fresh
fig, become crisp. Dried figs ship impeccably. But a fresh fig that's picked
before it's fully ripe and shipped a long way conveys the idea and some of
the pleasure.

For all figs' powerful reputation for sensuality, not everyone
sees the appeal. Some people think they're wonderful; others find them

inexplicable, which is surely a reflection of what they've tasted. For a sweet, juicy, flavorful fig, the variety as well as the place makes a huge difference.

The fig is a botanic oddity. The flowers are inside the fruit, which means that with some kinds pollination can be difficult. The edible species, *Ficus carica,* began with the wild caprifig, whose name means "goat fig"; apparently the small, dry fruits were eaten by goats. It was probably first domesticated in the Jordan Valley and spread eventually to the Mediterranean, where it found itself completely at home and seems to have diverged into delicious varieties. The varieties are sometimes divided into four groups: the caprifig, the common, the Smyrna, and the San Piero, which is better known as Brown Turkey.

The caprifig and Smyrna varieties are pollinated by particular tiny wasps, each native to a small geographic area; they don't bear fruit outside their home territory unless they're specially pollinated. Most figs bear an early crop, in late spring or early summer, from buds that formed the previous year. These figs, called brebas, are larger than main-crop figs but normally inferior, except in atypically hot weather. The main crop ripens from August into fall.

The important varieties in California are Calimyrna, which is a variety of Smyrna, and Adriatic, Brown Turkey, Conadria, Kadota, and Mission, which are all common figs. The green Calimyrna was originally the Sari Lop, from Turkey, a variety that's several centuries old; it's the most important commercial fig and the point of reference for quality. Larger than most, Smyrna figs are highly regarded for eating fresh, with a nutty flavor; dried, they're as sweet as candy. Other Smyrna varieties are the Marabout, from Algeria, and the dark purple Zidi, from Morocco.

The Adriatic (also known by other names, including Grosse Verte) may have something of a strawberry flavor. It's luscious and fragile; almost all Adriatic figs in California go for drying and fig paste. Brown Turkey has other names besides San Piero; a French one is Bourjasotte. Although not all Brown Turkey figs may be the same, the variety is rated by some as the best for eating fresh. Conadria, an introduction from 1956, is used for drying. Kadota is the same as the Italian variety Dottato, also used for drying. Black Mission figs, a piece of California history, were planted by the early

Franciscan missionaries. I like them dried better than fresh. Other admired varieties include Rouge de Bordeaux, Figue Noire de Caromb, and the striped Panachee, with its raspberry interior, and there are many more.

If you search cookbooks, you discover that fig recipes, especially ones calling for fresh fruit, are surprisingly scarce or absent altogether, even when the subject is the cooking of places where figs thrive. Chefs sometimes put fresh figs in a salad, and in high-end cooking, fresh ripe figs can appear with meats—duck, rabbit, guinea fowl, pork, ham. The raw fruit is merely finished for a few minutes in the juices of the pan, scarcely cooked. Similarly, for dessert ripe figs sometimes go into a hot baked tart shell and then spend a few minutes in a hot oven. Recipes for cooking fresh figs often call for what I think of as more perfumey flavors: anise, orange, liqueurs (especially orange ones), fortified wines, aromatic honeys (orange blossom, lavender, or lime tree), sometimes Port. They strike me as old-fashioned, oblivious to the danger that the fig's own flavor may be lost. Like dried figs, fresh ones are put with thyme. They're good caramelized. They go with nuts, citrus zest, and cream. Fig jam can fall flat on character and acidity, but it's always appealingly different from other jams.

Dried figs are cooked in white wine, red wine, or Port, and they can accompany pork, rabbit, pheasant, guinea fowl. The writer Diana Farr Louis describes *sykomaidha,* a sort of dried-fig bread made all over Greece; on Corfu, she found it wrapped in chestnut leaves and "made of chopped dried figs kneaded into a paste with ouzo and/or mastic liqueur, grape must, walnuts, orange peel, black pepper, and fennel seeds."

HOW TO PICK A RIPE FIG: From late summer into fall, sweet, flavorful main-crop figs appear at some warm-climate farmers' markets. Choose figs that are very soft but not damaged or overripe. Smyrna figs in wet weather will split slightly open; a drop of nectar appears at the hole in Brown Turkey and Mission. Avoid figs with a smell of fermentation. If you don't eat really ripe figs almost immediately, within hours of being picked, they start to deteriorate; if you want to keep them longer than that, you have to refrigerate them. A quartered fig is visually striking, and serving the fruit cut open shows that it isn't spoiled within.

My friend from Istanbul says, "I have never, ever seen anybody at home eat a fig with a skin." (He conceded that his mother sometimes eats certain tiny figs whole.) Some Americans never peel a fig, and some do, depending partly on the variety. Some like the dark skin of a Mission fig. You peel a fig by trimming off the stem end or cutting an × over it and pulling away strips.

COMPLEMENTS TO FIGS: Like melons, fresh, ripe figs go with paper-thin prosciutto. When they're put with meat, it's more for novelty than for taste. The best dessert complements are raspberries and cream, and the two can be combined by folding the sieved fresh berries into the sweetened whipped cream. Fresh figs go with light-flavored or floral honey, almonds, and pistachios. Some people enjoy them with anise or clove. Some people like them with blue cheese. Dried figs go with varied spices, caramel, stronger honey such as thyme, thyme itself, red wine, orange zest, dates, walnuts, pistachios, cream, and certain cheeses.

NOTES ON WINE: When fresh figs are prepared with flavorful complements, they're sometimes served with Muscat de Beaumes-de-Venise, Madeira, tawny Port, sweet sherry, or *vin santo.* I'm certain special combinations occur, but I'd rather concentrate on the fig. Dried figs stand up to tawny Port, *vins doux naturels,* and other oxidized wines.

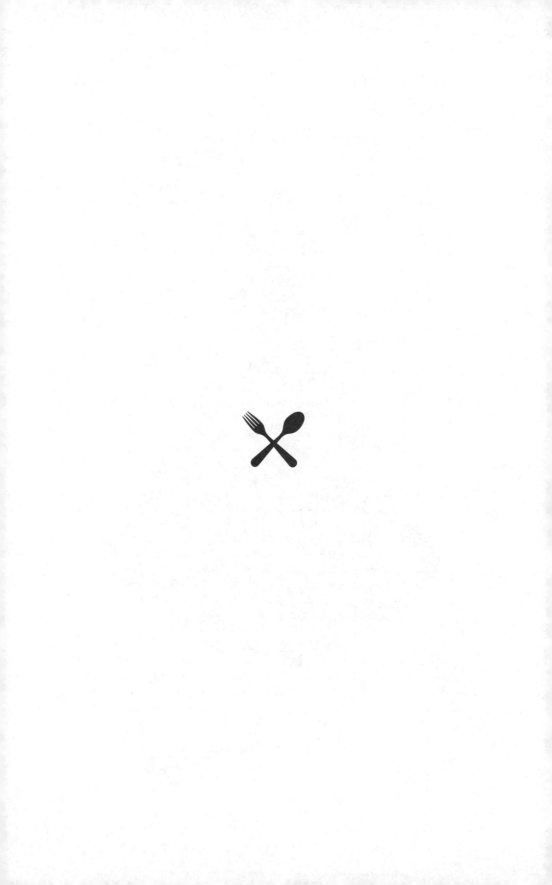

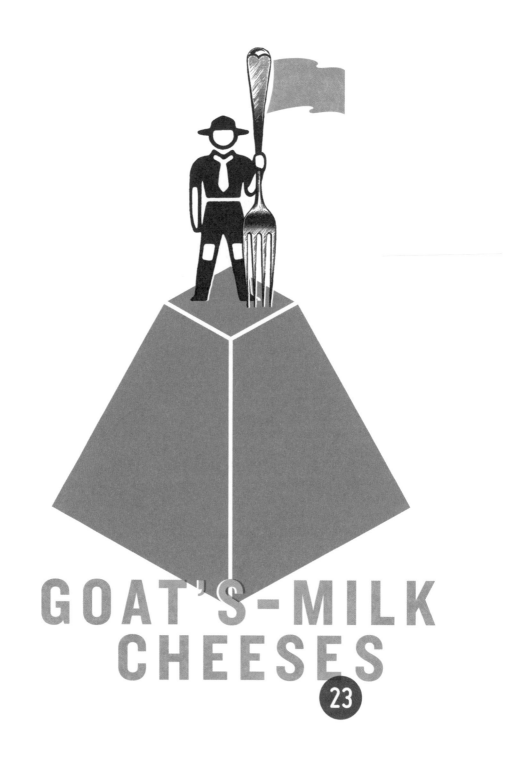

GOAT'S-MILK CHEESES

23. GOAT'S-MILK CHEESES, SMALL AND OFTEN LUSCIOUS

S mall, soft goat's-milk cheeses, typically round and flat, are one of the great pleasures of the table in France and everywhere they are now made. The newly formed cheeses, often from raw milk, are soon covered with microflora that form a bloomy rind and start the ripening, though some drier kinds have a plainer skin. Within two weeks, they're typically in an excellent state. The soft white interior gives an impression of fat, though no cream has been added to the whole milk. The taste combines a clean acidity and a dairy taste with something that might be called nutty; you may be aware of a touch of goat. Some cheeses are drier and firmer; others are lusciously creamy and even flowing. Although most production in France now takes place on a more or less large scale, many cheeses are still made on farms. Traditionally, they appear in French markets in early spring, after the does bear their kids and start to give milk, and they disappear again in late fall. Wherever they're made, they are the common cheese of that place.

They occur as far north as the Loire Valley, which has a concentration of fine examples, and they proliferate in the South. Some have official appellations. There are logs of Sainte-Maure from Touraine, rounds of Selles-sur-Cher from just to the east, pyramids of Pouligny-Saint-Pierre and Valençay and little drums of Crottin de Chavignol from the Berry, leaf-mounted Mothais sur Feuille from Poitou and the Charentes, Beaujolais from the same place as the wine, Cabécou from central and southwest France, Rocamadour from Périgord and Quercy, Charolais (which can also be pure cow) and Clacbitou from Burgundy, Rigotte de Condrieu from the Lyonnais, Picodon from the southern Rhone Valley, the chestnut-wrapped

Banon and the savory- and rosemary-coated Poivre d'Âne from Provence (which can be made with mixed milk). All these and many more.

"The goat is the cow of the poor," according to a French saying. A cow requires a certain abundance of pasture that results from a certain minimum of rainfall, but a goat or sheep can thrive in drier, wilder, less fertile territory, even foraging on brush. And goats, for their weight, give the most milk. Once, the peasants who raised goats could afford to eat meat only rarely. They ate cheese every day, sometimes at every meal. Making cheese was also a way to preserve food for winter, when the animals ceased to give milk. The small goat's-milk cheeses associated with peasants weren't found on aristocratic tables, nor until relatively recently were they served in great restaurants.

The ingredients once were only milk, sometimes rennet, and always salt, though today commercial cultures are often added. Unlike big wheels of cow's-milk cheeses, these small ones require no great quantity of milk, no copper cauldron, no fire to heat the curd, no big wooden molds, no press, no cool, moist cellar for ripening (though a good cellar doesn't hurt). Originally, the milk and curd were held in stoneware jars. The maker used a ladle to fill small ceramic molds pierced with holes to allow the whey to drain. And the new cheeses were turned out to dry and ripen on rye-straw mats. Sometimes in fair weather in Provence the small cheeses were ripened outdoors in the shade, protected from animals in homely cheese cages.

The small goat's-milk cheeses, although most are now made in plants that combine the milk of many farms, remain the epitome of a farm cheese. In France, a *fromage fermier* must be made on the farm, by those living on the farm, using only that farm's milk. Milk that isn't trucked anywhere can be maximally fresh, in perfect condition. It's used raw for superior results and to save on the labor and equipment of pasteurization. The taste of a well-made cheese reflects the specific location, its soil and climate, plants and microorganisms. The small goat's-milk cheeses are well adapted to farmer-artisans of limited means. The best farm cheeses are the best of all.

Raw milk carries the full aroma as well as some of the microflora that contribute to the flavor of cheese. Pasteurization damages texture; raw milk gives firmer curd. The sooner milk is set into curd, the better, still warm from the udder in the best of all possible worlds. Sometimes cheese used to be made twice a day, after each milking; very exceptionally it still is.

(It's a cheese connoisseur's lament that all too commonly in many parts of the world milk is collected from farms only every two or three days and is then trucked to a distant plant. The delay and refrigeration harm the good microorganisms and increase the possibility that bad ones will multiply and other undesirable changes will occur. As the milk waits inside a farm's bulk tank, it's mechanically stirred, to make the temperature even throughout and prevent the cream from rising, then the milk sloshes inside a truck tank and again when it's pumped from container to container at the plant. All that movement breaks some of the fat globules, which allows destructive enzymes to begin to turn the fat rancid.)

Where a cow's-milk cheese is somewhat yellow inside, goat's- and ewe's-milk cheeses are white, because those animals convert nearly all the plants' carotene to vitamin A, eliminating the yellow. Goat's milk is also slightly richer in fat than cow's, and ewe's milk is richer still in both fat and protein. Compared with cow's milk, both goat's and ewe's milk have smaller fat globules, and the milk lacks a certain protein that causes fat globules to stick to each other and rise, so the cream doesn't readily separate. The milk for traditional goat's-milk cheeses is always used whole. The different flavors of the cheeses from the three kinds of milk come mainly from their different fats, as they're acted on by enzymes during ripening. Beyond that, goat's-milk cheese has a sharper acidity, and the particular proteins in goat's milk tend to produce more crumbly cheese. Often in the past, goats and sheep were mixed in the same herd—sometimes they still are—and the milk was, and is, mixed together to make a single kind of cheese.

Once upon a time, there was no fixed recipe for a farm cheese, only a general form for the particular area, executed differently by each farmwife (it was almost always she who made the cheese). The taste also reflected the qualities of the particular milk, the season, recent rainfall, the details of making and handling the curd, salting and turning, the humidity of the aging room, the skill of the maker. Now many points of technique are fixed in the fourteen official French appellations for goat's-milk cheeses. (The old French Appellation d'Origine Contrôlée, or AOC, system is being swallowed up by the European Union's Appellation d'Origine Protégée, or AOP, system.)

Nearly all the small goat's-milk cheeses are made with a *caillé acide,* an "acid curd." Over eighteen to twenty-four hours at cool temperatures, the acidity in the milk naturally rises and that by itself will set the curd. The rennet of the past wasn't as consistent and reliable as today's commercial rennet, and now a small amount of it is usually added to speed up the process and give a slightly firmer curd, with less loss through the holes of the mold. For some cheeses, including industrially made ones, the curd is intentionally broken up, but filling the molds with a ladle, the oldest method, gives the moistest, most delicate cheese.

The new cheeses are turned in their molds two or three times a day for several days, then unmolded onto wire racks or perforated plastic mats. After that they are turned for several more days, sprinkled with salt on one side and then the other, as they firm and shrink, at cool room temperature. The *caillé acide* cheeses are ripened from the outside in by surface microflora. When the cheeses are made with raw milk using more natural methods, the varied kinds and colors of mold are determined by the surface moisture, pH, salt, and temperature. And a cheese made in the warmth and humidity of summer shows more varied wild microflora—gray, green, blue, black, yellow, possibly red. Being small and relatively thin, the cheeses have a proportionately large surface area, and they ripen quickly. Frequently, they are eaten while they retain the appealing contrast of a creamy outside with a very white, chalky core.

Refrigeration at any point will slow and can nearly halt the evolution of a cheese. The longer and deeper the chill, the less a cheese is able to recover afterward. For partly to fully ripened cheeses, a compromise temperature used by some makers is mere coolness, no lower than 50 degrees F (10 degrees C), which holds back the cheeses without stunning them.

The small goat's-milk cheeses are delicious at every stage, starting with the still-draining day-old rounds (before that, the curd itself is good, such as with honey for dessert). At around ten to twelve days, according to the appellation, if there is one, the cheeses may be sold under their official name. After two to three weeks, a tan rind has formed that is largely or entirely covered with white or blue-green or more colorful molds. Today the makers often add commercial cultures, selected for their whiteness, and those take over, producing a pure white coating. At this point, the cheese is about "half dry" (*demi-sec,* the French say) but still quite soft and about at its peak. Some cheeses taste peppery from the breakdown of certain fats. Gradually they become "dry" (*sec*), which really means only quite firm. As they continue to dry, they turn amber and gain the rich caramel flavors of an old cheese coupled with a strong peppery bite. Eventually they shrink to peppery orange disks as hard as hockey pucks—not for every day and not so much in demand, but in their way delicious.

Many cheeses, however, follow a different path from the start. Rather than being intended to dry, they are made extra moist and matured in a moist atmosphere, where they turn creamy and even flowing. After that they don't keep very long, but they are the most luscious cheeses of all.

All the kinds I've been describing, whether dry or creamy, are acid-curd cheeses. There is another sort. In the warmth of Mediterranean France, spoilage microbes could proliferate in the milk before the acidity rose, so instead the curd was set with a much larger amount of rennet in a much shorter time, often two to four hours. This *caillé doux,* "sweet curd," was also ladled into small molds. The cheeses ripened at first from the surface inward, but then they turned creamy throughout all at once from all the enzymes in the rennet, ending up with a thicker crust and an unusual, pleasing earthy flavor. Like the retreating Provençal language, these goat's-milk cheeses were nearly extinct by the late twentieth century. All that remain are Banon, Saint-Félicien de Lamastre, and here and there an individual cheese made on a holdout farm.

Fresh cheeses, being so mild, are lost among the stronger ones of a cheese course. They're best eaten as a snack, or at the beginning of a meal, or as the main part of a light meal. Not just fresh cheeses but small goat's-milk cheeses at various stages of maturity are excellent at the center of lunch or supper, along with a loaf of bread, salad, a glass of wine, maybe fruit for dessert. At such a meal, a single small, ripe goat's-milk cheese can be ideal—full of flavor and directly to the point.

It makes no sense to cook such a beautifully made small cheese. Even the French practice of serving an oven-warmed goat's-milk cheese on top of a green salad, dating from the 1970s, defies logic. The heat makes the cheese soft, heavy, and goaty and throws the entire taste out of balance, destroying the appeal. The delicate consistency of a hand-ladled goat's-milk cheese, something to treasure, is also lost when the cheese is mashed into bread or crackers. It's much better to eat it with a knife and fork.

These are a few of the more important small goat's-milk cheeses, plus one typically ewe's-milk interloper, from roughly north to south:

CHAVIGNOL or CROTTIN DE CHAVIGNOL (AOP) In and around the Sancerrois of central France, and especially around the wine village of Chavignol, raw goat's milk is turned into a very small, drum-shaped cheese with slightly bulging sides. The curd is "pre-drained" on cloth before it is put into molds, which makes even the young cheeses dry, firm, and somewhat shattering when cut. To qualify for sale in the US, some Crottins are aged for sixty days, much longer than usual, and they acquire a translucent outer layer and a more intense, frequently peppery taste. To preserve Crottins for winter eating, the cheeses are sometimes still *repassé:* packed together in stoneware pots, where an anaerobic transformation makes them truly powerful.

SAINTE-MAURE DE TOURAINE (AOP) The familiar goat's-milk log, about six and a half to seven inches (sixteen to eighteen centimeters) long, is widely made in the province of Touraine and, without the qualification "de Touraine," in other parts of France. The long mold tapers so the cheese will slide out, and a straw runs through the center to strengthen the log while it's still young and fragile. Often the cheese is ash-covered, which may hasten ripening by making the surface less acidic; it also gives a more wrinkled skin. If you cut a thin slice from a log and break it, you see the arc where one ladleful of curd met the next, proof of hand-ladling. When young, the cheese is smooth in texture, melting in the mouth. As the days pass, it turns drier and more crumbly, and the slightly acidic, nutty taste becomes stronger and more distinctly goaty. I like Sainte-Maure at about the third or fourth week.

POULIGNY-SAINT-PIERRE (AOP) This slightly truncated pyramid of raw goat's milk, about five inches tall (twelve and a half centimeters), is made in a small part of the central French region of Berry. The producers adopted the shape a century ago, modeling it on the village church tower, it's always said. After about two weeks, the more industrial versions are covered with white mold, while the more traditional ones have a partly blue crust and a fuller flavor. A similar but more cut-off pyramid called Valençay, also AOP, is made around the town of that name in the same region.

PÉLARDON (AOP) A model of the southern type of small goat's-milk cheese, the Pélardon is a round that originated in the Cévennes Mountains and is still made there and in adjacent parts of the Languedoc and Roussillon. Today's appellation encompasses a vast area of five hundred communes. To speed the setting of the curd and to seed the raw milk with organisms that ripen the cheese, farm-cheesemakers may add only whey from the previous making, not commercial starter. Unlike most of the small cheeses, for which there's a limited historical record, references to Pélardon go back almost three hundred years; the taste was always strong and peppery.

BANON (AOP) Made from raw milk in a broad area in the high hills of Provence and named for a small village there, Banon is one of the cheeses creamy enough to eat with a spoon. It's the best-known of the largely disappeared category of *caillé doux*. In the late twentieth century, Banon was still the most renowned cheese of Provence, and yet little of it was produced (and most of that was *caillé acide*) until the appellation was approved in 2003. Banon is aged for five to ten days, and then, what truly sets it apart, it is wrapped and tied in the tannic leaves of chestnuts, which slows drying but allows the cheese to breathe. Before it can be sold, the cheese must age for at least ten more days, but six weeks inside the leaves might be ideal, and it will keep for months beyond that. Inside the wrapping, Banon can reach a nearly collapsing state and grow strong. Although Banon doesn't become peppery, some people find the flavor challenging.

LE GARDIAN, also called TOMME D'ARLES and TOMME DE CAMARGUE (NO APPELLATION) This ultrafresh cheese is made in Provence near the mouth of the Rhone River. Since no official rules apply, depending on who's making the cheese, the milk may be goat, ewe, or a mix. Any kind is good, but Le Gardian is at its luscious best when made of pure ewe's milk. The cheese has no skin; its color is pure white outside and in, and its texture is perfectly smooth. You see trays full of the cheeses at markets, the white rounds sitting close together, half immersed in whey, each topped with a bay leaf and a sprinkling of Provençal herbs and black pepper. The cheese is never flowing but always creamy, almost slippery in texture— lightly resilient to the touch, like a Bavarian cream. In its home area, Le Gardian is not traditionally refrigerated, which would only harm the flavor; it's purchased and eaten within twenty-four hours of making, before the delicate flavor and lightness are lost.

HOW TO BUY SMALL GOAT'S-MILK CHEESES: Buy them directly from a good maker, such as at a farmers' market, or from a careful shop. The best season for milk and cheese as a rule is spring, when the soil warms and the flowers bloom, but good and even exceptional goat's-milk cheeses are made through fall. (Winter cheeses are sometimes made with frozen curd.) In a perfect world, cheese would never be refrigerated at any point, and uncut cheeses would remain unwrapped—cheese is living and needs to breathe. Yet some of the best shops, even in Paris, now display all their cheeses both chilled and tightly covered in plastic film. If the cheeses sell rapidly, the harm is less.

Very fresh goat's-milk cheeses, no more than a few days old and with little or no mold, have a simple, lactic flavor. They should taste clean but not one-dimensional; raw-milk ones have more depth, and they're really the only fresh cheeses worth eating on their own. Avoid the small, unripened goat's-milk cheeses made of pasteurized milk and covered with or mixed with herbs. The cheese itself is rarely good, and the herbs are often meant to hide shortcomings. It's better to buy a superior fresh cheese and add your own herbs, chopped just before serving.

Any of the small goat's-milk cheeses, however rustic, should appear neat. The rind of the bloomy rind sorts is often wrinkled, but it shouldn't be separating from the inside of the cheese (due to too-fast ripening at too-warm temperatures). It shouldn't be cracked and leaking, nor should the insides be so liquid as to be runny. Most surface molds these days are pure white from commercial microflora; more natural and flavorful goat's-milk cheeses are dominated by bluish molds and often show other colors.

Small goat's-milk cheeses in France are well-ripened in as little as two weeks. The drawn-out aging of some cheeses sent to the US produces a drier, denser cheese with more aggressive, often more peppery flavors; normally distinct cheeses tend to converge in taste.

Even the more aged small goat's-milk cheeses should taste clean, and a good ripe taste can sometimes be delicate. Bitterness, which can have many causes, is always a defect. And no cheese should taste strongly salty (in cheese, as in bread, extra salt is sometimes intentionally added to give an illusion of more flavor), but oversalting and undersalting are much less common than they once were. A cheese shouldn't be too dry or crumbly, depending on the sort. When all comes together, the small goat's-milk cheeses have one of the most complex, satisfying, and fundamental tastes of any cheese.

HOW TO KEEP AND, IF NEEDED, RIPEN SMALL GOAT'S-MILK CHEESES: The small, soft goat's-milk cheeses are likely to have matured at more or less natural temperatures, and even if they've been refrigerated during shipping and distribution and for a time in a shop, when you get them home, it's better to put them somewhere at between cellar and room temperature. If they sit out for any length of time in a warm place, the moister cheeses, especially, deteriorate. Hardest of all on cheese are temperatures and humidity that go up and down. Some shops specialize in ripening small goat's-milk cheeses and sell them in an optimum state, but often what you buy benefits from further ripening.

If the cheese is already ripe, or you have neither the time nor a cool place in which to ripen it, unwrap the cheese and then somewhat loosely close it again in its wrapper, which is often specially made for the purpose. If you aren't going to eat it in the next few hours, refrigerate it. Try to eat it within a day or two. Be certain to set the cheese out several hours beforehand; unwrap it, put it on a plate, and cover it with an inverted bowl to hold in humidity while it breathes and warms to cool room temperature.

If the cheese would benefit from further ripening, and you have time and a cool spot, say a corner of a cellar at about 55 to 60 degrees F (13 to 16 degrees C), then remove the cheese from its wrapper, set it on a plate, and give it a fine spray of water (or fling drops with your fingers). Cover the cheese with an inverted bowl to hold in humidity, and put it in that cool spot. At least once a day, lift the bowl to allow in fresh air and add another spray of water—enough to condense on the inside of the bowl. Every day or two, turn the cheese over. In two or three days, the rind may show a fresh downy coat of mold. The cheese may then be at its best, or it may require a few more days. Track the evolution partly by smell—there may be a strong whiff of ammonia but not too much if you lift the bowl daily and turn the cheese every other day. Mainly, though, check how soft the cheese has become by pressing gently with a finger. Unless you have experience, err on the side of underripeness.

COMPLEMENTS TO SMALL GOAT'S-MILK CHEESES: A just-made cheese, hardly more than turned out of its mold, likes a grinding of black pepper and dousing with just-chopped fresh herbs, especially chives and savory. Fresh cheeses also go well with walnuts and walnut oil. Olive oil, in which goat's-milk cheeses are sometimes immersed, doesn't hurt, although there's no synergy. US restaurants often disregard the nature of an individual cheese and what might truly go with it, serving slivers of diverse cheeses with a collection of dried fruit and nuts, chutneys and jams. The one sure-fire thing that makes cheese taste better is fresh bread. You do no harm to the texture of the creamiest cheeses if you mash them into the bread, but I so much appreciate the texture of any other sort that I find the idea of mashing the cheese into bread hard to understand. Eat the cheese with a knife and fork, alternating bites of cheese with bites of bread.

NOTES ON WINE: Small goat's-milk cheeses call for wines with refreshing acidity and moderate alcohol (less than 13 percent, to give a number). There's a romantic appeal to matching a cheese with a wine from the same place, and it often works. One of the great flavor trios is Crottin de Chavignol with a salad dressed with walnut oil and a glass of Sauvignon wine—cheese, oil, and wine all being made around the village of Chavignol near the town of Sancerre. But there's also a broad logic of what goes with what. *With an ultrafresh, moist goat's-milk cheese,* drink a fresh, fruity, young white or pink wine, even a very light fruity red, modest in alcohol. *With a creamy, flowing cheese,* choose a richer white, such as a Hermitage, a rich Alsace Pinot Gris, one of the richer Chenins, or certain rosés. A more fat-tasting, less acidic version of the cheese will counter a wine's acidity and make it seem richer. *With a drier, harder goat's-milk cheese* (certain Sainte-Maures, always Crottin de Chavignol), drink a moistening white wine—a light, not too ripe white Sancerre (made of pure Sauvignon Blanc in the upper Loire Valley appellation that includes prime territory for the variety), a Condrieu, a young Chablis, a Savennières or other Chenin Blanc from Anjou, a white Mâcon, various southern whites, including in principle Châteauneuf-du-Pape, but the southern wines have grown increasingly alcoholic. Or try a Finger Lakes Riesling from New York, which is always light. *With completely dry, hard goat's-milk cheeses* of the sort we scarcely see in North America and whose pungency is hard on wine, there are no good matches, and the best thing is the simplest white or rosé wine. The same is true of the leaf-wrapped, creamy Banon.

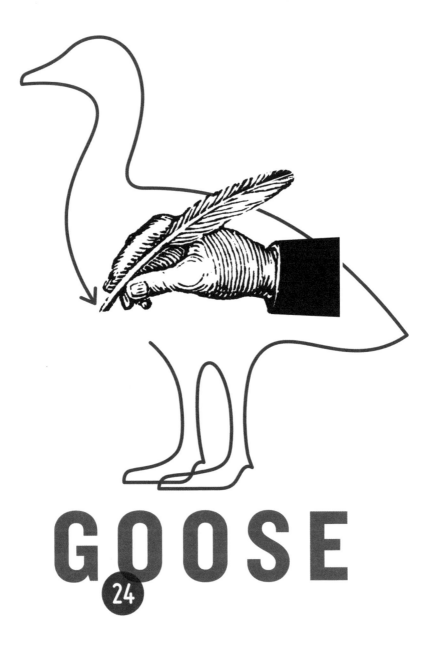

GOOSE

24

24. GOOSE

Compared with the birds we usually eat, goose is more highly flavored, more evidently bony, and more protected with fat. All the meat is dark and flavorful, but the fat is the wonderful thing, with its gutsy animal flavor and none of the refinement of good fresh butter or olive oil. Cooks who roast a goose for the first time are often worried by the large quantity of fat that appears in the pan, but the meat itself isn't fatty, and if it's carefully prepared, you don't end up eating any more fat than you do with other meat. Before the legs of a goose are fully cooked, the breast begins to dry and toughen. To avoid that, a goose breast, like a duck breast, is often cooked separately from the legs, to just rare or medium rare. Goose goes with sweet and acidic counterpoints, sometimes both together, including apples, prunes, and sauerkraut. In southwestern France, a center of goose eating, the main traditional cooking fat is goose. There and elsewhere goose is made into *rillettes:* the well-salted meat is cooked gently with its fat until it can be stirred to moist shreds. They're better made from goose than from duck or pork. Finest of all is the immortal form of goose, *confit*—real *confit,* made with enough salt to preserve and transform it. The cut-up goose is rubbed with salt, garlic, pepper, herbs, and spices, and the salt is given a day or two to penetrate. Then the meat is cooked slowly in its own fat and preserved under the same fat, supplemented if needed by lard, so it survives for weeks without refrigeration (though the cold is a good idea). Only after a month is the characteristic flavor evident. Duck and pork also make excellent *confit,* but not as special as the goose version. And goose meat is made into sausage, stuffed into the skin of the neck, cooked in goose fat, and put up with the rest (including the giblets) as *confit.* Still, the best part is the fat—*confit* fat is the most delicious fat of all for frying potatoes.

Fat keeps a goose warm and buoyant in water and carries it through the lean winter. Feeding for fat is taken to an extreme in the birds raised for foie gras, "fat liver"—honey-beige in color, extremely large, fatty, soft, mild, and highly delicious. The birds raised for foie gras have very thick, meaty breasts; on menus, half a breast from a foie gras bird is the *magret.* Geese gave the original foie gras. Duck foie gras, which some people like better, has largely replaced it, because ducks are easier to raise and their livers fatten more quickly. Low-priced foie gras requires large-scale, semiautomated methods, with the ducks tightly confined in individual plastic crates—if foie gras is cheap, you know you shouldn't eat it. I've seen the force-feeding on small farms in southwestern France, where the birds are outdoors every day. Taken as a whole, the treatment was much, much more humane than the way industrial chickens or pigs are raised. That's not to say it was right and good. Very exceptionally, foie gras is produced only in autumn without force-feeding by relying on the birds' natural urge to fatten themselves in preparation for winter. They eat at will. Obviously, the quantity of that foie gras will always be limited. But there's regular goose liver, which is delicious in the same way as other poultry liver.

A wild goose is sleeker and more horizontal than the upright domestic goose, with its large rear. Dozens of breeds exist in the West and more elsewhere, especially in China, where the goose was domesticated centuries before it was in Europe. Chinese and African geese are descended from the swan goose, a separate species. The wild goose native to Europe, the greylag, which is gray in color, gave rise to the European breeds. All the varied breeds are white or gray, or sometimes mixed in hybrids. While you may come across a farmer proud of a particular breed—Toulouse, Alsatian, Emden, Venetian, Chinese—no one breed seems to rise to the top.

What's more important for the meat is that, although geese eat mostly grain, they're outdoors on pasture. In any case, a goose, being weeks older than the other domesticated birds we cook, including most turkeys, is full of flavor, and it benefits from the tenderizing effects of braising, which allows varied accompaniments: bitter orange, sour cherries, boletes, olives.

Confit is the central flavor of *garbure,* a substantial cabbage soup from southwestern France, but the famous use for *confit* is in another dish from the region, *cassoulet,* which is named for the *cassole,* the ceramic vessel in which it's baked, a hand-thrown, wide truncated cone. *Cassoulet,* at least in theory, occurs in three distinct forms: those of Carcassonne, Castelnaudary, and Toulouse. Richard Olney, in *Simple French Food,* impeccably describes one version, unnamed but seemingly the one from Carcassonne:

> The beans are cooked apart, their flavor enhanced by prolonged contact with aromatic vegetables, herbs, and spices; the mutton is cooked apart, slowly, the wine and other aromatic elements refining, enriching, or underlining its character; apart, the goose has long since been macerated in herbs and salt and subsequently preserved in its own fat; a good sausage is famously allied to witchcraft. All of these separate products are then combined; a bit of catalytic goose fat—with the aid of gelatinous pork rind—binds them together in a velvet texture, and a further slow cooking process intermingles all the flavors while a gratin, repeatedly basted, forms, is broken, re-forms, is rebroken, a single new savor moving into dominance, cloaking, without destroying, the autonomy of the primitive members.

Before roasting, it helps to salt a goose inside and out a day in advance, a little more heavily than you might normally. And to let the fat flow out of the bird as it cooks, puncture the skin all over with a heavy trussing needle or a very pointed blade, without piercing the meat so juice will flow, too. Place the bird on a rack, assuming you use an oven, so it doesn't fry in its fat. (If you roast before a fire, be certain to place a dripping pan carefully below.) I don't stuff a goose or any bird for roasting, because in order to cook the stuffing sufficiently, you must overcook the bird. And I don't bring a beautiful whole goose (or duck) to the table, because I remove the two halves of the breast when they're done and then return the legs and carcass to finish cooking. Meanwhile, let the breast rest in a warm spot. When the cooking is done, save the fat, refrigerating it in a glass jar, so as to have the pleasure of it for weeks to come.

HOW TO BUY GOOSE: The natural season for fresh goose, when the birds are fattest and most meaty, is fall to the end of the year. A well-raised goose is unfortunately not an economical meat. Look for one that was raised out-doors and looks reasonably fleshy. At one of the few North American farms that raise geese, you may have to reserve well ahead. (It's much better to buy a well-raised frozen goose than none at all.) How many people a goose serves depends greatly on the bird in question—its quantity of meat in relation to fat and bone. A ten-pound goose might serve only six.

COMPLEMENTS TO GOOSE: Garlic and herbs (thyme, savory, oregano, rosemary, and the branches of highly aromatic dried Greek sage sold in Greek markets) enhance goose, especially in *confit.* Goose likes strong cooked greens, including spinach and chard. In the same way as pork, it goes with members of the cabbage family, from Brussels sprouts and turnips to sauerkraut and sweet-and-sour red cabbage. Also like pork, goose goes with apples, onions, prunes, chestnuts, and boletes. (The apples, onions, and chestnuts can be combined with the red cabbage: the onions are cooked in fat, then the cabbage goes in with vinegar or wine, a clove, a bay leaf; eventually the chestnuts follow, and finally the cut-up apples.) Goose is good with celery root, whose marked flavor can be made milder by mixing it with equal amounts of potato. Also good is salsify (though so little of it has a characteristic taste). Goose is excellent with dried beans. A braised goose with cabbage goes beautifully with dark rye bread. If you have a wild goose, then put it with *wild* wild rice (not paddy-grown). Roast goose likes freshly grated horseradish. One of the best of all foods is potatoes browned in goose fat.

NOTES ON WINE: Much depends on what accompanies the goose. Usually it benefits from rich, aromatic white wines, either dry or more or less sweet but with the acidity to balance both their own richness and that of the goose. The grapes might be Riesling, Pinot Gris, Gewürztraminer, or another variety grown in Alsace, an old region of geese-raising. Also good are Austrian and German Riesling, and I've liked a traditional Jura white. Reds go equally well, especially with a roast goose with a rare breast. Look to Pinot Noir or Syrah, traditional Brunello di Montalcino, old Bordeaux, gamier bottlings of Syrah and Shiraz, traditional red Rioja, and traditional Nebbiolo.

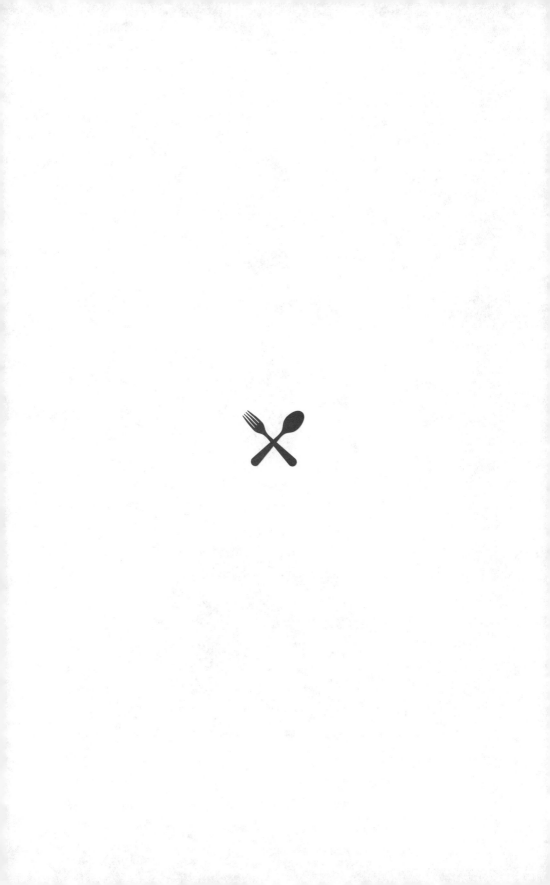

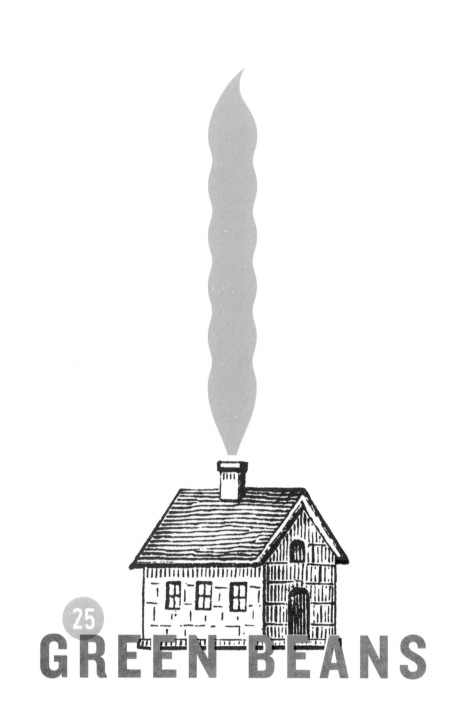

GREEN BEANS

The green-beaniest green beans are young, not more than about four inches long, taken straight from the garden, and they belong to one of the flavorful French *filet,* "thin," varieties. I can eat them with pleasure almost every day of their season. They have a lot more flavor than the two most-praised American varieties, Kentucky Wonder and Blue Lake (in either their low, bush form or the original pole-bean form). Cooked, the *filet* beans have a rich flavor, as vegetables go, sweet and nutty. Green beans, also known as snap or string beans, are *Phaseolus vulgaris,* together with wax, fresh shelling, and dry beans. They're sometimes called kidney beans, after the shape of their seeds, which are very different from the wide, flat ones of lima (butter) or fava (broad) beans (*P. lunatus* and *Vicia faba*). In a perfect world, you would always pick green beans in the morning before the dew evaporated and serve them at lunch rather than wait for dinner. Early in the season, they deserve to be their own course.

I've never seen green beans for sale that are as luxuriously young as those I pick from my garden; I usually include a few that are newly formed, threadlike. It takes a lot of young beans to make a pound, and they grow so quickly that they require daily hand-picking. For market gardeners, the cost in labor is so high that some don't grow them at all and nearly all those who do pick them big. After the beans are five or six inches long and the pods begin to swell on their way to maturity, the flavor changes noticeably. Fat, fibrous pods, bumpy with seeds, have much less flavor. But mature American varieties, boiled with cured pork for as long as three or four hours in the traditional Southern way, are a different vegetable and good in their own right.

Fashions in vegetable varieties come and go, if only because seed houses want new and different ones. I once grew rows of different modern *filet* varieties, some with old-fashioned strings and others with the strings bred out of them, so as to compare. I carefully tasted and chose a favorite, only to have it disappear from catalogs a few years later. And it wasn't any better than the old varieties Fin de Bagnols and Triomphe de Farcy (the beans of the latter are purple-streaked until fully cooked). Both of those are bush varieties that, wanting to twine just a little, throw up incipient runners. The oldest varieties of green beans have tough strings that don't break up with chewing. But young *filet* beans, even if they belong to stringy varieties, haven't yet formed strings.

Cooking heightens the flavor of green beans—full cooking until all the raw taste is gone. For years, I believed that most vegetables were better undercooked than overcooked. Yet for flavor, that's not true. No one likes mushy vegetables, but if you compare batches of green beans, you'll likely conclude that the most cooked batch has the best, strongest flavor—much stronger than that of beans retaining a shadow of crunch, no matter the variety. Some people advocate serving raw or barely cooked green beans in salad, but even for that purpose, fully cooked beans taste better. To test my changed views on doneness, I cooked batches of Fin de Bagnols and Rolande to three different degrees of doneness, and the most cooked batches of both had by far the most flavor, variety being irrelevant by comparison. (To compare the varieties, I tied handfuls of each in loose bags of cheesecloth, dropping them simultaneously into the same pot and simultaneously pulling them out. Both were excellent, with Fin de Bagnols being possibly finer.)

A brighter green color tends to mean better flavor, but any acidity in the cooking water dulls the color. Cooks have often added a little baking soda to make the water neutral or slightly alkaline, but too much soda gives a soapy taste and a pappy texture. Then there's the question of salt. To quote the talented English chef Heston Blumenthal: "You do not need salt in the water in order to keep your vegetables green. There, I have said it—I have committed the cardinal sin of questioning perhaps the single most unquestioned act in the kitchen." But, as he would agree, salt can play a useful role. Home cooks often add about a tablespoon of salt to a gallon of water (about five grams per liter), as if cooking pasta. Professionals add much more. Salt at seawater concentration speeds cooking, and with the shorter time the vegetable keeps a brighter color and loses less flavor to the water, as Harold McGee explains in *On Food and Cooking*. Seawater is very salty—3 percent salt, which is just over ⅓ cup per gallon (120 grams for four liters). Few home cooks may be brave enough to try that.

HOW TO BUY GREEN BEANS: No green beans are likely to be as wonderful as those you pick from your own garden, but bought beans are well worthwhile. At stands or farmers' markets, look for *filet* beans, the smaller and fresher, the better. Test for freshness by bending a bean to observe its rigidity and, if you're allowed, break it to see whether it makes a crisp snap. Beware of beans that are very long and thin—certain varieties stay thin even as they grow long and old and lose their good taste. Better varieties, if they happen to be named, include the more easily found Fortex or Maxibel and the less common Fin de Bagnols, Triomphe de Farcy, and Émérite. Or choose an American heirloom, such as Blue Lake or Kentucky Wonder.

HOW TO COOK GREEN BEANS: Pinch or cut off the stem ends and, if the variety is old-fashioned, also the tails, which can be a little tough. (With the tiniest beans, take just the stems.) Check to see whether there are strings: choose a larger bean, and break off a stem by pulling it down the length of the bean to see if it will unzip. If it does, string both sides either by pulling or by taking off a thin slice with a knife or vegetable peeler.

For best flavor and color, cook green beans fast. Put the whole beans into lots of rapidly boiling, well-salted water—enough water that the pot returns almost immediately to a boil after the beans go in and enough salt to season them as they cook. Replace the lid for a minute, which has no bad effect and gets the water back to a boil more quickly. Then uncover the pot so you can watch. I divide the beans by size into three or four piles and cook them in batches, removing them with a wide strainer. With smaller beans, start to check the doneness by tasting after two to three minutes.

Drain the beans well, return them to the hot pot, season further with salt if needed, and shake the pot over high heat to dry excess moisture, keeping the beans constantly moving. Add butter only off the heat so it doesn't turn to "oil," an ounce or more, cut up, to a pound of beans (60 grams butter to 500 grams beans), swirling so it forms an emulsion with any remaining water. Swirl the pot vigorously with two hands rather than mar the delicate vegetable with a utensil. The butter, in addition to flavoring the beans, keeps them from drying out. For salad, cook the beans close enough to serving time that they cool but don't have to be refrigerated. Drain them, but don't "stop the cooking" by plunging them into cold water, which takes away flavor.

COMPLEMENTS TO GREEN BEANS: Young green beans are easiest to appreciate with minimal accompaniments—butter, fresh, sweet (nonbitter) olive oil, salt, and little or no pepper. To compensate for any flavor shortcomings of the beans, after cooking them, add ripened cream (crème fraîche); butter or cream with Parmigiano; slivers of raw dry-cured ham; chopped onion or garlic or both, cooked in fat until translucent; chopped garlic cooked in olive oil and then, off the heat, mixed with chopped cured anchovies (beware overkill); aioli (green beans are part of the Provençal *grand aïoli*); or good canned tuna, along with just-sliced raw sweet onion and a lemon-juice dressing. Green beans go with many meats, maybe lamb first of all.

NOTES ON WINE: I've made some explorations, and I suspect that no wine really complements green beans, with their particular flavor and underlying sweetness. Butter helps wine go with the vegetable, and when there's Parmigiano or ham mixed with beans in a course by themselves, try a slightly rich white Burgundy. With a green-bean salad, a good dry rosé.

GREENS

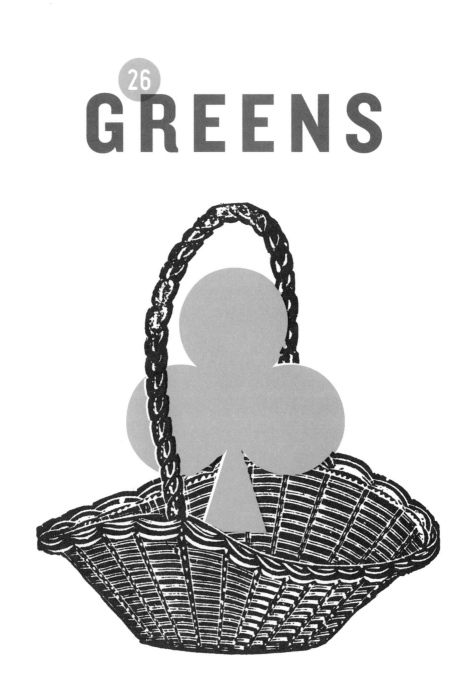

26. GREENS, STRONG AND SOMETIMES BITTER

Wild greens were once, of course, the only kind. Unlike cultivated greens, they're generally strong, bitter, and tough, all but the youngest. Certain species are mild enough to eat for just a short time in spring. It was only during the last few centuries that some leafy plants, such as kale and lettuce, were transformed by selection of the best into sweet garden vegetables. The old bitterness and toughness sometimes linger in part or resurface boldly in drought. After the cold months, when in many regions there was nothing green to eat, spring brings a focus on wild greens. Then, in the moisture and increasing warmth, the leaves are briefly mild and tender, delicious. The goodness may last only until the flower stalk rises. During that short time, the leaves are good with olive oil and lemon juice in salad. The more intense are better cooked at any season. Mixed with cheese, eggs, and herbs, they fill some of the wide, thin *torte salate* of Liguria. On Crete, complicated mixes of different wild greens, sweet, bitter, and aromatic, are cooked, mixed with cheese, and baked in a *hortopita.* Country people didn't flee from a certain amount of bitterness, which often brings compelling flavor with it. (It's not a green, but a prime example of the old rural embrace of bitterness is the tassel hyacinth, *lampascione* in Italian, a part of the cooking of the southern region of Puglia. When I first ate it, I found it incomprehensibly bitter. But it's a prized vegetable, cultivated now as well as wild.)

Around Nice, some of the early wild greens of spring have long been eaten as the salad we know by the Provençal word *mesclun,* "mix." According to the onetime mayor of Nice, Jacques Médecin, writing in 1972, the typical mesclun contained three main items: wild rocket (arugula), dandelion, and new lettuce, and "one can add a little cress and chervil." Then mesclun became popular, commonplace in restaurants, and the formerly wild rocket of spring and summer began to be cultivated in milder form year-round. Elsewhere in Provence, a *salade champêtre* (*salado champanello* in Provençal) might contain wild lettuce, spiny sow thistle, goat's beard, and bitter chicory, put with mustard dressing to go with game.

Where I live, there are wood sorrel (in the garden and the woods), sheep sorrel (lawn and garden), watercress (woods), purslane (garden), stinging nettles (open areas), lamb's quarters (garden), wild carrot (field and roadsides), milkweed (field), dandelion (field), ramps (woods), fiddle-heads (woods), and more. Weeds, living in the easier conditions of a garden, fall into a sort of middle ground. More of them are good for salad. Many of our North American weeds arrived together with the first Europeans, the seed being mixed with the hay for shipboard livestock.

You eat the tender tips of new milkweed before it turns impossibly bitter. Ramps, forest plants whose leaves resemble those of lily of the valley, have a pungent heat when raw; they can be cooked like greens and are at home in a mixture of them. I've always found it hard to catch dandelions early, before they become shudderingly bitter: the leaves can be no more than three or four inches long, with the flower buds still clustered at the base, not rising at all. The diverse kinds of sorrel are united by their clean acidity. Wood sorrel is relatively tiny, but its cloverlike leaflets and yellow flowers are beautiful in salad. I don't bother with sheep sorrel, so much smaller than but similar to garden sorrel. That grows several feet tall, with big arrowheadlike leaves; the young ones are tender during all but the hottest part of summer. (In earliest spring, they don't yet have any flavor.) Less exciting to taste but pleasing to look at are fiddleheads, the famous wild edible of spring where I live. In Vermont, they must come from the ostrich fern, and you have to catch them early before they unfurl. The pepper and marked flavor of stinging nettle are commonly set off by cream in soup. The feathery leaves of wild carrot, or Queen Anne's Lace, are always quite bitter. (And the root is wholly unimproved—hard, narrow, fibrous, and bitter. It seems a miracle that it could be related to a garden carrot.)

Purslane becomes a rampant garden weed if you let it go so as to have more to pick. (It spreads and then it sows itself and next year appears everywhere.) It makes an excellent high-summer salad, the succulent leaves providing a crunch and a refreshing slippery juice. Purslane of a slightly different variety is the dominant ingredient of the Turkish salad *yoğurtlu semizotu salatası:* snap the purslane leaves, taking as little stalk as you can; for dressing, mix full-fat yogurt with translucent slices of garlic, olive oil, salt, black pepper, and lemon juice; optionally, add finely cubed or shredded cucumber. Purslane turns tender with cooking and makes a good contribution to a mix of cooked greens.

Perhaps mistakenly, I ignore mustard and collards. In my garden, mustard quickly grows very hot, distracting in salads; I've liked cooked mustard and collard greens in the hands of other cooks, but they're not what I grew up with. My favorite cultivated trio for cooking is spinach, chard, and the tenderest beet greens. First in the pot, usually, goes finely chopped garlic, cooked gently to translucence in olive oil; then the greens go in with just the moisture clinging after they've been washed. Greens also appear in *caillettes,* from the South of France, one of the homiest and best forms of charcuterie. They originated with the pig killings of fall or winter, when some of the meat and perishable innards were combined with the wild and cultivated greens of that cold season—today typically spinach or chard or both. The well-seasoned meat-vegetable mixture is formed into balls, wrapped in caul fat, baked, and served, usually cold, as a first course.

Even cultivated rocket has an appealing skunkiness unless it's very young, raised in a hothouse, or grown in very fertile, moist soil. The sulfurousness is mainly in the raw leaf, which at the same time is peppery and sweet. Strong rocket is best in mixtures of greens, including cooked, or put into a salad with sliced ripe tomato to spread out the taste.

When you cook greens, especially with a little cured pork, the pot liquor is excellent. I eat it with grilled bread. If you don't cook the leaves in a soupy amount of liquid, then cooking them with fat, or afterward promptly coating them with it, keeps them from drying if they aren't served quickly. Greens tend to retain strong character compared with most other garden plants.

HOW TO BUY AND STORE GREENS: The beautiful qualities of fresh-picked leaves quickly disappear. Use them as soon as you can after you gather or buy them. Meanwhile, wrap them in a damp towel and keep them cold. Leaves are especially vulnerable to drying out and picking up off-flavors in a refrigerator, but it's probably the best choice.

COMPLEMENTS TO STRONG GREENS: Prime complements are salt and fat— butter, olive oil, nut oils, duck or goose fat, lard (keep animal fats from congealing by serving hot greens in a hot bowl or plate). Cooked greens also like garlic, onions, hot pepper, and cured pork. They like thyme, oregano, savory, and sage, though more than a touch hides the flavor of the greens. Black pepper is excellent. Cooked or in salad, they go well with roast pork, goose, and ham. And either cooked or in salad, they go with eggs cooked in the shell, from soft to hard. Cooked greens go in stuffing mixtures for pasta along with Parmigiano and ricotta or other fresh cheese. Balsamic vinegar points up a dish of cooked greens.

NOTES ON WINE: The astringency, as opposed to bitterness, of some greens "dries out" the appealing fruit flavors of a wine, but a refreshing minor white wine goes with a mess of greens in their liquor on garlic-rubbed, olive oil–coated toast.

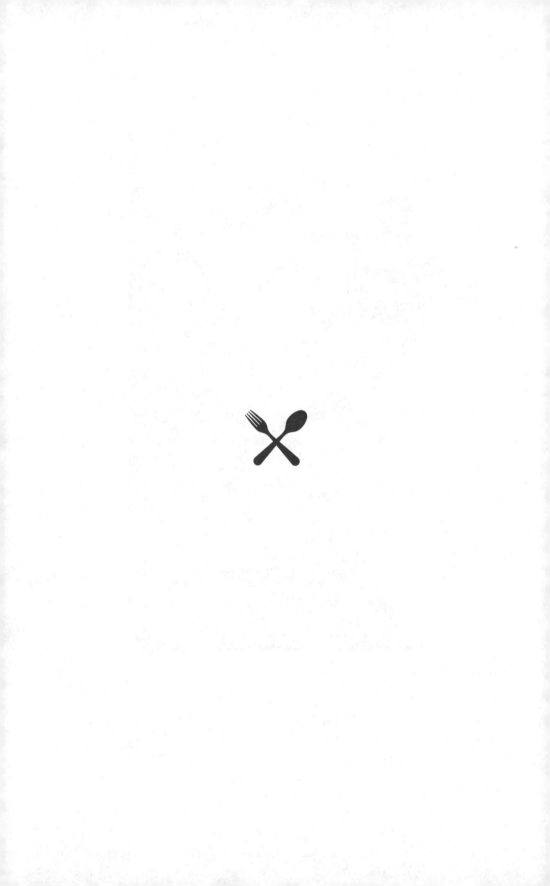

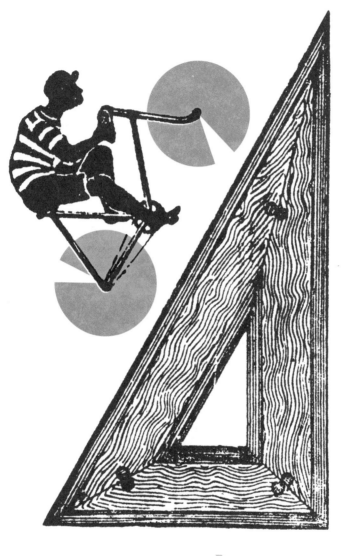

GRUYÈRE

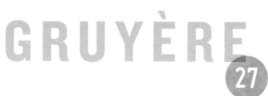

27

Gruyère is a mountain cheese—nutty, buttery, and *big*. In Switzerland, its land of origin, the average wheel weighs 77 pounds (35 kilos). In France, the average wheel of Gruyère de Comté weighs almost 90 pounds (40 kilos). Swiss marketers distinguish their cheese as "Le Gruyère," and Gruyère de Comté is always called just Comté. Both kinds are made in the Jura Mountains, which run mostly through Switzerland. The terrain, the cold climate, the poor mountain soils lying over limestone, granite, or the mixed stones of lower elevations, produce good forage for cattle. Comté is made in the old province of Franche-Comté, and Swiss Gruyère comes from five cantons. Each cheese has its Appellation d'Origine Protégée, or AOP, from the European Union. In addition, 15 percent of all French cheese is much-lesser plain "Gruyère" (which France honors with an Appellation d'Origine Contrôlée but the EU grants merely an IGP, or Indication Géographique Protégée, rather than a more prestigious AOP). Gruyère of whatever kind is related to but not the same as the holey "Swiss" cheese, called Emmentaler, or Emmental when made in France, which, as a rule, is much less interesting in taste. Swiss Gruyère and Comté today have no more than a few scattered, pea-sized holes, but they used to have eyes more like those of Emmentaler. (Holes up to the size of a cherry are permitted in Comté, and at least until recently it was possible to find a few wheels still made that way for those who like the old style. When the cheeses commonly had holes, they were aged at warmer temperatures conducive to bacteria that produced gas that inflated the eyes.) The cheeses were originally made big because it wasn't possible to get them frequently from the mountains to market, especially in winter. The milk of various nearby farms, all very small, was combined to make a single, relatively dry, hard cheese that would age well over long periods without drying too much and could be shipped over long distances. The result, at its best, is one of the world's great cheeses. In one wheel or another, depending on countless influences but mainly age, provenance, and the cheesemaker, you might find flavors of grass, hay, celery, cauliflower, mushroom, yogurt, melted butter, apricot, honey, citrus, nuts, meat stock, leather, pepper, sautéed or burnt onion, coffee, dark chocolate, or smoke.

Gruyère makes superb eating as is, and it's *the* cheese for cooking, with its adaptable flavor and wide availability. It goes into omelettes, soufflés, fondues, *gougères* (cheese puffs), and is excellent for browning on top of a gratin. (A sauce with enough cheese melted in it to have real flavor tends to become gluey, so the cheese is better put on top of a gratin. Anyway, classic *sauce Mornay* is so completely out of fashion that I can't remember when if ever I've had a properly yolk-bound cheesy one.) Younger Gruyère, say around six months old, melts better, and good young wheels can offer some depth of flavor. And because the younger cheese is less concentrated, you can eat more of it, making it the center of a simple lunch or supper, as the farmers do who produce the milk. Outside the producing countries, however, good young Gruyère can be hard to find—the best US shops specialize in aged wheels. In France, *vieux* Comté, from selected wheels twenty-four months old or more, is especially prized: stronger, nuttier, toastier, more caramel. Gruyère in Switzerland matures faster, and there a chef or shop might seek out exceptional fifteen- to twenty-four-month-old cheese.

Gruyère takes its name from the Swiss town of Gruyères (spelled with an *s*), historically a market town for cheese and cattle; it lies at the meeting of the plain and the mountains. The earliest reference to the cheese by name—or more precisely to a cheese made *"à la mode de gruière"*—occurs in Nicolas de Bonnefons' 1655 cookbook, *Les Délices de la Campagne.* But the cheese often cited as the ancestor of all big mountain cheeses is Sbrinz, from central Switzerland, whose descendants are said to extend even to the great Italian Parmigiano-Reggiano.

Cheese has the best flavor when the cows eat living plants and hay rather than grain or silage, which gives off-flavors and creates other problems. Silage is forbidden for any Gruyère. Ideally, the cows eat only what is raised on each farm, the grasses and varied plants of the locality growing in permanent hay fields and pastures; they give characteristic aromas to the cheeses. The best Swiss wheels are normally Gruyère *d'alpage,* meaning "from high mountain pastures." The Comité Interprofessionel du Gruyère de Comté, the association that manages the French appellation, made a scientific study of one section of the territory and found thirty-one plants contributing aroma to the cheese, first of all the commonplace dandelion, then garden burnet, caraway, lady's mantle, thyme, yarrow, mustard, and more.

Certain breeds of cattle are better adapted to certain regions, and cows that haven't been intensively selected for high yields tend to give more concentrated milk. For Comté, the milk comes from Montbéliarde cows. In Switzerland, the cows are typically the international Holstein, originally from the Netherlands, with a scattering of native Swiss breeds. The rules for producing milk and cheese, particularly for Comté, are detailed and ecology-minded, reflecting the tie between place and taste. Gruyère de Comté comes from thirty-five "industrial" plants but mainly from a system of about 135 *fruitières,* small cooperative cheese plants, often one per village, with no more than several employees. In Switzerland, 170 small dairy plants produce Gruyère.

The milk for Gruyère must be used within twenty-four hours and it must be raw. A very few Comté cheesemakers rely solely on wild flora, adding only the whey from the previous cheesemaking; in Switzerland, only whey and no other culture is permitted. Once the curd has set, it's cut into particles the size of a grain of wheat. Then comes the essential step that sets the big mountain cheeses apart: the curd is "cooked" in the whey to a temperature of just 125 degrees F (52 degrees C)—a little higher for the Swiss—which makes the tiny particles shrink and release more whey, so the curd is drier even before it's put in the wide molds and powerfully pressed. The heat also selects the flora that will ripen the cheese, destroying harmful ones and keeping those more tolerant to heat.

When the wheels of Comté are taken from the molds, salt is scattered by hand over the surface. Wheels of Swiss Gruyère are soaked in brine. The *affinage,* the aging, is generally a separate craft. The wheels, which rest on spruce planks, are periodically turned and rubbed with brine to form a hard crust and prevent molds from growing. The crust allows the cheese to breathe; very noticeably, the cellars are filled with the scent of ammonia. For almost all Comté, the dominant aging is cooler, an innovation of the 1980s by the late *affineur* Marcel Petite. Comté matures at just 45 to 48 degrees F (7 to 9 degrees C), which slows the evolution, reduces the risk of something going awry, and allows somewhat different flavors to develop, which Comté producers argue are more complex. Swiss Gruyère matures at a more traditional temperature of around 60 degrees F (16 degrees C).

The minimum age for Swiss Gruyère is five months, and for Comté four months. Most wheels of either one are sold at no more than eight or ten months. Age magnifies both strengths and defects. Each wheel has a different peak, when its good qualities are at their best and any defects aren't yet too apparent. Only a tiny portion of top wheels improve for more than a year. Old Gruyère is hardly the same cheese. After about twenty months, the flavors of *vieux* Comté are more animal (roast beef) and grilled onion. There's enough variation in taste that in France or Switzerland a good shop will stock wheels of two, three, or more ages.

Where a slice of young Gruyère is smooth and elastic, the aged cheese is hard and easily breaks. In the mouth, its texture ranges from floury to slightly granular and comes with a sensation from dry to fat, the creaminess or fattiness increasing over time. Some astringency can occur. There may be a suggestion of sweetness, and in mature Gruyère a small bitterness is acceptable. High quality, as usual, comes with a long aftertaste.

Besides Gruyère, some very good, big, mountain-type cheeses, mostly new ones, are made without an appellation, though the appellations remain the essential points of reference. Some of the other historic mountain cheeses made with cooked curd and pressed in wide shapes, like Gruyère, are:

APPENZELLER (NO APPELLATION, SWITZERLAND) This centuries-old cheese from northeastern Switzerland, rather than an appellation, has a registered trade name. The wheels, from partly skimmed raw milk, weigh just 13 to 18 pounds (6 to 8 kilos) and are regularly rubbed with *sulz,* a brine containing white wine, spices, and a wide selection of mountain herbs, each dairy plant having its own secret recipe. The wheels are aged for three to eight months. The taste is often tender and mild, recalling fresh milk, and at its best is very good.

BEAUFORT (AOP, FRANCE) From Savoie, in eastern France, Beaufort is one of the superb mountain cheeses. Raw whole milk from Tarine and Abondance cows is made into wide, flat wheels, weighing 15 to 22 pounds (7 to 10 kilos), with an orange surface and characteristic concave sides. (The equally fine, similar-looking Abondance, also from Savoie, is only half cooked and so not quite of the category.) Beaufort must be at least five months old. Ivory to pale yellow inside, it has a fresher, milkier taste than Gruyère.

L'ETIVAZ (AOC, SWITZERLAND) From the Vaudoise Alps, in southwestern Switzerland, L'Etivaz (the *z* isn't pronounced) is produced by almost seventy families who still practice transhumance, taking their cows to *alpage* at 1,000 to 2,000 meters, where each cheese is made by the farmer in the summer chalet. The milk is raw, the skimmed evening milk being combined with the whole morning milk, and only whey and rennet are added. The curd is cooked in copper cauldrons over a spruce fire, which gives the cheese a hint of smoke. The wheels, which weigh anywhere from 22 to 84 pounds (10 to 38 kilos), are aged for at least four and a half months, and each year up to a thousand wheels are selected to be aged in attics for at least thirty months. L'Etivaz shows no holes and has a deep yellowy-ivory color, with a texture ranging from tender to breakable, depending on age. Quality is variable and typically includes a peppery note.

SBRINZ (AOC, SWITZERLAND) Made in central Switzerland from raw skimmed milk in copper cauldrons, Sbrinz comes in very large, very hard wheels of 56 to 99 pounds (25 to 45 kilos), aged for a minimum of sixteen months. The yellow to golden-yellow surface covers an ivory to pale-yellow interior. Sbrinz is much closer to Parmigiano than to any of the other mountain cheeses, though quality isn't always top. The official description in the appellation rules calls for a "fruity, grilled chickory" flavor.

Summer cheeses are more yellow in color, and summer Comté is more fruity or flowery, more expressive, and often superior. Winter cheeses are paler and far more subtle, with more lactic, vegetal, nutty flavors, perhaps of coconut or cacao. But with Gruyère neither color nor season is firmly tied to better flavor. The least good summer cheeses are insipid or off-flavored, and the best winter ones are extremely good. Although the same considerations apply to the Swiss cheese, much less is made of the differences in age and season. And you can't make an equal side-by-side comparison of summer cheese with winter cheese; one will always be six months older than the other.

Some decades back, both Swiss and French Gruyère were more variable from wheel to wheel and overall more alike. Today Swiss Gruyère is cooked to a slightly higher temperature, and the wheels, rather than being sprinkled with dry salt, are soaked in brine long enough to become saltier. (Comté is one of the less salty cheeses.) Afterward the wheels of Swiss Gruyère are aged at warmer temperatures and mature more quickly, more at the pace of other great traditional cheeses. Typically, Swiss Gruyère has a somewhat more assertive character. Yet Comté, while more reserved, is just as complex. The best farm-made Swiss Gruyère is perhaps less controlled, with more often a thread of bitterness; the taste is more rustic, earthier.

HOW TO BUY AND KEEP GRUYÈRE: For cooking as well as eating, I've sometimes found good young Swiss Gruyère at a modest price, but the best, farm-made during the warm months of *alpage,* can be pricey, and the best Comté tends to come only from selected wheels. Gruyère of whatever kind isn't automatically special. For that, go to a shop that really knows Gruyère and, especially if you want aged cheese, one that has access to top wheels and cuts pieces to order. You'll certainly be offered a taste before you buy. Look first of all for an absence of defects and a long aftertaste, and then for positive qualities of flavor and texture. Younger Gruyère is the usual choice for cooking and easy melting, although an older cheese can be finely grated and mixed into a sauce or filling, and you can combine ages to gain complexity. For eating on its own, the age you prefer is a matter of taste.

Subtle differences occur in the milk and process from day to day. Each *fruitière* under its lead cheesemaker, mostly because of his or her technique and partly because of its farms and location, tends to produce cheeses with certain flavors and a certain level of quality. A few top dealers request Comté from specific *fruitières*. Some wheels of Gruyère acquire interior cracks, called *lainures*. They're generally considered a defect in a young cheese, but in an old one, while they don't add anything, they often coincide with superior flavor. As with other cheeses aged for long periods, small, crunchy crystals of transformed protein eventually form—a sure sign of age.

If possible, serve Gruyère on the day you buy it. With more mature Gruyère, within hours of its being cut and exposed to air, especially in a warm place, the flavors reach a peak and disperse. During the time before you serve it, keep Gruyère in its wrapper in a cool place (fat appearing like perspiration on the surface of a firm cheese is a sure sign of too much warmth). A cool cellar or pantry is ideal, but if you don't have a cool spot like that, refrigerate the cheese, remembering to take it out well before you eat it. Gruyère is most flavorful at about 60 to 65 degrees F (15 to 18 degrees C), which, according to the size of the piece, can take several hours to reach.

COMPLEMENTS TO GRUYÈRE: Bread is the most important, preferably sliced from a sourdough "country" loaf, either white or tan (the darker color coming from flour containing some bran). Fresh walnuts during their fall season go well with both young Gruyère and a fine aged one. (Some restaurants new serve cheese with a chaos of sweet competitors—preserves, honey, chutney. The last in particular, with its sugar, acidity, and complicated spice, buries much of the cheese flavor. The traditional cheese-with-sweet idea is less aggressive: Basque cherry preserves with firm Basque ewe's-milk cheese. And quince works with certain cheeses, a useful notion when there's no wine.) In cooking, Gruyère is complemented by eggs in an omelette and by—to offer a very specific example—cauliflower and medium to hard-cooked eggs in white sauce, with the cheese gratinéed on top.

NOTES ON WINE: Cheese begs for a refreshing drink. The old red-wine-with-cheese rule has been overturned, and nearly everyone agrees that most cheeses taste *much* better with white wine than with red. It's the tannin in red wines that makes them quarrel with cheese, and the cheese in turn diminishes or erases the fruit flavors in the wine. If you really want red wine, two cheeses that go better are Mimolette and old Gouda; a more mature red, whose tannin has joined the sediment in the bottom of the bottle, is easier with cheese. A middle-quality Pinot Noir, however, can find something in common with Gruyère. And with a younger Comté, try the Jura's red Trousseau and Poulsard. (As great as Switzerland's cheeses are, its wines aren't on the French level.) And creamier, not-too-strong Gruyère goes with Jura *crémant* (sparkling) wine. Better than any of these might be a *grand cru* Chablis. Good Champagne is the favorite choice of one top *affineur*.

With a well-aged Comté, the great cold-weather accompaniment is *vin jaune* made in the same region (in the appellations of Arbois, L'Étoile, Côtes du Jura, and the small, highly prestigious Château-Chalon). The wines' curious *rancio* flavors—rancid walnut, other nuttiness, caramel, curry—respond to more or less related flavors in the cheese. Beware that each wheel's set of flavors affects the wine and that only the finest aged Comté will speak to, rather than argue with, an old Château-Chalon. Not as special but less expensive are the similarly made but younger and less-exalted traditional Jura whites (from all the same appellations except Château-Chalon), which carry loud echoes of *vin jaune*. As to dishes, with a Gruyère soufflé, drink a Chardonnay such as Mâcon; with *gougères* (cheese puffs), drink a Chablis. With fondue, drink a traditional Jura *sous voile* white. (If a traditional cheese tends to go well with the traditional wine from the same place, that might be because they grew up together and shaped each other—the cheesemaker drank the wine, the winemaker ate the cheese.)

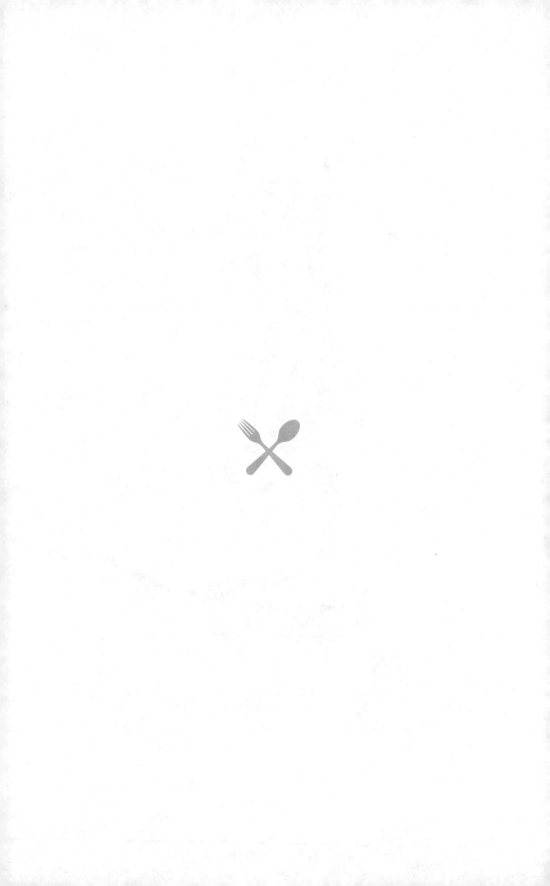

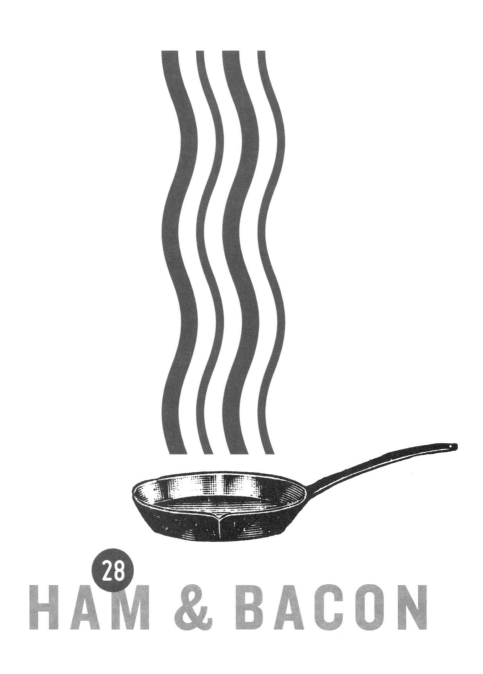

28
HAM & BACON

28. HAM AND BACON

A ham, as it ages, reveals the quality of fresh pork in the same way that a mature cheese reveals the quality of the original milk. A poor ham gets slowly worse, a middle-of-the-road one remains just that, and a good one gets better until, sometimes, it becomes great: sweet, clean, meaty, almost fruity, piquant, complicated. To tame the intensity and ensure tenderness, the pink-to-mahogany meat is sliced paper thin. In Italy, the white border of fat is treasured. It carries its own flavor and absorbs others, and where fat is mixed with lean, it softens the lean's intensity. A good ham takes about a year to become really interesting, and it may improve for months or another year after that, before it dries out and declines. A mere brined ham, as satisfying as it can be, never rises to the level of a dry-cured ham. Once, in almost every pig-raising place, curing hams was part of life on a farm. Pigs were killed in the cold of fall or early winter, which helped the meat to keep until the salt reached the bone and preserved it. Smoking, a further preservative, is often a more northern and mountain phenomenon, typical of German hams, for instance, and not Italian ones. Traditional dry-cured hams are aged through the seasons at rising and falling temperatures. Spain, with its powerful appreciation for ham, makes *pata negra* ("black hoof") hams from Ibérico pigs, including Serrano ("from the mountains") and the sought-after *jamón ibérico de bellota.* The last word means "acorn," referring to the food that fattens certain pigs in autumn. In Spanish shops you see rows of hams hanging from the ceiling hoof upward, often with a small metal cup attached to the lower end to catch the occasional drop of fat in warm weather. France has Bayonne and other dry-cured hams but not a widespread, deep-rooted appreciation. Italy does, with its *prosciutto di Parma, prosciutto di San Daniele* from Friuli, *prosciutto toscano,* and more. *Speck,* from the Tyrol, divided between Germany and Italy, is dry-cured, typically juniper-flavored, and smoked. And the pear-shaped *culatello di Zibello,* made not far from Parma, exploits the best, boneless part of the fresh ham, salted, then tied tight inside a pig's bladder and aged for an average of more than a year. By then, the *culatello* is covered with tan mold, the twine sags, and as much as any ham it looks primeval. Dry-cured hams don't require refrigeration; they're well preserved by salt.

In the United States, the tradition of dry-curing survives only in the South, where the outside of a ham is often covered with black pepper, sometimes hot red pepper (originally to protect against insects). The very best farm-cured Southern hams are at least as good as the great European hams. Years ago, when I would buy a Southern ham from time to time, I would always cook it, which was a lot of trouble. Then I realized the hams could be eaten raw like prosciutto, though for the proper translucent slices you almost need a slicing machine, but not quite—patience and a long, thin, very sharp knife accomplish a lot.

Commercial curers in the US South always used to buy mainstream pork, sometimes produced regionally, sometimes not. Recently, as the old local markets for country ham began to shrink a little, some producers sought a national market whose taste had been formed by Italian prosciutto. At the same time a few producers, for part or all of their production, began to seek conscientiously raised pigs, not least for the superior taste.

Everyday cooked brined hams from commodity pork, often very cheap, are made by injecting the meat with a weak brine that contains a lot of sugar. It adds water to the ham and makes a quick partial cure, but not enough to preserve the meat, which has to be refrigerated. That's not to dismiss all brined hams, which come from a long tradition. A little salt works wonders on pork, and in place of the effects of age, a brine can introduce herbs and spices. A good lightly brined German or French ham can be excellent. Since the meat is less salty, you can eat a lot more and make a meal of it.

Feed can also make a big difference to the taste. The once-famous Smithfield ham has long since lost its reputation. Under the original Virginia law of 1926, it was supposed to come "from the carcasses of peanut-fed hogs," which gleaned the fields after the harvest. With the efficiency of a machine harvest the practice ended, but those who've tasted hams from peanut-fed pigs say they had a much softer, yellower fat and a slightly different taste. When I've sampled hams from acorn-fed pigs, I've thought I detected a subtle nuttiness. In parts of the world where cows and pigs used to be raised on the same farm, the whey from cheesemaking went to the pigs. In Parma, the pigs were fattened on whey left from making Parmigiano cheese.

The breed affects the ham, though the way the pig is raised is more important (see "Pork") and not all the pigs of a breed are equal. The best-known breed for ham is Spain's *pata negra,* which is really a group of breeds. A US ham curer who has compared a few breeds finds that Berkshire ham has less nuttiness, more meatiness, and its fat leaves a buttery-creamy taste.

A ham, just to be clear, is made from the hind leg of the pig (hams are also made from wild boar, beef, deer, goat, duck, goose). The skin is left on, and all the surfaces are rubbed with salt, then sometimes buried in it, as if in a pile of snow. The centuries-old antioxidant saltpeter (potassium nitrate or nowadays sodium nitrate) helps to fix a brighter color, protects against botulism, reduces rancidity, and alters the ham's evolution so as to enhance the flavor. Often in the South the cure contains sugar. The fresh whole hams are packed in salt for fifteen days or more; once the time was commonly thirty and even fifty days. The salt draws out so much moisture that spoilage organisms can't survive. Preservation requires a minimum of 4 percent salt, but some hams run higher, often in the past much higher, making the meat impossibly dry, puckery with salt. Much more flavor develops in hams that lie near the minimum.

When hams are smoked, that's done at cool temperatures, so there's no chance of cooking them. The smoke, in the US typically from oak or hickory, has an antioxidant effect. Before the ham is hung up to age, the Italian technique is often to seal the part not covered by skin with a paste of fat and a little salt and flour.

Many hams are still exposed to natural temperatures and humidity, passing through the changes of the seasons. Some such exposure is required, for instance, under the rules for the *prosciutti* of San Daniele and Parma, which are aged in the hills, where air currents aid drying. Alternatively, artificial conditions aim at ideals that don't always occur in nature. (But do the indoor environments capture all the effects of climate in a particular place?) The inner fat and the thick outer cap keep the ham from drying too much as it ages. Enzymes act on the protein, breaking it down into highly flavorful forms. In a well-aged ham, white dots appear here and there in the meat, looking like grains of salt; really they are transformed protein, related to the same phenomenon in cheese. An array of aromas appears in a great ham. In a more rustic old-fashioned ham, made anywhere, a hint of rancidity is part of the appeal.

Most bacon, like most ham, is made quickly by pricking the fresh belly with needles and pumping it full of weak brine to make an instant cure, which isn't a cure at all, because the brine isn't salty enough. If the bacon isn't refrigerated, it rots. The taste is bland, and the brine usually contains phosphates, which prevent a stale taste and cause the meat to hold more water. That creates wet, floppy slices. For dry-cured bacon, the rind is traditionally left on, and the fresh belly is salted in the same way as a ham but for a much shorter time. The lean streaks are always the saltiest part, because salt won't dissolve in pure fat; it enters only the small amount of water held within the fat. As with ham, the saltiness of bacon shouldn't stand out so much as underline the piquant cured taste. After you taste meaty dry-cured bacon, the other kind just seems watery, hard to enjoy. In the South, you can still buy dry-cured bacon directly from some farmers, and a few commercial enterprises use hand techniques with excellent results.

Brined bacon, like brined ham, can be very good if it comes from a strong brine full of aromatic additions. I've had excellent brined bacon from a German butcher, though I'm not impressed by most small-scale US brined bacon. US bacon is smoked with various hardwoods, and some Southern smokehouses, rather than dry wood, use green, which gives a harsher, tarry, creosote flavor. A ham can tolerate strong smoke like that, since its surface is trimmed and discarded, but smoke from green wood easily overwhelms bacon.

For a few weeks after smoking, the flavor of dry-cured bacon settles and improves, but after that the bacon dries and loses flavor, and the surface fat, exposed to air, gradually turns rancid. Vacuum-sealing in plastic prevents drying and rancidity, but it's better to eat bacon within a few weeks and meanwhile keep it wrapped in paper, which allows it to breathe. If you fry old-fashioned dry-cured bacon with the rind on, then on the hot slice the rind forms a crisp, pleasantly chewy, gelatinous edge.

Bacon, broadly, embraces at least three forms: *pancetta, guanciale,* and *lardo,* to use the Italian words meaning "belly," "jowl," and "fatback." The first, in Italy, is usually unsmoked, cured with aromatic components, and rolled tight, so the slices reveal a spiral. The second, jowl, is the slightly lean-streaked, fatty cheek—more fatty than belly bacon but cured like it. And it tastes nearly the same, except the cheeks have a firmer fat that melts more pleasantly in the mouth. (Charcutiers prefer fresh jowl fat for a pâté or terrine, because it doesn't melt as readily and there's less danger of ending up with a little meat loaf swimming in fat.) The jowl, being more exercised than the belly, is sometimes said to be more flavorful, though I don't taste a clear difference.

"Salt pork" in the US once meant any cut of cured pork from the barrel, and then was applied mostly to fatback, used mainly as a flavoring in cooking. But as the US pork industry abandoned the old lard hogs and focused on leaner pork, fatback disappeared from the mainstream. Packages of salt pork in the supermarket are brined, *un*smoked pork belly. Now the old breeds are coming back on a small scale, but in the US cured fatback remains scarce.

The world's most famous fatback is *lardo di Colonnata,* from the marble-quarrying village of that name high above the Italian town of Carrara. *Lardo* doesn't mean rendered pork fat (that's *strutto*). Rather, the slabs of this fatback are cured in sea salt and a small multitude of herbs and spices, which must always include ground black pepper, rosemary, and coarsely chopped garlic. The *lardo* is layered with these in a marble coffer. A brine forms that excludes air, and the *lardo* matures for at least six months. Unlike dry-cured bacon, the *lardo* becomes more tender and the flavor improves. The taste is clean and fresh. Usually, the *lardo* is streaked with lean. But pure white *lardo,* trimmed of its rind and served in restaurants in paper-thin slices as part of an antipasto plate, melts on your tongue.

Lardo is wonderful as eaten around Carrara: thin slices on bread with tomato, onion, oregano, and black pepper.

Lardons—little sticks cut crosswise from thick belly slices, usually brined but sometimes fresh (never smoked)—are sautéed and combined with sautéed button mushrooms and cooked tiny onions to make the classic Burgundian garnish, especially for braised meats. It's an underappreciated, old-fashioned touch, and the *lardons* provide most of the taste. Before they're sautéed, they're first simmered in water to reduce the salt they'll add and to render the more easily melted (less-saturated) fat so it doesn't melt later and sit greasily on the surface of the dish.

You can roll thin slices of brined ham around one or two cooked leeks or a cooked endive, and cover them with béchamel and breadcrumbs to make a gratin. Cooked brined ham makes the well-sauced, closely related Burgundian pair *jambon à la crème* (which has more cream) and *jambon au chablis* (which has more wine). One of the best things made with brined ham, yet again from Burgundy, is *jambon persillé,* a charcuterie specialty in which chunks of ham are packed in a richly flavored gelatin made from pig's feet and filled with fresh parsley. Mild brined hams lend themselves to sauces with mustard or Madeira and to fruit accompaniments, including familiar apples and pineapple.

Great dry-cured ham is best appreciated when eaten by itself. But a slice of ham or bacon is enormously useful flavoring—the bouillon cube of old-style home cooking. And as many people have said, the best part of a great ham may be the bone that is finally left and gives up its flavor to soup.

HOW TO BUY AND STORE HAM AND BACON: In a store that sells raw ham in slices, ask for a taste. If you have the option, choose a ham that isn't boned and ham or bacon that has never been in plastic. If you know a reliable producer, look for the name (the US hams I've bought in recent years have come from Gatton Farms and Benton's Smoky Mountain). If you buy a whole ham, take courage and, in the area where you'll start to carve, pare away the surface with a strong blade. I make the actual slices with a narrow twelve-inch slicing knife, which allows longer strokes and smoother slices with fewer saw marks. Once you've begun to cut into the ham, unless you take more slices every day or two, the exposed moist meat may mold. If that's a danger, it makes sense to wrap and refrigerate a ham, though I've never done that. I do often drape the ham with plastic to hold in moisture.

Traditional dry-cured bacon comes with the rind on, which slows drying. A very little Southern country bacon is cured with the ribs in place, and if you have a sharp boning knife, you can order that as opposed to a "clear side." The ribs further slow drying, and there's good meat between them. As soon as bacon is sliced, it begins to lose flavor, so buy slab bacon and slice it yourself. I cut it, for straight, even slices, with a ten- or twelve-inch chef's knife, whose heft is useful for getting through the rind and any dry edges. Store dry-cured bacon in the paper it comes in. At room temperature, especially in warm weather, mold can appear. For that reason, I often refrigerate bacon, and to reduce drying I add an outer layer of plastic. Dry-cured bacon remains tender and holds its best flavor for only a few weeks.

COMPLEMENTS TO HAM AND BACON: Thin slices of dry-cured ham go of course with melon and fresh figs. Italians often eat slices of prosciutto wrapped around crisp *grissini* (breadsticks), but really good fresh white bread, even though it doesn't have the same crunch, tastes better, and dry-cured ham is impeccable with sourdough whole wheat and good dark rye. Ham likes other starches, too, that normalize its salt: potatoes, rice, beans. Salt pork, or nowadays often smoked bacon, is key to New England baked beans (the more traditional ones have little or no sweetening). Both dry-cured and mild brined ham go with parsley, celery, chestnuts, lentils, lima beans, mushrooms and Madeira (or Bourbon) in cream, Gruyère cheese (used to top a gratin), and Dijon mustard (excellent diluted with nothing more than heavy cream to make a sauce). Mild brined ham goes with leeks, cream, mushrooms, tomatoes, and sweet potatoes; it goes especially well with cooked greens and a little garlic or onion, maybe some hot pepper. Brined ham goes with cooked fruit: apples, peaches, apricots, and pineapple, that icon of mid-twentieth-century ham cookery (it's so familiar that I have a hard time knowing whether or not it's actually good). *Lardons,* from smoked or unsmoked bacon, are delicious in strong-flavored salads of spinach or frilly escarole (with a poached egg), and certainly they're prime with onions and mushrooms in the classic garnish.

NOTES ON WINE: The salt and fat of ham and bacon call for a light wine, optionally with a touch of sweetness, a wine you can drink a lot of—white, pink, or very light red. High alcohol isn't refreshing, and the tannin of most red wine exacerbates saltiness. Drink the same wines that go with other charcuterie, such as Edelzwicker or Sylvaner from Alsace, Vouvray or other Chenin from the Loire Valley, Riesling from diverse places, white or red Beaujolais, Lambrusco, or light "New Wave" California wines, and many more. A more serious combination with dry-cured ham is dry Fino or Manzanilla sherry. Turning to brined ham, with *jambon persillé* drink Beaujolais, with *jambon au chablis* drink *premier cru* Chablis. A ripe white Sancerre can work with ham dishes. And a cooked brined ham, prepared for instance in a Madeira cream sauce with mushrooms, can make a light red such as a lesser Burgundy, a red Sancerre, or a Jura or Alsace Pinot Noir seem better than it is.

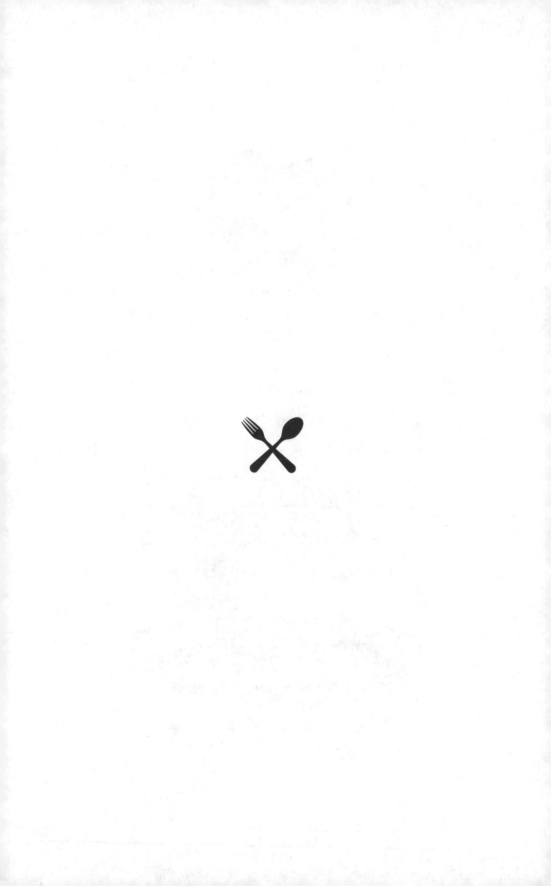

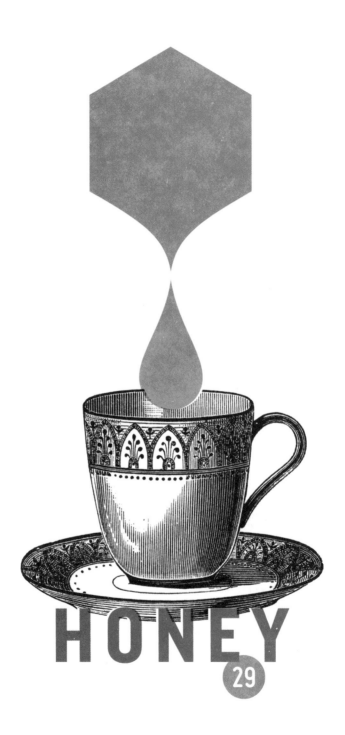

HONEY

29

29. HONEY

Honey, an older sweetening than cane sugar, has one of the most varied, delicious tastes of all foods, and it's possibly the food most obviously and directly linked to the place it comes from, sometimes to a short period of days and the particular plants then in flower. The "bee pasture," as beekeepers call it, extends for a mile to a mile and a half from the hives, farther only when nectar is scarce. The honey flows take place in fits and starts. In temperate climates, they occur mostly during a few weeks of spring and early summer and again in smaller quantities in fall. Clover, widely planted in fields, makes honey that's so familiar in taste it seems generic. Most beekeepers blend some or all of their honey together, giving it no more specific label than "wildflower," "spring," or "fall." But nearly all the very best honey comes mainly from a single kind of flower.

The bees of a colony tend to stick to one kind of nectar until it's exhausted, whether or not another excellent source appears nearby. It takes time and trouble for the beekeeper, but by observing bees and flowers, he or she can put empty wooden frames of honeycomb into the hives at the beginning of a flow from a particular plant and remove full ones at the end, before the bees start to work the next flower. That way the honey comes predominately from one species. Around the world, possibly a few hundred such single-flower honeys are made.

According to the source of nectar, liquid honey ranges from colorless through shades of amber to reddish-brown to near black, with a few greenish or bluish exceptions. Darker honeys, such as thyme, contain more minerals and traces of other components—generally, the darker the honey, the stronger the taste. But color and strength say nothing about how good a honey is. An underlying part of the flavor comes from the particular combination of sugars, often roughly equal amounts of glucose and fructose with some maltose, a few percent of sucrose, and tiny amounts of others. Offsetting the intense sweetness is a pleasing tartness from gluconic and other acids, which also help to preserve the honey. But the main flavor falls into the category of flowers, fruit, caramel, or all three, and with them many other sorts of flavors appear, sometimes strong ones. Most of the flavors responsible for the distinctive, often complicated character of each different honey come from the very minor constituents, reflections of a particular nectar. Some kinds of honey are very delicate (raspberry, acacia), some powerful (rosemary, lavender, lime tree), and some aggressive (chestnut, buckwheat). I like almost all kinds of honey, though I tend to be drawn to dark, even odd, ones.

The flavor of honey also reflects the weather. A single-flower honey may be more or less pure and intense as some flower either suffered or bloomed in unexpected profusion with a superior perfume. From year to year, the differences can be striking.

Nectar is mostly water and becomes honey mainly through evaporation. The bees accomplish that in the hive partly by fanning with their wings. Within days, the moisture declines usually to around 18 percent, though the honey for sale may be higher or lower in moisture than that, which can make a big difference in its consistency and ability to keep. But the result of the bees' work is considerably more complex than mere concentration, as the nectar passes in and out of the bees' bodies before it's deposited in the hexagonal cells of the comb. When those are full, the bees cap them with wax. Honey doesn't spoil as a rule, because it contains too little water for anything to live in it, but when it contains enough water, yeasts will ferment it—adding water is the first step in making mead.

In recent years, using bees to pollinate crops has become more profitable in the US, and some bees have been bred for their ability to pollinate rather than make honey. Large-scale beekeepers, who maintain thousands of hives and make arrangements with farmers, transport their hives on tractor-trailers, sometimes across the country, as different crops come into flower. Betweentimes, the bees may be fed sugar syrup, which used to be given only as emergency food if hives ran out of food at the end of winter. The hard treatment and exposure to toxic agricultural chemicals are responsible for Colony Collapse Disorder, in which up to 90 percent of a beekeeper's colonies die over the winter. So many variables are under suspicion that the cause may never be fully understood. Few if any conscientious beekeepers who operate locally on a small scale have had the problem. It's far better, for you and the bees, to buy honey from these beekeepers, who don't respond to pest and disease problems with chemicals and drugs. Their primary product is honey.

A good beekeeper takes only surplus honey, beyond what the bees need to survive the winter. He or she slices off the wax caps with a hot knife and puts the frames of comb in a centrifugal extractor. As it spins, a tiny stream of honey is hurled from each cell. A few beekeepers do nothing further; they don't even strain out the occasional bee parts, bits of wax, and other harmless particles. Once the honey is in jars, most of these float to the top while the rest settle to the bottom, so you can avoid them easily enough. Such unmanipulated honey has more flavor, and as a further sign of how natural it is, within a few months most kinds crystallize.

Honey is a supersaturated sugar solution, and when it contains more glucose than can remain dissolved in its small amount of water, the glucose forms crystals. Certain honeys, especially tree honeys, crystallize very slowly, and a few when pure contain a lower proportion of glucose and never crystallize at all. Those include acacia, tupelo, and thyme. Among the honeys that crystallize, some form coarse crystals and some have a more pleasing fine, soft texture, depending on the sugars in them and the speed of crystallization. Faster is finer. Beekeepers can ensure a smooth, fine, soft, and easily spreadable texture by stirring a little already finely crystallized honey into the liquid honey, which causes it to turn quickly. The consistency of this "creamed honey" is appealing, but I prefer a wholly unmanipulated texture, whether liquid, crystallized, or in between.

Big North American packers flash-heat their honey to very high temperatures and immediately cool it somewhat to reduce damage to flavor and color, but it's still hot and runny enough to pass through a superfine filter. The aim is to melt every tiny crystal and then remove every other minute particle, whether pollen, tiny air bubble, or anything else that could provide a seed for future crystal growth. The resulting honey remains liquid almost no matter how long the jar waits on a store shelf. But the heat deprives honey of some of its best flavors, leaving a flatter, simpler taste.

The most flavorful honey is not only unheated and unfiltered but still in the cells of the comb, sealed by wax, never exposed to air, never touched. "Comb honey is real honey, before man decides to spoil it," an old Vermont beekeeper once said to me. "Every time you do something to honey you change it a little." There isn't a lot of comb honey for sale, because it requires the beekeeper to go to extra trouble and because the honeycomb itself is fragile, easily damaged. The bees, too, have to work harder, making new wax and building new comb to replace what's taken. Yet comb honey has the finest flavor—fresher, cleaner, more distinct, *honier*. With honey, as with so many foods, what is treated least is usually best, though the simple approach often requires more knowledge and discrimination from the producer and the customer.

A few of the many fascinating honeys are:

ACACIA Despite its name, acacia honey comes from the false acacia tree (*Robinia pseudoacacia*), known in North America as black locust. It's hard to find a US example that's pure enough to show the characteristic flavor, but France and Italy produce a lot of good acacia honey. Typically, it's a pale straw yellow and remains liquid for a very long time, never crystallizing completely. Because acacia honey is low in acidity, it seems particularly sweet. The flavor, unusually refined and sometimes lost in combination with other foods, is gently floral, with hints of vanilla and something of new beeswax.

CHESTNUT The European chestnut (*Castanea sativa*) makes one of the most common European single-flower honeys, a medium to dark reddish-amber liquid. It crystallizes on its own, but often the nectar is mixed in the comb with honeydew (see next page) from the same tree, and then the honey crystallizes only partly or not at all. Chestnut honey from nectar is lighter in color, thinner, stronger and more bitter in taste, the bitterness masking any floral component. The powerful, complex flavors include burnt sugar, malt, coffee, boiled chickpeas, and overripe apple, which come with a light astringency and a long aftertaste. Many people don't like chestnut honey, but when it isn't too bitter, to me it's one of the best kinds.

HEATHER Various heather species give honey, all of it dark, often with reddish glints, all quickly crystallizing and strong-flavored. Italian heather honey comes mostly from tree heath (*Erica arborea*), which despite its name is often no bigger than a shrub. The liquid honey rapidly forms a soft mass of fine crystals. It tastes of caramel, or caramel with cream, with something of burnt wood and perhaps licorice. The darkest and most prized heather honey, which comes mainly from Scotland, derives from ling heather (*Calluna vulgaris*), also called true heather. Curiously, this honey sets in the comb as jelly. And it's often sold in the comb because, to extract it, each cell must first be stirred (done as a group with a mass of pins) or the honey must be pressed out of the comb. It gels again in the jar, and an unmixed example may never crystallize. The somewhat intense flavor is of caramel, cocoa, and leather. Ling heather honey is less acidic than some kinds and slightly bitter.

HONEYDEW Although bees make it, this strong, dark to very dark European honey comes not from nectar but, strangely, from what is called honeydew: tree sap gathered by insects, especially aphids. Bees prefer nectar, so honeydew honey is rarely anything like pure. It comes especially from European spruce (*Picea abies*), silver fir (*Abies alba*), and holm oak (*Quercus ilex*). The taste isn't far from that of chestnut honey, and the two are often mixed; I like it, but not everyone does. The rarer oak version has complex flavors of caramel, dried fruit, something spicy or licorice, coupled in my experience with a marked bitterness. The more common spruce and fir honeydew honeys are less bitter and more like malt, maple syrup, and condensed milk.

LAVENDER A specialty of Provence, where large amounts of lavender are raised for the perfume industry, lavender honey may come either from true lavender (*Lavandula officinalis*), which also grows wild, or from the hybrid lavandin (*L. officinalis* × *L. latifolia*), which is much more widely planted because it yields more essential oil. The pale liquid honey rapidly forms medium-fine crystals that look nearly white. Its flavor, like that of rosemary honey, recalls the leaves of the herb without having their herbal-resinous quality; the taste is intense, floral, full of ripe fruit.

LEMON One of the most special of all honeys is lemon (*Citrus limonum*), which was the universal favorite of everyone who happened by my house a few years ago when I amassed more than forty honeys for tasting. Lemon is usually heavily mixed with other citrus, but this was a distinctive example from near Salerno, in southern Italy. It was crystallized, very pale yellow, and it made any orange honey seem crude by comparison. The flavor was precisely that of a lemon blossom; the honey was the most elegant I've ever tasted.

LIME TREE Despite its name and flavor, lime-tree honey doesn't come from citrus at all but from the European tree more often called, in other contexts, linden (*Tilia platyphylla* and related species). Its dried leaves and flowers make a popular herbal tea whose flavor is similar to that of the honey. The liquid honey is very pale, sometimes with greenish lights; it's slow to granulate, when it becomes white to cream-colored with coarse crystals. The taste is strongly of lime, almost minty, fresh, somewhat intense, and with long aftertaste. (In North America, a parallel but rare honey comes from *T. americana,* or basswood; I've come across only one example.)

THYME The strongest, purest thyme honey (*Thymus* spp.) comes from Greece, where it's both common and highly valued. Some of the darkest, thickest, and very best (if it hasn't been adulterated) comes from the island of Kythera. Thyme honey was once my favorite of all kinds; now I find it impossible to decide. Even thyme honey from pastures in western Massachusetts and the Catskill Mountains of New York, where thyme is heavily mixed with milder nectars from other plants, has a distinctive reddish-brown color and strong characteristic taste. It takes a very long time to crystallize. The taste, not at all like the leaves of the herb, is pleasantly reminiscent of an old-fashioned herbal medicine, such as sassafras or horehound.

TUPELO The white tupelo (*Nyssa ogeche*), a small, crooked, deliquescent tree, is confined almost entirely to swamps and edges of rivers in an area of northern Florida and adjacent Georgia. But the tiny greenish-yellow blossoms yield large amounts of nectar for a famous Southern honey. The color is pale amber with, when held to the light, a subtle green cast. Unmixed tupelo will never crystallize. It tastes smooth, sweet, light, and has a subtle character that is sometimes called anise or herbal and to me is more like menthol. I've sometimes tasted in the honey a hint of the cinnamon candy Red Hots (which might be an impurity from another flower).

HOW TO BUY HONEY: Most kinds of honey, whether blends or dominated by a single flower, are extremely good as long as the honey has been minimally treated: not significantly heated, severely filtered, or otherwise altered. "Raw" honey has more flavor, assuming the word has meaning. A faint haze in liquid honey shows that it hasn't suffered from harmful filtration. With most kinds of honey, though, crystallization is normal and strongly suggests they haven't been mistreated. If you buy honey directly from a small-scale beekeeper, there's a greater chance it will be as fresh and good as it should be. If possible, taste before buying. Beyond those considerations, single-flower honey is often better and provides the most direct link to a place. Comb honey isn't practical for most purposes, but it has the most flavor. It comes in the form of "chunk comb" surrounded by liquid honey in jars or, better, as "cut comb," sold either in small plastic boxes or in special small square or round sections filled directly by the bees in the hive and untouched. New comb honey has the best flavor of all.

HOW TO STORE HONEY AND SUBSTITUTE IT FOR SUGAR: I leave honey at the ambient temperature of my kitchen shelves, which often changes. Most liquid honeys crystallize fastest at an average of 57 degrees F (14 degrees C), however. To discourage that, it's best to store honey below 50 degrees (10 degrees C); the crystals will form much more slowly and be finer. You can always liquefy honey by gently heating the jar in a pan of water, which will do little harm. Honey gradually loses flavor, but normally it never spoils, and you can keep and use it for years. Very occasionally, though, after a jar is opened, the honey acquires the smell and taste of a sour dishtowel; I've never confirmed the explanation, but I believe it occurs sometimes when liquid honey contains enough excess water for bacteria to work. Comb honey is protected inside its natural package, yet the wax is somewhat permeable, and the honey inside remains at peak for no more than a few months. With honey in a jar, for best flavor, use it within a year of its making.

Honey can replace sugar in a recipe, though the water, sweetness, acidity, and flavor in honey vary so much that any rule is imperfect. One formula is to use 25 percent more honey than sugar by weight and reduce the liquid in the recipe by three to four tablespoons per cup of honey. Heat drives off fine aromas, so don't use special honey in cooking.

COMPLEMENTS TO HONEY: The complements to honey depend on the particular honey, but very fresh cheeses and yogurt tend to go well with most kinds of honey. (Greek thyme honey wonderfully matches ewe's-milk yogurt.) Hard aged cheeses, such as Gruyère and various ewe's-milk cheeses, are better with light-flavored honeys; to cite a specific pair, Parmigiano goes admirably with acacia honey. These combinations work, but I confess I enjoy an aged cheese more on its own or with a glass of wine. Lemon and cream, separately or together, go naturally with honey. Raw and cooked fruits, such as peaches and apricots, go with light-flavored honey, and grapefruit goes with almost any sort of honey. If the fruit is cooked, it's better to keep all the honey's freshness and flavor by adding it raw afterward, such as to rhubarb (if you allow that it's a fruit). Very strong, dark honey, such as buckwheat, goes well in spice cakes, such as gingerbread and French *pain d'épices,* and in dried-fruit-and-nut cakes, such as Italian *panforte.* Nuts in general complement honey: ground hazelnuts in cake, whole almonds in nougat (*turrón, torrone*), pistachios or walnuts in baklava, sesame seeds in halvah. Both toast and fresh bread, with or without butter, are ideal complements to honey.

NOTES ON WINE: Straight honey is too sweet for even the sweetest wine, and the flavors of strong honey compete with those of the wine. But when honey is a mere component of other things (a cake, a tart), it can be flattered by a sweet Muscat, Gewürztraminer, or other floral wine whose flavors are related to but different from those of the honey.

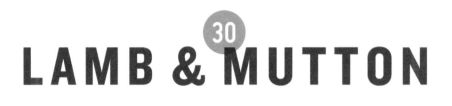

LAMB & MUTTON

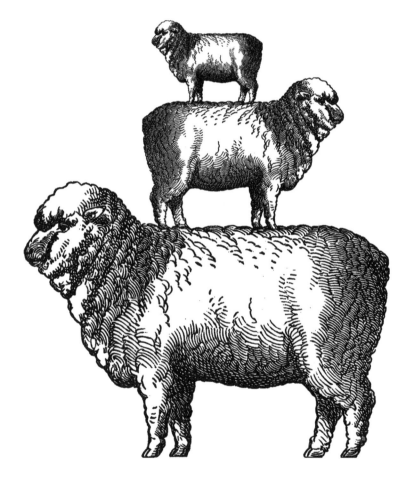

30. LAMB AND MUTTON

Lamb is a primordial meat of spring, though now available year-round, and good lamb is tied to pasture. Sheep are highly efficient grazers that thrive outdoors. Lambs belong with their mothers, nourished by their milk. After only a couple of days, lambs begin to nibble at grass. If they're allowed to remain with their mothers, they consume mostly milk, until the balance is tipped at anywhere from six to twelve weeks, shifting wholly to grass at anywhere from eight weeks to eight months. Even in winter, sheep, including lambs, need only hay, with perhaps an option for shelter and a little corn in the coldest weather. Lambs can be fattened entirely on pasture without grain (there's less work for both people and machines) if they have steady new growth. On an increasing number of small farms, they're rotated every day or few days through a series of carefully managed paddocks. The best pasture and hay contain as much protein as grain. A farmer once commented to me that in April and May, when the weather is warming and plants are growing fastest, his lambs are "so fat it's amazing; they're ready in a month. Those are the best to me."

Suckling lamb, about four to six weeks old, is very pale, tan, gradually becoming tinged with pink. It's tender, and some people enjoy it very much, but like kid of the same age, it doesn't have much character. (To add depth, a shoulder of *abbacchio,* as suckling lamb is called in Rome, is sometimes cooked with lard, sage, and rosemary and served with anchovy sauce.) For flavor, it's cooked to at least medium. As lambs get older, their meat becomes more pink and the flavor is more interesting. Eventually it turns red. For simplicity's sake, lamb is usually defined as being less than a year old. After that, it's mutton. Typical US-raised lamb is six to eleven months old. But the best lamb taste might lie somewhere between three and six months. And for the best combination of flavor, juice, and tenderness, that meat is cooked rare to medium rare.

Older lamb is often said to taste "muttony"—strong, even pungent, especially the fat, which makes many Americans avoid lamb altogether. Sometimes the grass diet is blamed. Like beef, much lamb is finished on grain, which produces more and harder fat, both outer fat and marbling. The fat comes from the carbohydrates in the grain. The marbled red meat with more saturated fat is often older and has a stronger, meatier taste. Feeding the animals corn increases fat, but other things being equal, it makes a more neutral taste. For the farmer, feeding them grain allows much more control: you know just how much protein the animals are getting.

There are more breeds of sheep than of any other livestock, though cattle come close. For better-tasting lamb, the meat should come from a breed or cross that does well on grass, rather than a special fast-growing cross. Farmers and chefs don't talk about particular breeds that give better lamb the way they do with pork and beef. But for milder-flavored lamb, it's essential that the meat come from one of the mutton breeds, as they're still often called, rather than a wool breed. The sheep valued for wool have much stronger-flavored meat, associated with the wool's lanolin, the waxy material that helps sheep shed water. US meat breeds are generally British in origin, such as Cheviot, Dorset, Hampshire, and Suffolk. There are also Katahdin and Dorper, called hair sheep, which molt in spring and don't need shearing. A Pennsylvania farmer I recently spoke with dismissed the idea of top breeds with better taste: "If the lambs gain well on grass and they muscle well, the taste takes care of itself."

Farmers and chefs agree that lamb, more than beef, tastes of what it eats. In France, there are varied geographic kinds, reflecting the pastures of each place, but the names hardly matter; more important, wherever you are, is to eat what's local and good. Most distinctive is *pré-salé* ("salt meadow") lamb, raised in Britain and especially Brittany and Normandy in France, such as by Mont-Saint-Michel. The sheep advance and retreat with the tides, eating the grasses and other salt-tolerant plants of the coastal marshes. The marine taste is often said to include iodine. A French chef once told me, "You taste the grass, you taste the salt—it's a completely different taste from other lamb."

After slaughter, quick chilling tightens and toughens the muscles. To prevent this "cold shortening," the carcasses should first be held at 55 degrees F (13 degrees C) and then go into the chill for what one hopes is a week of dry-aging and, with more mature lamb with a thicker fat cap, up to two weeks or more. The longer period may not be important, but it adds something. The usual wet-aged meat in plastic has unpleasant, sour-tasting juices around it; dry-aged meat is nutty. For a chef, the problem with buying whole animals from small farms is inconsistent texture, fat, connective tissue, and size, and unequal portions. Animals that run have tougher muscles, which perhaps up to a point is good.

Mutton, the sheep counterpart to beef, was once one of the most admired meats, and the best chefs have never thought otherwise. I hardly know it, but in the US it's beginning to come back into fashion. (In Britain, a hogget is from one to two years old; only after that is the meat considered mutton, a somewhat more common item in Britain than in North America.) Better mutton is two or more years old and comes not from a ewe but from a wether, a castrated male. If he isn't castrated, the meat will be too intense. (Lambs that aren't castrated grow faster; they're slaughtered too young for it to matter to the taste of the meat.) According to one old haute cuisine account, five-year-old wethers are best, but keeping animals that long is expensive and today unlikely to happen. Mutton is cooked just a little more than lamb, to about 135 degrees F (57 degrees C). In Britain roast mutton is traditionally served with red currant jelly, but black currant is supposed to be better, with its strong, slightly musky side to complement the near gaminess of the meat.

The prestige cut of lamb is the rack, the six to eight ribs next to the shoulder, when they aren't broken into chops. Next comes the loin; the whole loin is the festive saddle. When the loin is cut into chops, it produces little porterhouses. Then comes the leg. The leg and rack or chops are best cooked rare to medium rare for maximum juice and tenderness. (The papery fell, in young animals, is a light membrane over the fat that covers the whole animal. It's very minor in young lamb, but in theory, it's left on the large roasting cuts, to protect them, and removed from small ones, such as chops, because it shrinks in cooking and pulls and distorts them.)

Shoulder chops are uselessly tough, but the shoulder makes excellent ground lamb to go with eggplant in moussaka, in Arab *kibbe* (usually meatballs), and in sausage. Lamb lends itself to spice. A braised shoulder is one of the best dishes. To be succulent, a braise must be heated slowly and then cooked well below a boil. That's sometimes done in earthenware pots, which conduct heat poorly and thus more evenly. The shoulder is more likely to hold its juices if it's braised whole on the bone, but then carving is messy. Somewhat like a roast, a braise benefits from a rest, as the temperature falls and a little of the flavorful juice is reabsorbed into the meat. A *navarin printanier,* a French spring lamb stew, is named for the *navets,* the turnips that join the other young vegetables ready in that season, including new potatoes. (A *navarin* originally called for mutton.) *Blanquette de veau,* braised shoulder and breast, with its pale egg-thickened sauce, is a classic of French home cooking.

The shanks are the most flavorful part of a lamb, and very succulent if they're carefully cooked, either braised or otherwise cooked very slowly, so the tough connections turn gelatinous and tender. Shanks especially go with garlic. I once braised a pot of lamb tongues, some of the best tongue I've eaten. My favorite kidneys are lamb, and lamb sweetbreads are excellent. I love the Marseille specialty *pieds et paquets,* "feet and packages"; the feet are cooked for hours with squares of tripe closed around chopped lightly cured pork with garlic and parsley, all in an aromatic tomato-wine sauce.

No meat is better than a roast leg of lamb. A leg logically shouldn't, but in the US often does, include a section of loin. Cut fully long (uncommon today in the US), it includes the whole shank, and then part of the pleasure is the variety in taste. Most of the meat is rare, but the narrow shank conveniently ends up well-done. For easy carving, you need the long shank to hold on to or, if the leg is young and small enough, to attach a French-style clamp, a *manche à gigot,* to use as a handle. For years, before putting a leg to roast, I removed the aitch bone (pelvic bone) to make carving easier; then I realized that even if that part of the leg is tightly tied, the cuts lose enough juice during roasting that the easier carving isn't worth it. The most flavorful, juicy, tender range of doneness is rare to pink—125 to at most 140 degrees F (52 to 60 degrees C). *Gigot d'agneau de sept heures,* a "seven-hour leg of lamb," is simmered very slowly with aromatic vegetables, herbs, wine, and stock until it is spoon tender. And a leg is sometimes baked on a bed of beans or potatoes, which benefit from the juice and fat.

Roasting, *real* roasting, requires intense, dry radiant heat, ideally from an open fire with the meat turning before it. A conventional oven, with its relatively moist heat coming from all sides, *bakes* whatever is put into it. The metal walls rarely get hotter than 500 degrees F (290 degrees C), while, as Harold McGee explains in his highly useful *On Food and Cooking,* the glowing coals reach about 2,000 degrees F (1,100 degrees C) and the energy radiating from an object that hot is forty times greater than it is from a 500-degree one. The metal appliance cooks not just by radiation but by convection and conduction (if the meat sits on the bottom of the pan).

To turn the leg of lamb before the fire, one of the oldest and best jacks is a string hanging from a nail and tied to the shank, so the meat slowly twirls. You have to give it a spin from time to time, or the meat will stop and burn on one side. A horizontal spit requires more force to turn it.

Because you roast in front of and not over a fire, the meat has little or no taste of smoke. The intense heat comes from one side only, and because no surface of the meat is exposed to the fire for long, the interior cooks relatively gently and evenly. Remove the meat from the fire or oven when it reaches approximately 120 degrees F (50 degrees C), depending on how rare you like it. Afterward the still-penetrating heat will raise the center a further 10 degrees or so. The leg must rest for twenty to thirty minutes, depending on its size, or the juices will run out when you carve.

The surface should be a rich brown, with crisp fat, and yet the outermost meat, when you slice it, should form only a thin layer of brown; beneath it the succulent interior should be cooked as evenly as possible to no more than medium rare, for maximum juice. It will always be least cooked at the bone. The usual tactic is to first brown the meat with high heat and then cook it more slowly, something that occurs naturally as a fire dies down. For a darker, crisper surface, some of the most careful cooks have always basted with pure fat and no juice, whose water would cool the surface, though other cooks like the mixed fat and juices because they create a flavorful dark gloss.

HOW TO BUY LAMB: According to your taste, look for more tenderness from younger lamb or for stronger flavor from older lamb. And in animals that haven't been raised on their mothers' milk, look for grass rather than grain finishing. (Heavily marbled meat from a lot of grain is unnatural for lamb, and the flavor isn't typical.) Buy lamb, if you can, directly from a farmer whose methods you know, or, probably better, from one of the new wave of butcher shops that specialize in meats from particular farms, which may have more carefully slaughtered and aged meats and have an actual skilled butcher behind the counter.

COMPLEMENTS TO LAMB: It likes garlic, olive oil, onions, tomato, anchovies, olives, capers, rosemary, red and white wine, lemon, curry (and optionally raisins and blanched almonds), saffron, clove, cardamom, and other spice, and lightly crushed juniper berries. Lamb is complemented by beans of all kinds—green, fava, tender newly shelled beans, and dried beans, especially *flageolets*. It goes with eggplant, bulb fennel, carrots, sweet green peas, spinach, chicory and escarole, braised cabbage, and turnips (such as in a gratin, with a roast). Rhubarb is often mentioned, but I don't find a special sympathy. Potatoes browned in pan drippings are particularly delicious. Lamb goes with mango chutney. (I've mostly avoided condiments in this book, because relying on them can lead to an unthinking sort of cooking, but they're often excellent. I grew up eating lamb with mint sauce, made quickly and easily by adding chopped fresh spearmint leaves to a sugar-water-vinegar syrup. I have a sentimental attachment to mint sauce with lamb, but I don't know whether I would like the combination if I came across it now for the first time. It's a wine killer.)

NOTES ON WINE: A young, flowery white wine goes with lamb braised with vegetables in white wine, and a more substantial white goes with very young, pale roast lamb. Light reds go with braises. But lamb in general complements a more substantial, mature red wine, and first to be mentioned is always Cabernet Sauvignon, particularly Bordeaux. More mature examples of lamb with stronger flavor also go with Burgundy and Rhone wines, traditional Brunello di Montalcino, old Bordeaux, traditional red Rioja, traditional Nebbiolo—wines that go with game.

LEMONS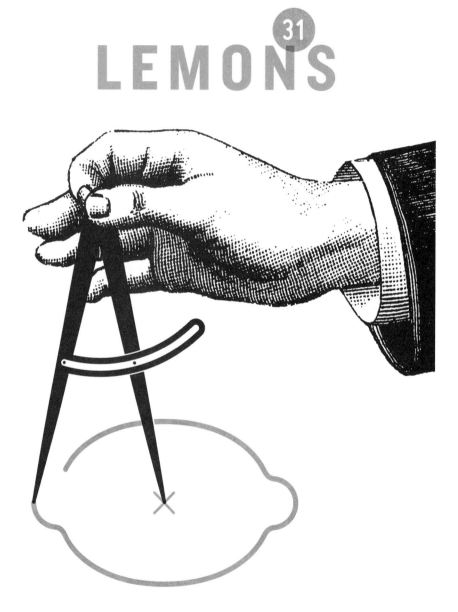

The marvelous depth of flavor of a lemon comes largely from the zest, but the juice is the most cheerful, enlivening part. (An ethereal side of lemon flavor is strikingly apparent in lemon-blossom honey.) Lemon juice is the most complementary form of acidity for lifting taste in general. Normally you add the juice when the cooking is done, so the fine acidity isn't driven off. You need enough acidity but not so much that the lemon flavor is identifiable. I've heard of a chef who goes through a case of lemons each night, and none of his diners realize. And sometimes the aroma is the main point. I certainly don't stop cooking if there's no lemon in the house—other kinds of acidity are also good—but I almost always have lemons. They're a year-round fruit, because they keep and there are several harvests from fall to early summer and sometimes in summer itself, depending on the location and variety.

US lemons, grown mainly in California and Arizona, almost all come from two good, nearly indistinguishable varieties, Eureka and Lisbon. Many if not most of these lemons, however, are picked underripe. They're more acidic and keep better, but they lack ripe-fruit aroma. Often they're picked when still green and then turned yellow by ethylene gas (something that otherwise occurs on the tree as the gas is slowly and naturally released by the fruit). Then mass-market lemons are coated with wax to keep them from drying out. The most distinctive and best-known US variety is Meyer, which isn't as strong in acidity as a regular lemon. Its ancestry surely includes orange or mandarin, shown in the color of the ripe skin and in the taste. To me, Meyer is also spicy. It's most useful where lemon is the dominant flavor, such as in a lemon tart.

In Italy, heading south from Naples along the coast of the Sorrentine Peninsula to Amalfi, you see miles of terraced hillsides with lemon groves protected by wooden frames. Straw mats are put over them to protect against wind and cold. The Limone di Sorrento, with its bumpy skin, is known for aroma as well as juice; it comes from the Massese lemon, in the Femminello group of varieties. The Limone Costa d'Amalfi is raised from the variety Sfusato, meaning "tapering." Some of the Italian varieties have been planted by specialist growers in California.

The fruit that comes closest to the lemon is the citron, a self-pollinating form of citrus that's older than lemons and oranges. It looks like a lemon but in much larger, cruder form. The flesh is nowhere near as sharp and juicy, although it's equally respectful of other flavors. The point of a citron is the thick peel, not so bitter as a lemon's and very fragrant, so it's often candied. (The usual commercial candied peel has little flavor apparently because it's made from firm, unripe fruit.) In Amalfi, the peel of the variety Sfusato, the same name as the lemon, is sometimes eaten thinly sliced as a salad.

As with other fruits, the blossom end of a lemon has more acidity, sugar, and flavor than the stem end, and the juice is always much more aromatic when you squeeze it at the last moment. That's part of the logic of serving wedges with fish or deep-fried food. On the streets of Naples, from a stand garlanded with plastic fruit, I've bought a bright cup of mixed orange and lemon juice pressed to order for perfect freshness. As an experiment, if you squeeze lemon juice and put it overnight in the refrigerator, and the next day compare it, blind, with freshly squeezed juice, you may think the overnight juice tastes fresher. It has little aroma, but it seems much stronger, all sharp acidity laid bare.

Lemon peel is full not only of flavor but of pectin, so lemon marmalade has no trouble setting. The flavor is in the oil of the zest. Fermentation alters and boosts that flavor in North African– and Levantine-style salted lemons. With a fresh lemon, it's important not to grate too deeply, or you get the bitterness of the pith. It's fairly easy to cut away all the peel from a lemon (or other citrus) with a chef's knife so as to have no white and only flesh. First remove a slice from the top and one from the bottom, cutting deep enough to reveal a full circle of flesh, then set the lemon on end and cut away the peel from top to bottom in swaths.

Lemon sauce uses the fat of butter, cream, and cheese to tie the tart juice to the pasta. Similarly, broth, butter, and cheese tie the juice to the rice in a lemon risotto (a nontraditional dish). The lemon juice–fat combination is also key to *vitello tonnato* (chilled veal in tuna sauce). Mediterranean *avgolemono* ("egg-lemon") sauces and soups thin the acidity with egg. Lemon curd is an emulsion of butter with lemon juice, zest, egg, and sugar (a good ratio is three lemons, three eggs, and ¾ cup or 150 grams sugar to five tablespoons or 75 grams butter). A lighter combination is lemon custard made with cream, something that often fills a tart. Even a lemon soufflé contains butter to balance the lemon.

Pure lemon flavor is probably best presented in lemonade or lemon ice made from freshly squeezed juice. For the ice, there's no set formula, but the concentration of sugar determines the texture: sweeter is softer. With any ice, rather than worry about the texture, aim for the taste you want—the balance among flavor, acidity, and sweetness—and close to serving time, either further freeze or else thaw the ice, as needed, to make it harder or softer. Then break up the coarse crystals to make it easy to eat, though this yields a flaky texture. I like an ice that's not much more solid than liquid. If you start to chase after a great lemon ice, ordering it often at *gelaterie* and restaurants, you find a wide variation in quality, and the biggest difference is freshness.

HOW TO BUY AND STORE LEMONS: Choose a lemon by holding it in your hand and squeezing. A softer one is riper and juicier. If you want the zest, be certain to buy organic lemons, and smoother skins make grating the zest easier. Lemons don't improve after they leave the tree, but they keep well at cool temperatures, even perfectly well for a week on the kitchen counter.

COMPLEMENTS TO LEMONS: It's easy to list the things improved by lemon. Fish and seafood like the clean sting of lemon juice, as well as the flavor. Lemon juice goes with artichokes, asparagus, broccoli, lettuce, avocado, chicken, beef, and fennel in salad, and it helps to compensate for bland fruit. In most of these uses, though, the lemon is the complement. True complements to lemon are butter, cream, olive oil, walnut oil, garlic, parsley, dill, cilantro, rosemary, cumin, ginger, and mint. In dessert, lemon is complemented by sugar, honey, coconut, pistachios, poppy seeds, and chocolate.

NOTES ON WINE: Lemon is no friend to wine, especially when there's enough juice to make food taste acidic. It helps if the wine itself is somewhat acidic and has concentrated flavor. To jump to a specific example, with lemon chicken you can short-circuit the problem with a dry Alsace Gewürztraminer. Generally with sour foods I serve a very simple white or red and I don't worry.

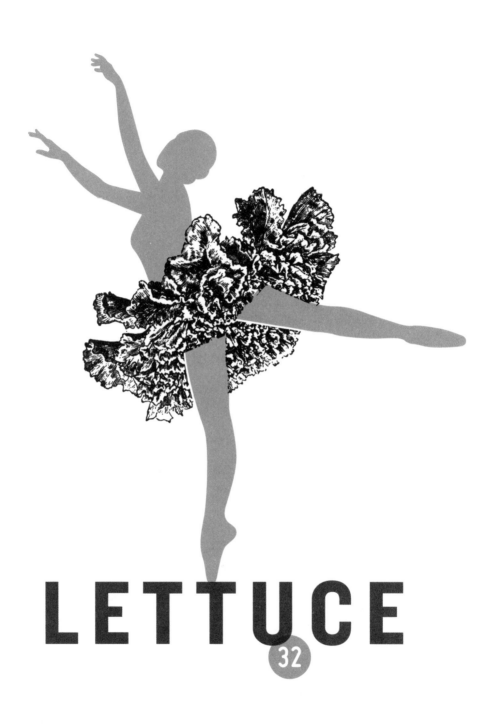

LETTUCE

32

P robably nothing is more important to a meal than salad, and in salad nothing is better than tender young lettuce (*Latuca sativa*), with its lively, wet crunch that contrasts with other foods. It's always refreshing, and the best lettuce comes with a distinct green, nutty flavor. Only a tiny minority of varieties produce lettuce like that, and any good new ones come and go from seed catalogs so quickly as to frustrate a gardener. Certain superior heirlooms, however, are consistently available. They have both good flavor and good texture, from soft to crisp. Of the several dozen varieties I've grown over the years, I especially like three.

Among the looseleaf family, I always grow Oakleaf, whose foliage has the familiar wavy outline of its namesake. Some looseleaf varieties have curly, frilly, or blistered leaves with rough textures, but not Oakleaf. Its open heads, like those of the rest of the looseleaf family, lend themselves to repeated cutting of individual leaves as they grow and regrow. Ignoring that potential, I slice off the whole heads at the ground so as to have the tender, partly blanched inner leaves. Oakleaf usefully withstands cold and light frost, although compared with other varieties it goes to seed more quickly in heat. Italian Lingua di Canarino and Catalogna are similar if not identical. A few newer Oakleaf cultivars I've tried have generally had darker green color and in some cases bigger heads, but they're not obviously better. I am impressed with the burgundy-spattered look of Flashy Green Butter Oak—red and variegated lettuces have been known for a very long time. All the Oakleafs seem reliable; they have good flavor and a tender, mild crunch.

The romaine family, also known as cos or long-leafed lettuce, is both flavorful and heat-tolerant. It's sometimes said that romaine should have a subtle, refreshing bitterness, but in my northern climate it's no different from other varieties. Romaine's characteristic tall, concave leaves have strong ribs. "The reason for this is simple," says the perceptive gardener and historian William Woys Weaver in *100 Vegetables and Where They Came From*. "The lettuces were used as an edible scoop or spoon when eating tabbouleh-like foods." The alternative name of cos is often said to come from the Greek island of Kos, but it's perhaps more likely to have come from the similarly pronounced Arabic word for lettuce. The French name *romaine,* meaning "Roman," apparently entered English after this lettuce passed from Italy through France, arriving at the papal court at Avignon in the fourteenth century. My favorite romaine is also the most flavorful lettuce I grow: the handsome, red-speckled Forellenschuss, whose coloring suggests the speckled trout of its name. Weaver says it's a dwarf form of Spotted Aleppo, which was carried from Syria to Europe in the eighteenth century. For salad, since I usually have an abundance of lettuce, I discard all romaine's darker green outer leaves, which are somewhat firm and tough, and I cut out and discard the thicker ribs of the remaining leaves. They're naturally somewhat blanched, and I like the lettucey flavor.

Butterheads, which include the varieties often called Boston in the US, form loosely closed, cabbagelike heads. In theory, butterheads have a buttery texture, but most of the ones I've grown have had limited flavor, and their leaves develop thick, brittle skeletons that give a dull, watery crunch not far from that of the insipid Iceberg. (In fact, that's a nineteenth-century heirloom, one of the big, tight crispheads, and some gardeners praise it. But when I grew Iceberg, it tasted just like the supermarket kind.) Not every butterhead has a brittle crunch. My favorite of all lettuces is the Boston type named Tennis Ball (specifically, the black-seeded one sold by the Seed Savers Exchange), which dates back to at least the eighteenth century. It's remarkable for having soft, thin leaves with the most velvety texture of any lettuce, and it has as much flavor as other similar lettuces, if not more. The variety is at its best soon after the heads have begun to form and before they grow at all tight. Tennis Ball was named not just for its size, which may have increased through selection since the early days (the mature heads in my garden are nearly as large as the usual Boston), but for the firmness of the heads as well. In salad, this lettuce needs a light dressing that won't mask its delicate flavor, and because its texture is lost in a mix with other varieties, Tennis Ball is best on its own.

Good flavor and texture come not just from variety, but from age, climate, season, weather—from soil with sufficient moisture and from somewhat cool temperatures. Where it's possible to grow lettuce outdoors in winter, the leaves turn leathery (they can be better than no lettuce at all), and in the mass market such heads have particularly poor flavor. At the other seasonal extreme, summer drought prematurely ages lettuce: it goes more quickly to seed and, depending somewhat on the variety, the strong bitterness of wild lettuce comes back, just as under any conditions older heads can turn bitter. The bitterness is concentrated in the white sap that gives lettuce its name (from Latin *lact-,* "milk"). In very hot weather, even with plenty of rainfall, the mature heads surge upward, seemingly over-night, producing thick flower stalks (which, if you like, you can peel and eat). Lettuce leaves can be too old to eat, but they're never too young.

HOW TO HARVEST OR BUY LETTUCE: Lettuce is one of the easiest crops to grow, and if you do plant it, try to harvest it before it loses moisture and aroma to the heat of the day. In stores and at farmers' markets, choose let-tuce, like most other produce, that isn't old or bruised but whose leaves look tender, healthy, and filled with moisture, as if they were still growing.

HOW TO STORE AND CLEAN LETTUCE: Lettuce tastes far better on the day it was cut, but an intact head will keep fairly well for a couple of days wrapped in plastic and placed in the refrigerator; tighter heads last longer than looser ones. (You can create your own "supermarket" lettuce by stor-ing a just-picked head in the refrigerator for a week.) Don't wash lettuce until a few hours before you eat it—never a day ahead—or it will lose most of its flavor. Once the leaves are free of grit and you've spun them or other-wise gotten rid of most of the surface water, either tear the leaves or slice them with a sharp blade (a dull one crushes and makes dark cuts) into sizes that will mix easily with the dressing. Wrap the lettuce in a clean towel, place the bundle in a salad bowl big enough to allow thorough mixing, and refrigerate until serving time. The leaves will become crisper, and most of the clinging drops of moisture will disappear so they won't dilute the dressing.

COMPLEMENTS TO LETTUCE: The chief complement to raw lettuce is fat, especially very fresh and not too bitter olive oil. (The freshest, most fruit-tasting olive oil is also more or less bitter, which is good with flavorful lettuce only if the bitterness is offset by enough fruit flavor.) Also delicious with lettuce are fresh nut oils (if they don't have too strong a roasted flavor from the ground nuts' being strongly heated before pressing), especially walnut oil with just-squeezed lemon juice. Dijon mustard hides the best flavors of oil and vinegar, but now and then a judicious addition is excellent in vinaigrette for lettuce. Or mix together Dijon mustard, rich cream, lemon juice, salt, and pepper with, optionally, a crushed clove of garlic; this dressing soon thickens, so thin it as needed with a little water. After whisking a vinaigrette to form a temporary emulsion (it's more lasting with mustard), promptly dress the leaves, tumbling them until they are evenly coated. Especially with delicate leaves, don't let the dressed salad wait and wilt. There are many more complements to lettuce, not least finely cut chives and sliced or chopped hard-cooked egg. Rather than any dressing, one of the best complements to whole tender leaves is warm juices from a grilled steak. Apart from using lettuce in salad, it's classic and excellent to cook some tender young lettuce with green peas (and lettuce is sometimes braised in stock, which is good, but generally there's no reason to cook it).

NOTES ON WINE: The acidity of a salad dressing throws off the taste of any wine, and anyway there's no reason to drink anything with salad.

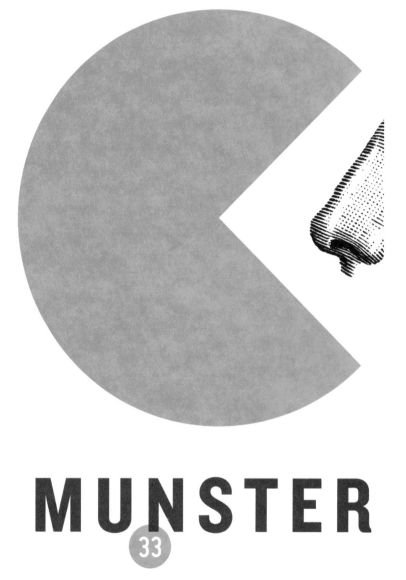

MUNSTER

33

33. MUNSTER AND OTHER
STINKY CHEESES

Munster is one of the best and, at its ripest, one of the stinkiest of cheeses. Its wild and fruity aromas, challenging and beloved, are sometimes called garlicky. The flat, soft, smooth rounds of Munster, under its Appellation d'Origine Protégée (AOP), come in two sizes: roughly three and a half inches in diameter by an inch or more tall and roughly seven inches in diameter and somewhat thicker. (According to the rules, the small is seven to twelve centimeters in diameter and the large is thirteen to nineteen centimeters.) The smell and orangy color originate with the regular "washing" of the slightly moist surface with brine—really it's wiped or brushed. (The transformation has always been attributed to "red mold," or *Brevibacterium linens,* an organism that's invisibly present on our skin; it proliferates in certain wet conditions. But recent research has found hardly a trace of *B. linens* on the ripe cheese, so its role, if any, is open to question.) If the cheese becomes too ripe or is kept tightly wrapped for too long, especially at warm temperatures, it can cross a line and become distasteful. Otherwise the smell of Munster and other stinky cheeses can be fairly tame. And curiously, the smell of any washed-rind cheese is much stronger than its taste. One of the great, unlikely flavor combinations is the marvelously rich, tangy deliciousness of a ripe Munster together with a glass of sweet Gewürztraminer wine.

The cheese is made in the provinces of Alsace and Lorraine in eastern France. More precisely, it comes from the Vosges Mountains, which lie partly in each province. The summits of these mountains aren't high and sharp but worn and rounded, and starting at about three thousand feet (nine hundred meters), you find seasonal farms and summer pastures, called *chaumes.* They provide superior food for cattle—wild grains such as red fescue and bent grass, but also aromatic plants such as wolfsbane, mountain pansy, caraway, and especially *fenouil des alpes* ("alpine fennel," or spignel), which contribute subtle flavor to the milk. Munster is an oddity among mountain cheeses. They're typically huge, hard, and durable, like Gruyère, and yet Munster is small and moist. It ripens quickly from the outside in, the chalky interior turning entirely creamy in just a few weeks. Even the high Vosges farms are relatively close to towns, where the moist, short-lived cheeses were and still are quickly sold.

Munster, a corruption of the Latin for "monastery," is the name of a small Alsatian town, site of the onetime monastery of Saint-Grégoire, founded in the seventh century. It's said that the cheese, like so many others in other places, was first made by monks. Those at Munster may well have produced cheese from the start, but there's no evidence that the present creamy, washed-rind Munster came into being until much later, possibly two hundred years ago. The same cheese made on the other side of the Vosges, in Lorraine, was called Géromé, the dialect name for Gérardmer, the market town where the cheese was sold. But the cheese from Alsace had the bigger reputation, and the name Munster eclipsed that of Géromé, although Munster-Géromé remains an officially recognized alternative name. Nearly all Munster comes from the four dairy plants in Lorraine, which are industrial in scale. Alsace has just two plants, both of them small and good and run by the Haxaire family, which make about 7 percent of all Munster. Another 5 percent is still made on farms, about ninety of them, mostly in Alsace. Typically now these are *fermes-auberges,* earning part of their income from serving traditional food and accommodating overnight guests. Most of the cheesemaking farms move their cows in May to the high *chaumes.*

The milk for the cheese comes mainly from Holstein cows, the highly productive dairy breed, originally from the Netherlands, that has largely replaced other dairy breeds throughout Europe and North America. Traditionally, the milk for Munster came from Vosgienne cows, whose population of 125,000 at the start of the First World War had fallen to just 3,000 by the 1970s, though it has returned to a stable 10,000. Vosgiennes are largely white, but their sides are covered with distinctive broad, ragged areas of black or sometimes dark red, and they have dark ears, muzzles, and eyes. Well-adapted to life in the mountains, they are kept by about a third of the farm cheesemakers. Vosgiennes give moderate yields of high-quality milk for cheese.

All the world's cheeses were once ripened by local organisms that lent each kind its particular characteristics. These souring and ripening microflora were naturally present, entering the milk from the atmosphere of the barn and cheesemaking room and by way of the equipment. In places, that still happens to some extent. But today large dairy plants, as well as many small ones, pasteurize the milk, eliminating the life within it. And modern dairy regulations, demanding such things as nonporous surfaces and constant cleaning, have made the dairy environment so clean that for several decades even raw milk has generally required an added commercial starter. The laboratory cultures, however, contain a narrower range of organisms that are somewhat different from those in the wild.

Each farmwife in the Vosges always had her own variation on the Munster recipe. The outlines today are fixed by the appellation rules. The milk, either raw or pasteurized, is warmed, rennet is stirred in, and within an hour the curd has set. (The Alsatians eat the just-made curd with sugar, crème fraîche, and kirsch—the traditional dessert *Siasskas*.) The curd is cut into large dice, which lose less whey than finely cut or broken curd, so the cheese itself remains moist. The molds today are plastic, stainless steel, or the traditional fir. The last used to be made on each farm and have all but disappeared; the wood holds heat better, giving a more even temperature and better draining, and it may harbor useful bacteria. Inside the molds, the curd settles, unpressed, as the whey flows out. The cheeses are turned several times within the molds while they become firm enough to hold their shape. They're sprinkled on both sides with salt and, once out of the molds, they're turned daily so they dry evenly and are exposed to air. Yeasts and other microflora begin to grow on the surface, lowering its acidity so the red mold can more easily spread. About half the farm cheeses, while they are still white and new, are bought and ripened by professional *affineurs*.

The more industrial producers add commercial strains of red mold, while on farms it comes from sources such as the wooden shelves of the ripening room. After four or five days, the rind is washed every day or two with brine. Larger operations use machines with soft plastic brushes, but if you wipe each cheese with a hand dipped in brine, you know exactly how it's evolving. The washing prevents the growth of a bloomy rind, like that on Camembert, and it nourishes the red mold, producing a single color all over. The minimum age is fourteen days for the small cheeses and twenty-one for the large, but either size takes about another week to become really creamy. (There's no fixed time for that, and in a traditional ripening room without artificial cooling, the cheeses ripen faster in summer than they do in winter.) As with all cheeses, the microorganisms responsible for flavor produce different substances at different temperatures. Too cool, and the compounds are simpler and the flavor is less interesting. Too warm, and the taste is more tart and chalky. Washed-rind cheeses matured at around 50 degrees F (10 degrees C) have a fuller, richer, more buttery flavor.

Taken together, each farm's equipment, methods, and location make its cheese unique. You see that even in the color. When Munster from different farms is collected by an *affineur,* and all are washed and ripened together in the same *cave,* they end up with slightly different colors. Those from one farm may be more yellow-orange; others may be more red-orange, pinkish, or rust-colored. Some Munsters are firm to a fault, even stodgy, but the softer ones can have a buttery texture. The creamiest, when they're cut, begin to flow a little.

The world holds many washed-rind cheeses with different characteristics, although outside France few cheeses are washed enough to give them such a marked combination of stinkiness and creaminess. Münster, with an umlaut, is made in Germany; the relationship between the two, if any, isn't clear, and I've come across only uninteresting mass-produced examples. Italy has just a few washed-rind cheeses, the best-known being the mild Taleggio, which is sometimes very good. From the mountains of Extremadura, in Spain, come various washed-rind *tortas.* Switzerland makes excellent washed-rind cheeses, which are often drier and larger than the French ones; the best are farm-made—somewhat rustic and variable, sometimes a little bitter. (Bitterness is generally a defect in cheese, but a trace can be a fair trade for exceptional flavor.) The official appellations are important in giving a cheese a clear definition and upholding quality, but there's been a recent proliferation of excellent nonappellation farm cheeses, washed-rind and other kinds, in Germany and Switzerland. Some of the strong, flowingly creamy Swiss ones include as part of the name *Fladä,* which means "cow pie." You may come across Stanser Fladä, Försterkäse, or Beermat, the last of which, as you might suspect, is washed with beer.

France alone produces about one hundred different washed-rind cheeses, including Maroilles, from a swath of the north, Langres, from Champagne, and Livarot, from Normandy, all with AOPs. Two more washed-rind cheeses, one French and one Swiss-French, each with its special qualities, are:

ÉPOISSES (AOP, FRANCE) Strong in odor and always flowingly creamy, Époisses, from Burgundy, has its own particular complication. It's the only AOP cheese that combines a washed rind with a *caillé lactique,* a "lactic curd," meaning it's set with very little rennet at a cool temperature over eighteen to twenty-four hours, enough time for the lactic bacteria to produce generous acidity and set a curd without much rennet. The acidity limits the growth of harmful organisms, which was important under the highly variable conditions of the past. But a lactic-curd cheese is fragile. Époisses is washed at first with either brine or plain water, and later with brine or water mixed with stronger and stronger additions of *marc* (eau-de-vie distilled, like grappa, from the pressings left over from wine). You can't apply full-strength marc to the newly made cheese or the alcohol prevents the red mold from growing. But once the mold is established, the marc dries the surface (just as rubbing alcohol dries your skin), firming the outside of the cheese, which, as it ripens, might otherwise collapse. And the marc adds its own flavor. "It's difficult to ripen. One has a moist cheese and one *washes* it—it's crazy!" Jean Berthaut once said to me. It was his parents who revived the cheese in the 1950s, saving it from extinction, and he continues to make it in the center of the village of Époisses. A related washed-rind cheese, Soumaintrain, originating not so far away, is slightly larger and often excellent. (Aisy Cendré, also from the area, is washed and then aged in ashes, which seems to me to add nothing.)

VACHERIN MONT-D'OR (AOP, SWITZERLAND) and MONT D'OR or VACHERIN DU HAUT-DOUBS (AOP, FRANCE) Under these three names, Vacherin is made in the Jura Mountains on either side of the French-Swiss border and is a luscious favorite at the end-of-the-year holidays. The taste can be dull, but certain examples soar. The size is anywhere from about four to thirteen inches in diameter by about two and a half inches tall (eleven to thirty-three by six to seven centimeters). Being soft and weak, the cheese is bound by a strip of spruce bark (just as the similarly tall but stinkier Livarot is held together by rushes, or nowadays by paper imitations), and the bark adds a detectable flavor. The tender Vacherin is sold with the further protection of a spruce box. When the cheese is fully creamy and ready, the top rind is carefully removed (French cheese sellers normally do this), and the Vacherin is served with a spoon.

HOW TO BUY WASHED-RIND CHEESES: The state of a washed-rind cheese, more than most kinds, depends on how long ago it left the *cave* where it was ripened and what if any care it received after that. Unfortunately, some of the washed-rind cheeses for sale in North America have seen better days. Buy either from the maker, from a specialist *affineur,* or from a purveyor who chooses well and sells the cheeses fairly quickly. Other things being equal, choose a cheese made from raw milk (*lait cru* in French) and on the farm (*fromage fermier* or similar words in French), which may have been ripened, probably to advantage, by a specialist *affineur.* The more industrial cheeses, made using commercial strains of red mold, are distinctly orange in color. The shade of a farm cheese is more variable, though consistent at each farm. Most cheese shops won't sacrifice a washed-rind cheese for tasting, but if you do get a taste, look for sweet, fruity flavors; the cheese shouldn't be bitter, marked by ammonia, or have any suggestion of an off-flavor. (I avoid the cheeses of certain larger makers, who use a commercial red mold that gives a smell I can only call fecal.) Some people prefer a milder or younger washed-rind cheese and others a more evolved and pungent one. Many like an in-between state—a creamy outside with a firm white heart. If you can't taste or even see the state of the cheese, then, if you're allowed, gently feel it inside its wrapper. A firmer cheese, as long as it isn't dried out, can be in better condition. A softer, moister washed-rind cheese is potentially more luscious, though more likely to have suffered—a very moist, fully ripe, flowingly creamy washed-rind cheese doesn't survive long. When in doubt, it's safer to buy an underripe cheese, and then if you're ambitious, you can ripen it further yourself (see next page).

The best Munsters of the year, though not exported to the US, are made from May onward from the milk of cows in high pastures, but winter cheeses from cows fed mountain hay can also be very good. Munster is made, ripened, and sold in France all within a few weeks, though most of the cheeses arrive in US shops well after that (more quickly by air, more slowly by ship). Some Munster producers use wine or eau-de-vie to wash some cheeses, though these can't be labeled Munster, and some Époisses producers use wine to wash some cheeses, though they can't be labeled Époisses. Such nonappellation cheeses can be very good. When buying Munster, two names to look for are Haxaire, a family of *affineurs* that also makes the cheese, and Fischer, a strictly *affineur* family, both of which export only pasteurized-milk cheeses to the US.

In contrast to Munster, an Époisses inside its box, beneath but not touching its covering of taut, clear plastic, is more paprika red, its skin is wrinkled, and it glistens from its washings. (A plastic film may not be ideal, but this one is pierced with tiny holes, as you can see if you look closely; it slows the loss of moisture without trapping too much ammonia and other gases.) Look for the shine and an unbroken rind holding together a sagging shape, which suggests full ripeness. The best seasons for Époisses from cows on pasture are May through July and October through December. Of the three dairy plants making Époisses, my preferred producer is Berthaut, although it uses pasteurized milk; in the region you may find a good farm producer (as I write, there's just one). A Langres, by contrast, is less intense, and its surface is duller from fewer washings, though it, too, wrinkles and sags as it ripens. (An AOP cheese with just three producers, Langres is washed but not turned, and as it ages a "*fontaine,*" or dish, forms in the top. Under the appellation, the *fontaine* must be at least 5 millimeters deep; as time passes the depth increases, but that tells nothing about the goodness of the cheese. The orange coloring, optionally, can be increased by the traditional coloring annatto. In Europe, look for Langres from the Schertenleib dairy and for raw-milk cheeses from Ferme du Modia.)

You can tell something about ripeness by the appearance of a Vacherin, but not much about flavor, and I don't know the name of a producer who consistently excels. You have to rely on a cheese seller who selects well.

With most Swiss washed-rind cheeses, just as with Munster, look for a slightly moist surface. Beyond that, it's hard to tell much by appearance. Try to find a shop that sells farm cheeses—a shop that knows what it's buying and sells the cheeses fairly quickly.

HOW TO KEEP, RIPEN IF NEEDED, AND SERVE WASHED-RIND CHEESES: Serve a washed-rind cheese within a day or two of buying it, unless it's underripe or slightly firm by nature. Meantime, if you have no moist, cool cellar perfect for cheese, keep the cheese in its wrapper and in the refrigerator. (Refrigeration is the enemy of good cheese, except perhaps the oldest and driest kinds, but few of us have an alternative if we want to keep cheese much longer than half a day. Anyway, almost every cheese for sale in North America, even the most handmade, has already been refrigerated for a time.)

Three or four hours before you serve the cheese, unwrap it and set it somewhere at about 50 to 60 degrees F (10 to 16 degrees C), so it will show its full flavor. If you have only a warmer place, set the cheese out for less time. If there's a draft or any risk of drying, cover it. If it already looks dry, then first mist it with water from a spray bottle or fling drops from your fingers.

If a washed-rind cheese hasn't been kept too cold for too long and its evolution too much suppressed, you can revive it yourself. You can even, if need be, ripen it further—not a little Époisses but a smooth whole cheese at least the size of a Munster. You need high humidity and a temperature of about 50 to 60 degrees F (10 to 16 degrees C). Set the unwrapped cheese on a platter, cover it with an inverted bowl to hold in humidity, and once a day over a few days turn it and lightly rub just the top and sides with a wet hand, so you have a dry surface that won't stick to the platter. What seems to be required more than skill is restraint, in the amount of water and the number of washings.

Soft-ripened cheeses, including washed-rind, can have an unpleasantly grainy, even partly crunchy, surface, whose flavor and texture can detract. But the rind of a cheese that was ripened fairly quickly, such as the best Munster and Époisses, and afterward not refrigerated for too long, is delicious and only adds to the pleasure of the stinky experience. As with other cheeses, the rule is: Taste the rind, and if you like it, eat it.

COMPLEMENTS TO WASHED-RIND CHEESES: The bread to go with pungent washed-rind cheeses can be anything from a baguette to dark whole rye. In Alsace, the venerable accompaniment to Munster is potatoes in their skins, said to be the preference of true connoisseurs. Munster is often served with caraway seeds, and in some instances the seeds are mixed into the curd during the making. The combination works, but the spice cancels out part of the Munster taste. (If you're in Alsace, it's useful to know that the common word in the region for both caraway and cumin is *cumin*.) Sometimes today, Munster and other washed-rind cheeses are used in cooking, such as in the filling for a custard tart, along with leeks and potatoes, which makes a good combination. But a washed-rind cheese in prime condition is special enough that I hesitate to cook it.

NOTES ON WINE: One of the sublime food-and-wine combinations is a fully ripe Munster with sweet Gewürztraminer from Alsace, the region of the world that produces the most refined, aromatic wines from the grape. An alternative, not quite as special, is sweet Alsace Muscat. As produced in the region, sweet wines from the two varieties share a rose aroma. Less dramatic complements to Munster are sweet Alsace Pinot Gris, Pinot Blanc, and Riesling. And with cheese many people, because sweet wines are less refreshing, like a barely sweet white wine. (With Munster, it's safer to stick to wines from Alsace. The whites typically have sufficient acidity, coupled with clean, clear aromas, although whether a wine is slightly sweet or completely dry is frustratingly impossible to tell from the label. Few of the region's producers use new oak, which would compete with the innate aromas of the wine or food.) The key with the sweet wines is to balance the intensity of the cheese with that of the wine, its flavor as much as its sweetness. A more intense cheese requires a more intense wine, but a wine with too much flavor and sugar makes a mild washed-rind cheese seem austere. And a very sweet wine will make even the strongest washed-rind cheese unpleasant and bitter. At the table, if you find that the wine and cheese are out of balance, save the wine for afterward.

Red Burgundy is often recommended with Époisses or Soumaintrain, but any red wine, even a light, low-tannin Pinot Noir, gives the cheeses a bitter, acrid taste. (A better Burgundian cheese for red wine is the mild Cîteaux, which is washed only a little, making it a mixed-rind type.) As a rule, no fully dry white wine complements washed-rind cheeses, but with Époisses or Soumaintrain a rich white Burgundy can be good. A safe white option with washed-rind and for that matter most cheeses is Champagne, which perhaps not coincidentally is the regional match for Langres. Vacherin, a lighter and easier cheese, goes with the lighter Jura whites, fresh light Beaujolais, or Champagne. And in place of wine, beer is traditional and excellent with many washed-rind cheeses.

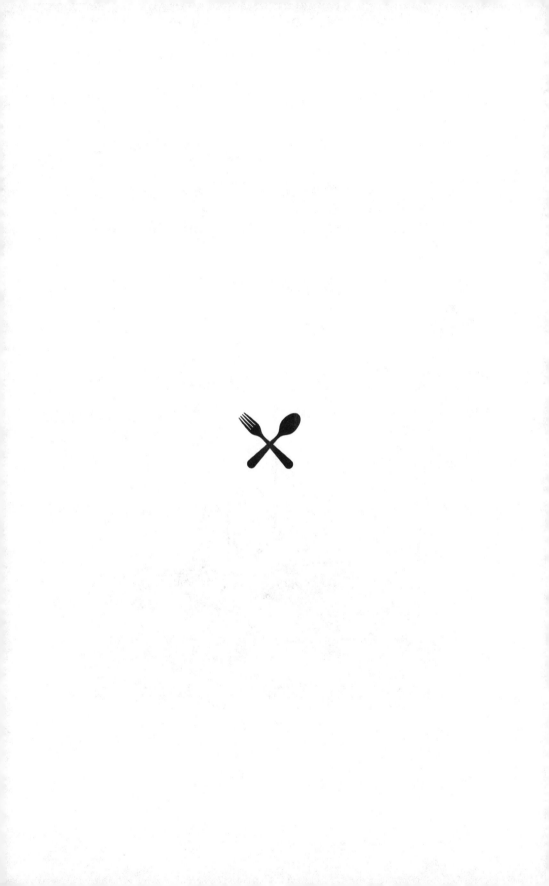

OLIVE OIL

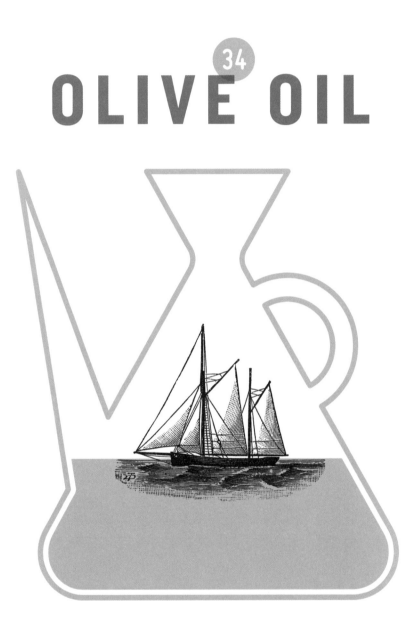

34. OLIVE OIL

The best fresh olive oil has a marked fruit flavor that suggests cherries and vanilla. The olives are picked early in the season at their peak of ripe fruit flavor, and within hours they're pressed, using impeccably clean equipment. Clean matters, because fats easily absorb whatever aroma or flavor they're exposed to. A sign of quality is a degree of bitterness and pepper. The oil is unrefined; its texture is luscious; it disappears on your tongue like butter. Carefully protected from heat, light, and air, it retains much of its fresh flavor until the next harvest and beyond. The uses of this best, most delicious oil are beyond counting—it's my fat of first resort, highly flattering to vegetables. The superior taste is perceptible even when you use the oil in cooking, although you can appreciate it far better when you add raw oil after cooking.

Over and over, we're told to buy extra virgin olive oil, which isn't wrong, and yet by itself that advice is useless. First, there's concern that some producers find ways to pass off lesser oil as extra virgin. Then, even with the most honest oil, the grade tells you only the state of the oil at bottling and says nothing at all about its condition weeks or months (or a year or more) later when you take it from a store shelf. Most of the extra virgin olive oil I've ever bought in North America, even pricey bottles, was already at least partly rancid from old age or abuse. You have to know your source. I've heard people say, maybe because they don't know the best fresh taste, how much they like the rancid, vegetal one, because it's more "olive."

In truth, these days any competent olive grower who wants to produce extra virgin oil knows how to do it, barring bad luck with weather or insects. Mere virgin oil has all but disappeared. The only other major retail category now is the largest one, plain "olive oil," which results when a grower aims mainly at quantity or when problems get the best of him or her and do real harm to the olives. Then the oil must be refined: its rancidity is chemically eliminated, which takes away all flavor and leaves the greasy texture typical of supermarket cooking oils. Afterward a little decent oil is added to provide some flavor, and then the refined oil qualifies for sale as "olive oil."

Producers of good olive oil often speak proudly of its low "acidity." Their use of the word, passed on by retailers and food writers, leads consumers to look for an acid taste in olive oil, something it never has. "Acidity" is shorthand for "free acidity," which is a scientific way to say rancidity. Olive oil is composed almost entirely of fatty acids—fat, in plain English. Some of this fat becomes free when its original link with other fat is broken by enzymes or combination with oxygen. That occurs when olives are eaten into by the olive fly or when the fruit becomes too ripe or is otherwise damaged or deteriorates before pressing. And it happens later on to the pressed oil if it's exposed to light, heat, or air or simply grows old. As defined by the International Olive Council, extra virgin olive oil contains no more than 0.8 percent rancid fat, measured as oleic acid, which is the chief fat in olive oil. The maximum allowed for certification as extra virgin by the California Olive Oil Council is 0.5 percent. Many good producers, wherever they are, achieve less than 0.2 percent. It's important to buy olive oil with low free acidity. Just remember that the oil in the bottle in front of you, depending on what happened to it, may no longer meet the standard.

Different kinds of olive oil, coming from different olive varieties grown in different places, have different flavors and consistencies, from light to viscous. Some oil by nature is more bitter, and some is entirely sweet; some tastes very strongly of fruit. When professional tasters evaluate oil, they work blind and clear their palates with water and apple slices. They gauge the fruitiness, sweetness, bitterness, and pungency—the peppery bite. They look mainly for defects but also for a range of possible good aromas: fresh almond, apple, raw artichoke, chamomile, citrus, eucalyptus, exotic fruit, fig leaf, flowers, new-mown grass, green peppercorn, green unripe fruit, herbs, olive leaf, pear, pine nut, berries, bell pepper, tomato, vanilla, and walnut.

The olive tree may have originated in what is now Turkey 14,000 years ago, and it thrives around the Mediterranean in warm, dry, eroded locations, particularly where there is limestone. Olive trees also grow well in more temperate, fertile places and as far from the Mediterranean as Australia, California, and Chile. More limestone soil gives oil with more bitterness and pepper, and more acid soil gives less. Heavier soil produces more body, and sandier soil and more rainfall make lighter oil. The trees survive down to about 18 degrees F (–8 degrees C); higher, cooler locations have few insect pests or none.

The trees never grow very tall, but they can live hundreds of years, gaining massive trunks or multiple ones. A few trees are believed to be two thousand and even four thousand years old. As with other tree fruits, the trend with olives is toward high-density, irrigated plantings in which the trees are set close together in rows, like bushes in a hedge. They lend themselves to mechanical pruning, spraying, and especially harvest, which saves a lot of labor. The machines also allow olives to be picked quickly at an optimum state. The high-density plantings aren't the most beautiful, and they may or may not be the most profitable in the long term, but the oil can certainly be good. It's difficult to make equal comparisons, but high-density plantings may yield less-intense oil. Great oil, so far, comes only from mature, traditional, nonirrigated trees.

The qualities of oil from a particular spot reflect climate even more than soil, and concentrated fruit perfume is probably tied above all to places with the right day-night temperature swings in October. A Tuscan agronomist, an olive specialist, once told me, "The ideal is *not* too much rain but cold nights, not freezing but cold"—from 5 to 15 degrees C (41 to 59 degrees F) at night and 20 to 25 degrees C (68 to 77 degrees F) during the day. "The aromas concentrate."

It used to be that olives were picked only after they had turned black, but the best fruit flavor comes from olives harvested still green or just changing color. Depending on the location, the modern harvest of green fruit starts at the end of October and is over by mid-November. (Not just the desire for fruit flavor but the warming climate has been pushing the harvest earlier.) The window for peak flavor, depending on the variety, lasts from perhaps five days up to fifteen or a little more. Hand-picking, as opposed to shaking the trees with a machine or beating the olives from the branches with poles, prevents damage to the tree and fruit, but to gather all the olives by hand during their moment of ideal ripeness, you need a lot of pickers. The olives on a tree don't all turn at once, so there's a mix of colors—green, reddish, and violet-black. Some people argue that, for the best quality, each variety must be picked, pressed, and bottled separately.

The olives picked at an early point of ripeness have not only more aroma but more polyphenols, loosely called tannins. The polyphenols are essential antioxidants that help to protect the oil against rancidity and loss of aroma (just as they protect the flavor of wine). The polyphenols also give the oil its bitterness and pepper, including sometimes a harsh rasp in the throat. It's not the quantity of polyphenols that benefits the oil but which ones they are. The *piccante* (peppery) ones are much more important for conservation than the bitter ones. But olive oil experts value both bitterness and pepper as part of a good taste.

Once picked, the olives should be pressed as soon as possible, within a few hours, while they are still at their peak. Some producers have their own mills to ensure the speed and quality they want. The olives are first reduced to a paste, pits and all. A number of good mills still use the traditional granite wheels turning slowly in a circular trough, and the stones have certain advantages. But they're harder to keep clean, and they expose the paste to a lot of air, which takes away some flavor and causes some fat to oxidize. Most mills around the world now use faster stainless-steel machinery, and the trend among the best producers is to protect the olives and oil from oxygen throughout the process by using enclosed machinery and even in some cases by displacing air with nitrogen. However the paste is made, it's then kneaded so the oil will absorb more aromas and flavors and so it will come together in bigger droplets that are easier to separate.

Nearly all the old vertical presses have been replaced with centrifuges, which exploit the lighter weight of oil compared with water. For flavor, it's important that these machines don't heat the paste, and they require added water, which washes away some of the aroma and polyphenols essential to good oil. The less water, the better. The first oil to run from an old-style vertical press or from a very slowly turning centrifuge is the "flower" of the oil—the most delicate part, usually mixed back in with the rest of the oil.

The color of the just-made oil, nearly opaque from all the fine material in suspension, can be a luminous chartreuse. Its flavors are *very* delicious—a revelation the first time you taste them. But the strong pepper and bitterness distract from the fruit and aren't in themselves pleasant. They ruin sweet lettuce. The old way to hide much of the pepper and bitterness, but not the fruit, is to make bruschetta: to pour the new oil on toasted bread. And cooking diminishes or eliminates the harshness and bitterness. A very little cloudy Italian *olio nuovo* is flown immediately to the United States, and some California oil is sold in a similar new state. But most imported olive oil doesn't reach North America until April, when the challenging tastes have begun to subside. I've had oil that a year later had lost its fruit flavor and yet retained an aggressive bitterness, but normally by then the harshness and bitterness have mellowed, leaving behind much of the delicious fresh flavor.

Cloudy new oil can be superb, and within a few months the fine particles inevitably settle, after which you can decant clear oil. That's the oldest way to get it, still used by certain good producers, although a little imperceptible material remains. Passing the oil through a filter removes some peroxides (undesirable products of oxidation), so the oil lasts longer, and it removes the finely dispersed trace of watery material that subtly turns rancid and hides good flavor. In wholly unfiltered oil, a sediment can form in the bottom of the bottle and decay and completely ruin the taste. One of the first forms of filtration, and maybe still the best, is to let the oil flow by gravity through fluffy white cotton. That's slow and exposes the oil to air, though you can use nitrogen to protect it. At the opposite extreme, too-aggressive filtration strips away flavor. It's not a big mistake to buy unfiltered oil, if it doesn't show sediment, but keep it carefully cool.

Like almost everyone, I praise the oil from olives harvested early. Today it's made from new plantings around the world and from very old ones; it comes from trees in some of the most ancient producing areas, such as North Africa. A new mass-market flow is beginning to appear from high-density plantings in Chile. And yet oil from early harvested olives, with a distinct fruit taste, hardly existed in commerce until the 1960s and became dominant only in the 1980s. Only then did the now-common practice of treating raw olive oil as a condiment begin to spread. It used to be that you could taste clean fruit flavors only in the very first pressings of each harvest, when the olives were less mature and the equipment was still clean. The harvest took place mainly in January and February, after the olives had turned fully black and were fairly soft, which increased the yield of oil and made it easier to extract with the technology of a wooden press.

Provence was a holdout. As recently as 2000, hardly more than a handful of growers there produced modern oil. Most picked the olives completely black and then stored them for a few days in a warm place so the fruit would become *coufi,* an old Provençal word, the same as French *confit,* which literally means "preserved." The black fruit underwent a fermentation that further softened it and took away any trace of pepper or bitterness. The technique gives a golden oil with a fattier texture and a flavor that has always reminded me of painter's linseed oil—not a compliment. More positively, the difference is compared to that between fresh and dried fruit. But the *coufi* olives can also give echoes of rancidity and other clear negatives. (Well-made black fruity oil is low in free acidity, but because of its nonconforming flavors it qualifies as merely "virgin.") The old-style oil is called *fruité noir* in French, "black fruity," and the modern oil is *fruité vert,* "green fruity." I like the green oil much better, and it constitutes most of the oil made in Provence by far, yet I would miss the taste of the traditional oil in old-fashioned Provençal cooking.

Some producers in Provence now make a little old-style oil from olives that become *coufi* in a closed container without access to oxygen, which creates a clean version of the black fruity flavor. The aromas are earthy—of cured black olives, cocoa, cooked artichoke, mushroom, and perhaps truffle—and the taste is more distinctly, narrowly *olivey,* like cured black olives. Cooking tames the flavor, placing it in the background. Traditionally in Provence, almost the only uses of raw oil were in vinaigrette and aioli, the Provençal garlic mayonnaise. An exception was and is chickpeas, for which there's a Provençal liking in salad and in hot puréed soup; the former is dressed with raw oil, and the latter is traditionally garnished with it, and in both cases there's an uncanny link in taste.

Olive oil, especially modern green oil, tastes strongly of the place where the olives are grown and of the variety. Each traditional area has its own varieties and likes its own oil. A few of the important areas are:

PUGLIA The heel of the Italian boot always used to produce much more olive oil than any other Italian region, though it's now rivaled by neighboring Calabria. Puglia has four olive oil denominations (Dauno, Terra di Bari, Colline di Brindisi, Terra d'Otranto) and divisions within them. Two widely planted varieties are Ogliarola, which is higher yielding, and Cellina, which is finer. There's well-made Pugliese oil, though I don't find it has a lot of character.

CALIFORNIA Quality has risen enormously in California in recent years. The Mission variety, planted around 1800 and considered native, isn't special. But much good oil is now made from European varieties, primarily Tuscan, and those of us who live in the US can order ultrafresh oil directly from some of the best producers. Their oil can cost as much as top Tuscan, although some good, fresh California oil from high-density plantings has been selling for much less.

CATALONIA The olive groves in this region of northeastern Spain are dominated by the Arbequina olive, to the exclusion of almost every other variety. It makes mild, light-textured olive oil with delicate fruit flavor. (I'm wary of most Spanish oil because the main Spanish olive, the Picual, has an aroma that is politely described as herbal but in truth is like cat pee.) Arbequina oil is entirely sweet—completely free of bitterness, with no more than a slight pepperiness—though with its low tannic content, it keeps less well. Its delicacy suits lettuce and fresh fish, foods that are easily overwhelmed by strong, bitter oil.

GREECE Olive cultivation is ancient in Greece, which has diverse regions and varieties, although for now very little of the best oil leaves Greece. It can be clean, light, subtle, delicately fruity, though generally without bold fruit and pepper. Fine oil comes from southern Crete, mostly from Koroneiki olives. The variety of the northern Peloponnesus is Kornea. Kalamata oil, made from the olive of that name, is smooth. Oil from the region of Sparta, from the Koroneiki olive, has more bite. Still more bite comes from the oil produced from Koroneiki in the rocky limestone of Mani (in the Peloponnesus and the southernmost extremity of mainland Europe)—steep, with rare rainfall and rarer application of fertilizer (as a rule, only manure). Yields there are low, and the oil is aromatic and pungent. Methods are organic, though the oil may not be certified, because the people were always poor and the land is too steep for the equipment used to apply chemicals. The harvest begins in November and runs through January.

LIGURIA The Italian Riviera, with its soothing climate and mainly limestone soil, produces a mere 1 percent of all Italian oil, and yet Liguria has always been known for its mild, sweet, light-textured oil. The lightness comes mainly from the famous Ligurian olive, the Taggiasca. Most of the oil is green and modern, especially sweet, with delicate fruit flavor. But some olives are still harvested black, giving a more old-fashioned, mild, sweet Ligurian taste. (Now extinct is *biancardo,* the very pale, delicate, ephemeral oil that used to be made from olives harvested in March and even June.)

PROVENCE Only the Mediterranean fringe of France is warm enough for olive trees, and most Provençal oil is modern in style, with an appealing, slightly restrained fruit and only moderate bitterness and pepper. Two varieties whose names sometimes appear on bottles are Picholine and Aglandau (also called Beruguette). Much of the oil comes from the limestone appellation of Les Baux, where both modern green and more traditional black-fruity oil are made at the cooperative's four-hundred-year-old Jean-Marie Cornille mill. All the olives today are harvested earlier than they used to be, and even the traditional oil has some pepper.

SICILY The best oil I've tasted has been Tuscan, and yet a highly discriminating Tuscan producer I know believes Sicilian oil is the best of all, certain ones having clear tastes of artichokes, for instance, or sun-dried tomatoes. I don't go that far, but I admire Sicilian oil. If you don't know producers, look for oil with a DOP (Denominazione di Origine Protetta), including Monti Iblei and Valdemone.

TUSCANY A disproportionate quantity of the world's top olive oil comes from Tuscany and its aromatic native varieties—Correggiolo, Frantoio, Leccino, and Moraiolo—which have been carried to other parts of the Old and New Worlds. The coolness of Tuscany's limestone hills intensifies the fruit taste. The oil is typically thick-textured, rich in fruit aroma, and its strong tannin enables it to keep unusually well. The vivid pepper and marked bitterness, which can be remarkably aggressive in the young oil, normally coincide with intense fruit. I've always suspected that the aromatic quality of Tuscan oil, including the selection of varieties, originated with a special Tuscan appreciation for the fruit taste from an early harvest. When in the late twentieth century the world market opened for top-quality oil alongside top-quality wine (a Tuscan grower typically had both grapes and olives), the Tuscan sensibility quickly influenced other olive-growing regions. The very best Tuscan oil has a quality I can only describe, to borrow a word used for great wine, as "noble."

Among all the uses of olive oil, the most luxurious is deep-frying in outstanding fresh oil used just once, which makes a costly meal. Not that olive oil is better for the purpose than lard, tallow, or seed oils, only that the taste of fresh olive oil is part of the world's wonderful diversity of fat. Usual deep-frying temperatures are no hotter than 350 degrees F (175 degrees C), safely below the smoke point of extra virgin olive oil, which depending on the example is often well over 400 degrees F (200 degrees C). The fresher the fat of whatever kind, the higher the smoke point and the better the taste. But it's a bad idea to deep-fry in cloudy new olive oil, because the suspended particles burn. And the heat of frying degrades any fat, so each succeeding batch burns at a lower temperature. On another topic of freshness and purity, in making mayonnaise lots of people worry that uncut olive oil will give too strong a flavor, and certainly it's hard to find a use for mayonnaise made with strong, bitter oil. But I reject the idea that good food should be made with heavily processed ingredients, such as greasy refined oil, which deprives us of a sense of the real thing. For mayonnaise, I use a mild, light, fresh olive oil.

A last note on olive oil, which underlines its nature. At the end of a meal in Puglia, it's traditional to eat sweet, tender vegetables—raw celery, chicory tops, new fava beans in spring, fennel, radishes, cucumbers—with olive oil as a *postpasto,* in preference to dessert. The sweet freshness and flavor of the oil have everything in common with the taste of sweet produce fresh from the garden.

HOW TO BUY OLIVE OIL: Those of us who live far from a producing zone, to make good oil more affordable, often use a less-expensive one for cooking and a more special one to add raw as flavoring afterward. Keep in mind with oil that the enemies of deliciousness are heat, light, air, and time. The original quality represented by the grade will have been lost unless the oil has been treated well all during its trek from the mill to your kitchen and table. Especially, the oil must have been kept consistently cool. Greener oil generally has more fruit flavor and lasts longer, and it may be fresher. But the green color comes partly from leaves that are inevitably mixed with the olives by the pickers and then not completely removed at the mill. More leaves give a deeper green, and some less scrupulous growers add leaves to ensure the color they want. The chlorophyll isn't just a pigment but also an antioxidant that helps to protect the oil.

A retailer can be excellent, but the person in charge of olive oil must know and love it—must confirm the quality by tasting when the oil comes in and again from time to time if it doesn't sell rapidly. (Store conditions aren't ideal for keeping oil.) Quality is usually much higher if, rather than buying a blend from a region or country, you buy olive oil that comes from a single property. (Best of all is identifying a great producer and buying directly, but few of us can do that.) Individual estates are more likely to aspire to high standards, but even so you have to know which the good ones are. When faced with unfamiliar Italian bottles, look for oil from one of the better Tuscan or Sicilian DOPs. Some importers sell directly. Or you might come across a special fresh bottle in a small Greek market. All bottles should show clearly the year of harvest, but few do. It suggests especially high quality when a label specifies the day of harvest and pressing, because flavor can differ noticeably even from one pressing to the next—a reflection of the section of trees picked, the steadily advancing ripeness, the time that elapses between picking and pressing, or some variable at the mill.

HOW TO STORE OLIVE OIL: Keep olive oil sealed from air and in a cool, dark place, though not so cold that the oil congeals and can't be poured. Generally, use olive oil within a year of the harvest, although very good oil, with plenty of polyphenols and well cared for, will last two years with no sign of rancidity. Once a bottle is opened, even fairly fresh-tasting olive oil, especially if it's a year or more old, loses noticeable flavor within two weeks.

COMPLEMENTS TO OLIVE OIL: Excellent, fresh-tasting olive oil complements an endless number of foods, and most of them set off the oil in return. Olive oil is especially complemented by garlic, anchovies, salt, and bread, fresh and toasted, and by raw vegetables in salad—obviously lettuce, with its affinity for sweet oil, and not least raw fava beans, which need only olive oil and not a vinaigrette. (When you do make a vinaigrette, use four to five parts or more excellent oil to one of vinegar, so the oil stands out. Old formulas call for less oil, probably because once upon a time the oil used was rarely very good.) Among the many cooked foods that benefit from a final flavoring with raw oil are most meats, especially lamb and grilled beef, most if not all vegetables, especially tomatoes, zucchini, and cooked greens (chard, spinach, collards, optionally flavored with garlic, ham, or both), and clear vegetable soups.

NOTES ON WINE: None.

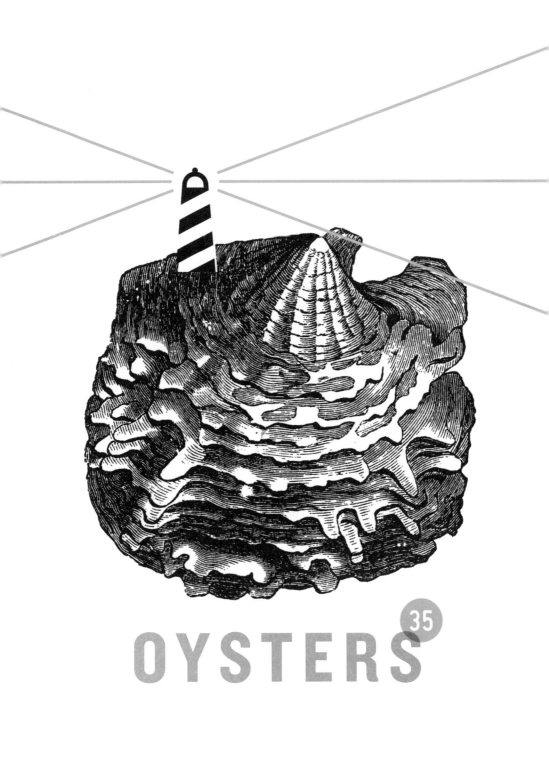

OYSTERS

35. OYSTERS, RAW

Oysters just taken from the water have a clean taste of the sea—no matter how often that description is repeated, it remains the best. No taste is more fundamental. Each kind of oyster in each bay, inlet, and river mouth has its own particular flavor, heavily influenced by what and how much the oysters have been eating lately. They need a mix of fresh water and salt water, for the minerals washed from the land and for the phytoplankton from the sea. An average oyster, to obtain its microscopic food, might filter fifty gallons of water a day. The largest species, the Pacific or Asian oyster, can filter as many as eight gallons an hour. The taste of any oyster reflects the season and weather, the tides, water temperature, and minerals in its stretch of water. More oceanic—saltier—water tends to make a skinnier, saltier oyster. Sweeter water containing more food tends to make a fatter, tastier one. But slower growth in saltier water intensifies flavor and can produce a superior oyster. Besides, different species taste different. A dozen or so are raised around the world, mainly five in North America.

As a rule, the oysters that we eat raw from the shell are cultivated, but not in the sense that anyone feeds them. Both wild and cultivated oysters filter their food from natural waters, with nothing put in or taken out. In contrast to other kinds of aquaculture, because shellfish aren't fed and because they filter the water, they automatically improve its quality. Whether wild or cultivated oysters are superior depends on precisely where they come from, the conditions in that location, and the skill of a farmer at exploiting them. Mainly the oysters are put where they have plenty to eat and plenty of room to grow. You can usually tell a wild oyster, because it hasn't had much room and its shell shows that it was chipped off a larger clump of oysters. Farmers may start the oysters in one location and finish them in another. Some farmers raise them in beds directly on the bottom, while others keep them higher up in the water on floating trays or inside containers such as baskets or bags; the latter is more expensive, but the suspended oysters grow faster.

Shallow water where fresh meets salt almost inevitably supports a thriving population of oysters, if the water is reasonably clean and nothing intervenes. The waters surrounding New York City were once filled with countless acres of oysters, billions of them, as was San Francisco Bay, before powerful changes were made to both. Oyster beds in many places have been lost to filling, dredging, silting, overharvesting, and pollution. The biggest source of oysters in the US was once the huge, shallow Chesapeake Bay, where a few years back the famous Chincoteagues and other oysters were almost eliminated by the parasite-caused diseases MSX and dermo. In the peak year of 1884, twenty million bushels of oysters were dredged from the bay; a recent figure was merely 350,000 bushels (and yet that was a significant increase over the lowest point in 2004). Many bay and other East Coast oysters are still wild. They usually go to shucking houses, while the cultivated ones, with their better-formed shells, go to oyster bars and restaurants. In the US, more oysters now come from Puget Sound in Washington than from anywhere else. Happily, after two centuries of bad news, a small revival is taking place in many waters on both coasts. As interest in eating raw oysters has risen, it's easy to come across diverse kinds of the highest quality and freshness.

Most oysters are named, sometimes highly specifically, for the place they come from, and as more producers have gone into the business, the names have multiplied until there are several hundred or more, including registered trade names. On the Pacific Coast, heading south from Alaska, just a few of the better-known names are Rocky Passes, Fanny Bays, Quilcenes, Samish Bays, Hood Canals, Skookums, Totten Inlets, Thorndyke Bays, Westcott Bay Flats, and Hog Island Flats. On the Atlantic, heading north from the Chesapeake Bay, there are James Rivers, Kent Islands, Cape Mays, the famous Blue Points (named for a projection on the south shore of Long Island, but long a collective name for oysters from Long Island Sound), Widow's Holes, Moonstones, Watch Hills, Whale Rocks, Prudence Points, Barnstables, Buzzards Bays, Cotuits, Wellfleets, Wiannos, Katama

Bays, Spinney Creeks, Pemaquids, Glidden Points, Caraquettes, Tatama-gouches, Bras d'Ors, Malpeques, Pickle Points, Raspberry Points, Red Points, Sea Cow Heads, Saltaires, and Sunnysides, the last seven coming from Prince Edward Island, a prime source. That's not to speak of the many oysters raised in Europe and elsewhere, some of which are flown to North America.

Oyster lovers are naturally drawn to the local kind. Warm-climate oysters, such as from Florida and Louisiana, are delicious when you're there, but they're milder, less salty, and generally softer, giving an impression of more fat. A firmer texture and cleaner taste come from oysters from colder water, which are slower-growing and typically stronger in flavor. In cold water, it can take an oyster five to seven years to reach a size that in a warmer location takes just three. In North America, "cold" might mean all of the Pacific Coast and the Atlantic Coast from Cape Cod northward. And because colder shores are usually more northern and tend to be less populated, the water is often cleaner. There's also a relationship of cold to sweetness, which in a fat oyster is associated with the substance glycogen, stored in the meat in preparation for winter.

When you open a fresh raw oyster, with its complicated pearly coloring, the smell is marine, from mild to strong, sometimes including iodine. The texture can be firm, almost crisp, or smooth, creamy, fatty, melting. The saltiness can be anywhere from mildly briny to sharp. A plump oyster is generally called "fat," and often it's "sweet," too, in the sense of less salty, since a fatter oyster usually comes from less salty water. But some fat oysters give an impression of actual sweetness. Different people perceive oyster flavor slightly differently. Possibilities include mineral, metallic, coppery, steely, tinny, creamy, nutty, and buttery. Tasters make comparisons to grass, fruit, citrus, kiwi, melon, and cucumber. Whatever the effect, no element of taste should dominate the rest.

Once upon a time, before there was refrigeration, it may have been considerably safer to avoid eating oysters in the *r*-less (summer) months. Besides worry about illness from bacteria during the warmest time of year, that's also when oysters spawn and aren't appetizing. But now some cultivated oysters have been bred not to spawn. (Since they don't reproduce, they never become established in the wild and must always be seeded.) Today we ignore the old *r* rule. We trust the producer and the government to test and shut down the beds when bacterial or other problems arise, although it's not a perfect system.

For taste, however, the best season for eating oysters is certainly linked to water temperature. When it falls below about 42 degrees F (6 degrees C), oysters become dormant. On the Atlantic from Cape Cod northward that occurs around early December. The oysters are at their peak—best-fed and fattest—from October to the end of the year, when the operations shut down for winter as ice makes harvesting difficult and uneconomical. The colder the location, the earlier the peak and the later the oysters start to eat again in spring. Where the water doesn't get cold enough to send the oysters into dormancy, they can be harvested through the winter. In Puget Sound, for instance, the season runs from September through April, with the peak coming in December and January.

Oysters grow faster if they're continuously submerged and feeding, rather than exposed at low tide, when they shut tight. And they grow faster if they're spread out so they don't compete for food. They also acquire a more typical shape with a deeper cup—referring to the half shell that will hold the raw oyster and its liquor. The more tightly the shells close, the better the oysters keep once they leave the water. The Eastern oyster, native to the North American East Coast, is the species with the tightest shell. Tighter shells also occur when oysters are tumbled in the water by waves and currents, which strengthens the adductor muscle that pulls the shells together. (The same muscle in a scallop is much larger and constitutes all that is commonly eaten.) A British Columbia producer I spoke with raises his oysters in deep water for speed and better meat and then "beach-hardens" them along the shore, where they open and close with the tides.

From most to least common, these are the five important species in North America:

THE PACIFIC, OR ASIAN, OYSTER The biggest, fastest-growing, most widely farmed of the world's commercial species is the Pacific,

Crassostrea gigas, originally from Japan, where it has been cultivated for centuries. Today it's the common oyster in Europe, and
on the West Coast of North America the oysters as a rule are Pacifics, often called "gigas." Around the world, Pacifics are so well
adapted and have become so widespread that they are considered
invasive. The shape, generally oblong and somewhat cupped, is
irregular and variable depending on where the oysters grow. Although they aren't ranked at the top for flavor, when carefully and
slowly grown they make some of the finest oysters. They're meaty
and have typical flavors of melon and cucumber; often they're
called sweet. Pacifics keep only a short time after harvest, holding
good quality for less than a week.

THE EASTERN, OR AMERICAN, OYSTER The only oyster native to the
Atlantic Coast, *C. virginica* is found from the Canadian Maritimes
to the Gulf of Mexico. In these days when oysters are shipped
across borders, rather than use the confusing name Eastern or
American, the trade sometimes calls them "*virginica*s." Some today
are also raised in the Pacific. The shape is typically elongated and
somewhat cupped. Less meaty, and saltier than other species,
Eastern oysters are also stronger flavored than most. I like them
best of all. Eastern oysters shut the tightest and keep the longest—
two months or more in the low 40s F (5 to 7 degrees C), but for
flavor the maximum time might be a week in summer and two in
winter.

THE EUROPEAN OYSTER The native species along coasts from Norway to the Mediterranean, cultivated notably in France, is *Ostrea
edulis,* also called the Belon, after the short river of that name in
Brittany that has long been known for its oysters. Compared with
the Eastern oyster, the European is smaller, with a more circular
and flatter—less cupped—shell. After their shape, European oysters are often called "flats." Yet especially after disease hit the species in the 1920s, it was partly displaced by the Portuguese oyster

(*C. angulata,* dumped overboard in 1868 from a ship in the Gironde Estuary, which leads to Bordeaux). It suffered again from disease in the 1970s and in the 80s, when it was nearly eliminated. (There are still only limited preventive measures.) By then the Portuguese, too, had been attacked by disease and the Pacific oyster had been brought in to replace it. Pollution and higher water temperatures due to global warming may also have had an effect. Cultivation of flats persists in Europe but only in minute quantities. Many more are raised in the United States, where disease hasn't affected them. The first time I tasted a European oyster, the intensity made me think of a cured anchovy yet somehow without the fishiness. But when flats are raised more quickly using suspended culture, the taste is milder. Compared with other species, the flavor is more often flinty, even metallic, with iodine. For my taste, the European is second in deliciousness to the Eastern oyster. The shells are softer than those of other species, with more flexible, crumbly edges, so they don't close as tightly. Europeans are the most perishable oysters after harvest, providing good eating for at most several days.

THE KUMAMOTO OYSTER *C. sikamea,* not much bigger than the Olympia, the smallest North American species, originated on the southern Japanese island of Kyushu in Kumamoto Bay, where, thanks to pollution, the oysters are all but extinct. Happily, fifty years ago some Kumamotos were transferred to Humboldt Bay in California, and today they are cultivated in various West Coast locations. They're available year-round, even in summer, when Pacifics and Olympias are spawning. The shell of a Kumamoto, compared with that of its close relative the Pacific, is rounder, the ridges that emanate from the hinge are more pronounced, and the cup is deeper, holding a small but full-bodied oyster. Kumamoto flavor is mild, with the same melon or cucumber flavor and sweetness as a Pacific. Because of the small size, mildness, and sweetness, Kumamotos are often proposed as beginner's oysters. And yet they're no less admired and excellent. They keep slightly better than Pacifics, for at most a week.

THE OLYMPIA OYSTER The only oyster species native to the West Coast, and not often seen for sale outside the state of Washington, *O. lurida* is considered by some to be the finest oyster of all. Its cupped oval shell is only the size of a silver dollar. The smallness and slow growth make the Oly expensive. Although its natural range is from British Columbia to Baja California, in all that area few wild Olys are found, for the usual reasons of pollution and overharvesting. In Puget Sound in the first half of the twentieth century, algal blooms caused by outflow from pulp mills nearly eliminated the rich oyster beds. Producers today concentrate on the much larger and more profitable Pacifics. With human help, however, Olympias are being reestablished in Puget Sound, which is the source of most of the Olympias for sale. Their meat is firm, sweet, delicate, refined, and distinguished by a coppery aftertaste, at least in oysters from Totten Inlet, in the southern part of Puget Sound. The strong taste somewhat recalls that of a European oyster. And like Pacifics, Olympias have a component of melon or cucumber, which some people perceive as celery. They keep for perhaps a week.

HOW TO BUY IN-SHELL OYSTERS OR ORDER AT AN OYSTER BAR: Oysters are at their best the moment they're taken from the water, and really top quality, depending on the species, lasts no more than a day or two—a hint of fishiness completely undoes the taste of the sea that is the entire point of a raw oyster. Try to eat European oysters (flats, or Belons) within a couple of days, and most other oysters within four or five days; Eastern oysters (*virginica*s) may be good for a week. Oysters keep longer at times of year when the water is especially cold and bacterial counts are low, and when they're kept very cold after harvest.

Oysters are fattest and tastiest—at peak season—from October through December from the Maritimes to Cape Cod, a little later in the mid-Atlantic states. In Puget Sound and in Tomales Bay in California, for example, although the oysters are mostly bred not to spawn and the season is year-round, they're slightly less good in summer, fatter in fall. On the Gulf Coast, oysters are a little fatter in winter, but the warmth and lower salinity mean the oysters largely taste the same year-round. It can be ideal to buy oysters directly from a good producer—after the date of harvest the most important thing is the producer. Some ship directly to retail customers, though the weight of the shells makes overnight shipping costly. Equally good sources can be a fishmonger, oyster bar, or restaurant that really knows oysters and has rapid turnover, and then you can taste a selection of varieties.

Faced with a display of oysters closed in their shells, you can tell a little something from appearance. Dry shells are bad, and if any oysters are gaping, it's time to leave. If you see some being opened, check that they contain a lot of meat for the size of the shell. If you know what's local or in peak season, choose that. At an oyster bar with an unfamiliar selection, it's ideal to be able to describe your taste to a knowledgeable shucker behind the counter, who can give you what you like. To cite two rough opposites, you might ask for firm, briny, metallic oysters or mild, nutty, soft, and creamy ones. Nowadays a typical serving of medium-sized oysters is half a dozen, but it used to be a dozen, and many oyster lovers will eat more than that.

One way to judge whether an oyster bar or restaurant cares about oysters is by the way they're opened. A good shucker is neat—doesn't serve oysters with cracked shells, hasn't spilled all the liquor, doesn't nick the meat with the knife, and in freeing the meat from the shell doesn't leave it looking like "scrambled eggs" (in the disgusted words of one producer). John Bil, of Prince Edward Island, a champion oyster shucker whose depth of knowledge never fails to impress me, glances momentarily at each oyster as he opens it and occasionally tosses one aside because the meat is too dry or not as opaque from good feeding or just doesn't look the way it should for its kind. It's key that the person opening oysters knows how each kind should look, in order to reject any individual that falls short.

HOW TO STORE IN-SHELL OYSTERS: During the hours before you eat them, keep oysters cold, about 40 degrees F (4 degrees C), not in water but with damp towels over and under. Hold them in a refrigerator or in a cooler on ice with the drain opened. When an oyster is too cold, you can't fully taste it, but a thorough chill underlines the sea taste.

HOW TO OPEN AN OYSTER: Shuck oysters only just before you eat them. If you're a novice, besides watching an expert at work, it's essential to have a good oyster knife or you may become too frustrated to get the knack. Some designs are badly inferior, and some metal is poor, the blade bending or the tip breaking after only a few shells. The steel should be extremely tough, hard but not brittle, and the handle should be comfortably rounded. The test of an oyster knife is opening thousands of oysters. The North American brand with the best reputation is Dexter-Russell; among the patterns, I use a Boston no. 22.

Some pros, particularly on the West Coast, open the oyster's rounded edge, while others go in at the hinge, which is what I do. With most oysters, it may be easier. First, with a towel, brush clean the hinges and sides, wherever the knife will enter. Place the cupped half of the shell down, and grip the oyster firmly in a heavy towel, folded double or triple to protect your hand in case you slip with the knife. Keep the oyster more or less level, so it retains the juice after it's opened. Push the tip of the blade directly into the hinge, a spot that may take practice to locate. Move the knife just slightly up and down or side to side, or rotate it just slightly back and forth. When the tip of the blade has penetrated an eighth of an inch or so, twist it back and forth while continuing to push, so as to pry open the shell—some oysters open much more easily than others. Once the hinge is slightly open, rather than thrust the blade deep to fully remove the shell, which might cut or dirty the meat, reenter at the side. Keep the point in contact with the top shell as you scrape the blade against it, cutting the adductor muscle, which holds the shells together. Discard the top shell, still aiming not to spill the liquid, and free the oyster from the bottom shell: cut the adductor where it is attached beneath the meat. (The French style, however, is to leave the muscle in place and the oyster attached.) Last, use the blade to remove any dirt or fragment of shell, wiping the blade clean on your towel. To keep the meat clean, touch it with the knife as little as possible.

In telling how to open an oyster, I've given the standard instruction to keep the shell level so as not to spill the juice. When the oysters are ultrafresh and not too salty, most oyster lovers think the liquid adds to the taste. One oysterman calls it "nectar." And yet some French connoisseurs discard that liquid and consume only what re-forms as the oyster briefly waits, on the theory that the new liquid is fresher, while other French connoisseurs reject any liquid as being as salty and boring as seawater. Taste and decide for yourself—I enjoy the liquor. (A few refined oyster eaters don't chew the slippery raw oyster, or they hardly chew. They just swallow. But chewing is the only way to fully experience the taste.)

COMPLEMENTS TO RAW OYSTERS: Raw oysters are for minimalists. Nearly all the classic accompaniments detract, if only a little. You can prove that to yourself by trying a dozen oysters with and without each of these: lemon juice, freshly grated horseradish, cocktail sauce, and *sauce mignonette*. The last is red-wine vinegar mixed with crushed black pepper and shallots, finely chopped at the moment of serving. Most *mignonette* has been sitting for hours or days—the shallots are old, and the sauce is completely distasteful—but even a freshly made one doesn't enhance an oyster.

One classic item is an exception to the no-accompaniments rule: plain buttered rye bread, without seeds. It does no harm. From a very different realm, the Bordelais combination of raw oysters with grilled spicy sausages gives an appealing contrast of cold with hot, raw with cooked. You eat an oyster, then a bite of sausage, then a bite of bread, follow that with a swallow of wine, and again and again. Originally, the oysters would have been flats, the more flavorful native European species, and maybe they're the only kind that makes the combination really great. Austin de Croze, a gastronome who recorded French dishes in the first part of the twentieth century, cited an alternative to the sausages: grilled rib-eye steak with a rich, long-cooked shallot-vinegar sauce—a bite's worth of meat for each oyster. (His metric amounts convey the proportions: to go with a 750-gram steak, slowly cook 250 grams finely chopped shallots with a liter of vinegar, until the liquid is almost entirely gone and the shallots have been reduced to purée.)

NOTES ON WINE: The common advice is that the wine for raw oysters should be acidic enough to play the role of lemon; thus, the theory goes, you drink a Muscadet, a New Zealand Sauvignon Blanc, a Sancerre. But one fall in tastings over a period of weeks, I found that the notion of drinking a more acidic wine, like the idea of the lemon itself, was somewhat mistaken. The wine almost never flattered the oyster (and the lemon juice never did). Besides the role of acidity, the wine's flavors and concentration were very important. And what kind of oyster are we talking about? Their different flavors, intensities, degrees of saltiness, and sensations of sweetness and fat all affect the wine. More flavorful oysters naturally call for a more flavorful wine. (Exceptionally, you come across recommendations for red wine, but even the lightest red, in my experience, is too dry and tannic for oysters, and the tannin can create metallic and fishy effects.) Crossing all the complications of wines with those of oysters might take years of tasting, with travel in season, to really understand, and then a short fanatical book to present them.

With oysters, good Chablis may be not only the safest but usually the best choice. The wine's mineral, even steely, aromas echo those of the oysters. And the stronger flavors of better Chablis work well with European flat oysters having a more iodine component. What works best is the best Chablis—a *premier* or *grand cru* bottle from a top producer (François Raveneau, René and Vincent Dauvissat, Laurent Tribut, William Fèvre).

Dry Champagne, blanc de blancs (made solely from Chardonnay grapes), is another common choice, and it's fairly safe, though it may not provide synergy. What's needed is a bottling with less flavor of fruit and more of yeast-bread-toast. (Similarly, the more fruit-flavored and floral Rieslings and floral Chenins aren't at odds with the shellfish, but, rather than the flavors interacting, they only coexist.) In sparkling wine, the gas that forms the bubbles is itself somewhat acidic, underlining the wine's clean crispness. The Paris sommelier Philippe Bourguignon, whose *L'Accord Parfait* remains by far the best book on matching food with French wine, recommends with Belons an old Champagne or a "vinous" one.

Some wholly dry Alsace Riesling qualifies as acidy and mineral enough for oysters. I've liked white Graves and Pessac-Léognan (the latter appellation contains the famous old Graves properties, from the time when the two appellations were one), which are the classics to accompany the small, spicy grilled sausages mentioned above. I've also liked traditional white Rioja (from López de Heredia, for example—there isn't that much traditional Rioja) with more flavorful oysters, including Maine flats. And while the old recommendation of Muscadet may not be special, a good one isn't bad with most oysters, and excellent bottles of Muscadet from organically grown, hand-picked grapes go for a song, compared with many wines that are much less interesting.

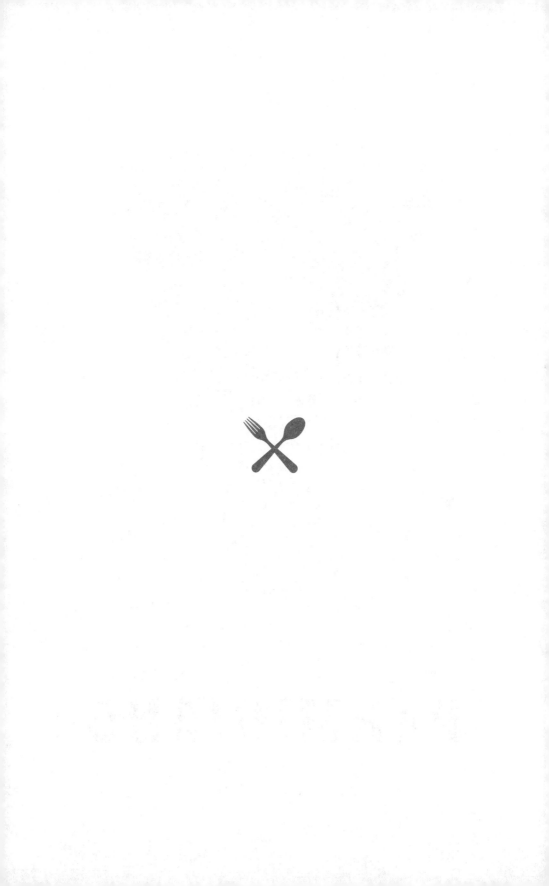

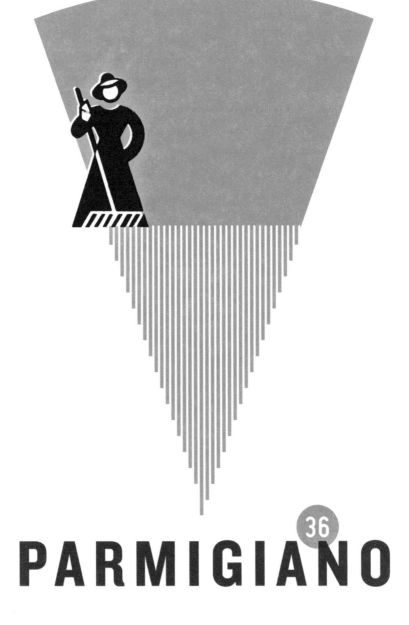

PARMIGIANO 36

36. PARMIGIANO-REGGIANO AND OTHER GRATING CHEESES

There's no more refined cheese in the world than Parmigiano-Reggiano, which blends with a wider range of foods than any other aged cheese. Besides its use as grating cheese, genuine aged Parmesan, to use the venerable English name, is excellent on its own, standing up easily as the single cheese of a cheese course. Under its Denominazione di Origine Protetta (DOP), Parmigiano-Reggiano is made in enormous quantities in a large area of mostly plain, encompassing the city of Parma, in the northern Italian region of Emilia-Romagna. The wheels must weigh a minimum of 30 kilos (66 pounds), and, as with other large cheeses, the milk for Parmigiano comes from cows. As early as the twelfth century, the area began to produce a cheese something like it: the curd was broken into bits and then heated to release as much whey as possible and produce a big, firm, dry cheese suitable for transport and long keeping. The broad type is called *grana,* "grain," named for the rough, grainy surface of the split cheese. From an early date, perhaps the beginning, *grana* was commonly grated. Today *grana* is produced in a huge section of northern Italy, where, besides Parmigiano-Reggiano, much is sold as Grana Padano (or, within that label, Trentingrana), which is typically a lesser cheese sold at a much lower price than the best Parmigiano. Yet Parmigiano can be a better value, considering that the concentrated flavor goes a long way. Parmigiano so dominates its swath of northern Italy that in much of the area it's the only traditional cheese.

There's a lot of talk these days of *terroir* in cheese, meaning that the taste reflects the place where the cheese was made, but the huge Parmigiano-Reggiano zone encompasses such diverse climates and soils that it's hard to point to unified effects of place. Mainly, the taste comes from the method. But an important influence is always what the animals eat. No silage is permitted for Parmigiano, and at least half the diet must be hay or grass (more than that is required for certain European cheeses). The best part of the zone for forage, and therefore milk and cheese, begins at the southern edge of the plain, about six miles (ten kilometers) from Parma at the closest point. From there the hills ascend to the Apennines and have wetter, richer pastures. The richest, anywhere, are south-facing. Mountain Parmigiano can handle longer aging, perhaps in part because more of the farms raise some cattle of the old breeds.

The world's dairy breeds evolve, slowly in the past and these days more quickly, selected for particular traits and at times crossed. During the twentieth century many Western dairy breeds declined or disappeared altogether, swallowed up or displaced by other breeds, primarily high-volume Holsteins. That happened in the Parmigiano zone, too, until it seemed that the original cattle might become extinct. They are the *vacche rosse,* "red cows," officially called Reggiana, and the closely related white breed Bianca Modenese, also called Bianca Valpadana. In the 1950s, there were 140,000 red cows and about the same number of white. By 1980, fewer than 1,000 red cows were left and not even that many white. Today, after a period of revival, the number of red is stable at about 2,500, but the white has continued to decline. A few dairies make wheels of Parmigiano from the milk of only one breed or the other. The traditional cattle are hardier and longer-lived, and their milk contains a more elastic form of casein (part of the protein) called KBB, which allows the curd to lose more whey and makes softer Parmigiano, as you can readily tell when you taste and compare. The red and white breeds give less milk than Holsteins, but their milk contains more protein and results in more cheese. That by itself isn't enough to offset the smaller quantity of milk, but the cheese of the traditional cows is also higher in quality and commands a higher price. Thus red and white cows turn out to be more profitable than Holsteins. Outside the area, though, their cheese is scarce.

Before it is turned into cheese, the raw evening milk rests overnight in shallow pans, where the cream rises. In the morning, most is taken off for butter and other uses. The skimmed milk is mixed with the whole morning milk in giant copper cauldrons. The only starter added is tart whey, full of lactic bacteria, from the cheesemaking of the day before. The milk is warmed to 86 to 91 degrees F (30 to 33 degrees C), and a tiny amount of calf rennet goes in. In a dozen minutes, a delicate curd has set. The cheese-maker breaks up the curd with the long-handled *spino,* a giant stainless-steel whisk with thin, sharp blades, which leave tiny bits of curd floating in whey. For twenty to thirty minutes, the curd is "cooked"—heated slowly to 131 degrees F (55 degrees C), which shrinks the tiny pieces so they release more whey. Finally, in a moment of drama, a cheesemaker gathers up the curd from the cauldron in a huge cloth, leaving behind the whey. The curd is divided between two circular molds, once always wooden and tightened with ropes. The molds are packed tight and compressed. Unlike that of most hard cheeses, the curd for Parmigiano is so dense and cohesive that it isn't mechanically pressed. After a few days, the new cheeses are put into brine, where they soak for up to three weeks.

Aging takes place in vast warehouses at a rather warm 68 degrees F (20 degrees C or so). Under the DOP rules, the wheels must be a year old, but the best age well for two years, and a very few top wheels improve for up to three years as their aromas become finer and more complex. Time magnifies defects as well as strengths, and there is a point when even the best cheese is as good as it will ever be and then it starts to decline.

There are, of course, other Italian grating cheeses besides Parmigiano and Grana Padano, some of them superb, and not all made from cow's milk. Good ones are much more difficult to find outside Italy than good Parmigiano. Much Italian *pecorino*—ewe's-milk cheese—made for grating is uninteresting and even rough in taste, but a little is great. Particularly fine are certain examples of Pecorino di Pienza *stagionato* ("aged") from the Val d'Orcia in Tuscany (albeit made from pasteurized milk). It's so hard to compete with the Italian grating cheeses that comparably good North American ones hardly exist. The best I've found were goat's-milk grating cheeses with the butterscotch edge that comes with age.

Up to a point, more fat gives more flavor to cheese, and it slows dry-ing, which allows longer aging. And yet for Parmigiano, some of the cream is skimmed. That was once true of many cheeses, and it continues for Par-migiano because there must be a balance between the fat and the casein in the milk or the hard, dry cheese will lose fat. Protein and fat are highest in fall milk, and thus the fall cheeses are the richest and most suited to aging. In a perfect world, you would look for a cheese made in fall from the milk of Reggiano or Modenese cattle living in the hills and eating outdoors on south-facing pastures.

Young Parmigiano-Reggiano can recall fresh-cut grass and hay, fresh fruits, sometimes pineapple, certain cooked vegetables, yogurt, butter. At a middle age running up to twenty-four months, a cheese may recall melted butter, citrus fruit, nuts, and meat stock. After thirty months, a cheese is stronger and slightly saltier, with more prominent flavors of nuts, along with suggestions of dried fruits and spice. Any good Parmigiano has a clean taste and a long aftertaste. The top wheels aren't creamy and easygoing but sour and sweet at the same time, with the sweetness appearing as caramel.

HOW TO BUY PARMIGIANO-REGGIANO: Try to taste before you buy—in a shop in Italy a taste is automatic. Buy a piece including rind (never, it may go without saying, buy already grated cheese). Preferably turn to a seller who particularly understands Parmigiano, knowing when wheels are at their peak and selecting well. Such a seller will almost certainly offer two or three wheels at different levels of quality and price. It's best if the cheese is cut to order, which may never happen outside Italy, and if you're lucky, the wheel will have just been opened. On the side of a whole wheel, you can read the age: the month, in Italian, appears in three letters, followed by the year in two digits, such as OTT 11; above them is the number of the plant. The wheel also shows the seal of the Parmigiano-Reggiano consortium (or the red- or white-cow one). Top, bottom, and sides, all the rest of the rind is covered with the name "Parmigiano-Reggiano," over and over, formed of small dots.

There's nothing remotely wrong with well-made younger Parmigiano, a little more than a year old, but with the very best cheese older is better, two and, very exceptionally, three years. More-aged cheese contains tiny, whitish crystalline grains, which are bits of transformed protein that crunch softly in your mouth, a favorable sign.

In North America, wheels of Parmigiano-Reggiano are normally cut open and reduced to retail-sized pieces with a power saw, which creates a large amount of sawdustlike "grated" cheese. The traditional Italian tactic yields a much more attractive result: a stubby, spadelike blade, in a skilled hand, scores the circumference, perforates the scored line, wedges the cheese apart, and further divides it into pieces. The exposed surface looks like split granite. Emilian shops and market sellers open their own wheels and pry off flakes for customers to taste. Parmigiano is among the more durable cheeses, but it's best to buy no more than you will use within two or three weeks.

HOW TO STORE AND SERVE PARMIGIANO-REGGIANO: The rind protects the whole wheel, but an exposed piece holds its flavor better in the cold. Wrap it well in plastic and refrigerate it. Avoid the pebbly texture that comes from "grating" a cheese with the blade of a food processor; hand-grating results in a light, loose texture that gives more flavor and mixes more easily. For maximum flavor, grate the cheese just before serving, or put the whole piece on the table, wrapped in a napkin, along with a grater. For Parmigiano served as a course on its own, pass a plate of freshly flaked pieces or else a large wedge stuck with a small Parmigiano knife (miniatures do exist) or another short, strong blade.

COMPLEMENTS TO PARMIGIANO-REGGIANO: Some of the most familiar and best are garlic, onion, mushrooms, bulb fennel (raw or cooked), butter and olive oil (such as in pasta dishes), walnuts (as in pesto), basil (pesto again). Parmigiano goes in soups, risotto, and pasta. Some people say that grating cheese doesn't go with fish and seafood, but in Italy they're often combined in pasta dishes, and they usually taste good. (How well does cheese go with fish in general? Usually not well, but grating cheese works when the fish is combined with tomato and other strong flavors.) Shavings of it make an excellent, big-flavored combination with raw rocket (arugula), put on red meats or on pizza just taken from the oven. A luxurious, special combination is small pieces of Parmigiano with drops of traditional balsamic vinegar.

NOTES ON WINE: I love a big meal with a cheese course, but for many people a whole course is too much, and with a meal of any size a taste of Parmigiano can be just right. But what to drink with it? Some people opt for Champagne, which isn't a mistake. In Emilia, a common choice is the local sparkling red Lambrusco. A lesser Chianti won't work, but a mature, full-flavored one will, and so will more concentrated, mature Nebbiolo wines. The Italian red most often recommended, though, is Valpolicella. Regular plain bottlings generally lack enough flavor to stand up to the cheese, but better examples of Valpolicella Classico Superiore work, and success is most likely with one of the two concentrated forms of Valpolicella, Amarone or Recioto, which are made from semidried grapes. Those wines need plenty of fruit flavor, and beware that some Recioto has too much sugar. The modern versions of these wines work, but the flavors of an older traditional bottle are more fun. I hesitate to break the trinity of bread, cheese, and wine, but eating a little of the concentrated cheese and sipping the strong wine, you can do without bread.

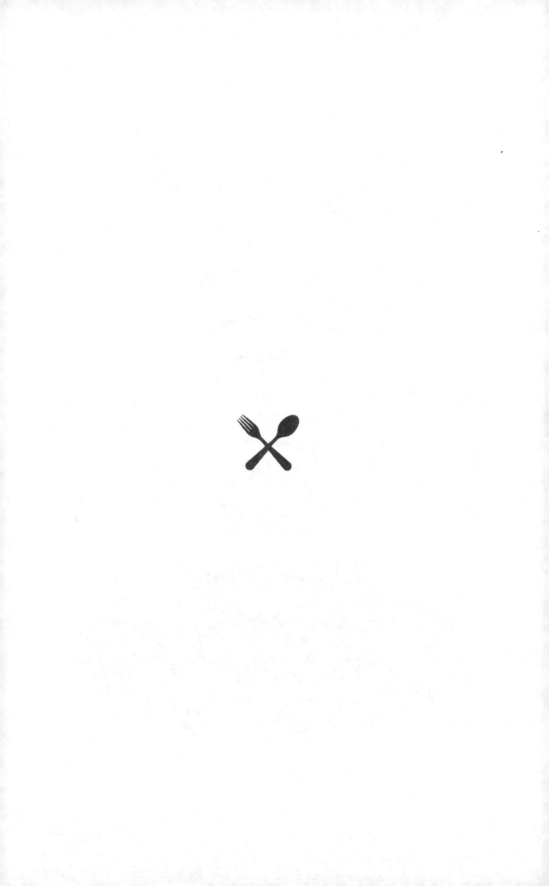

PASTA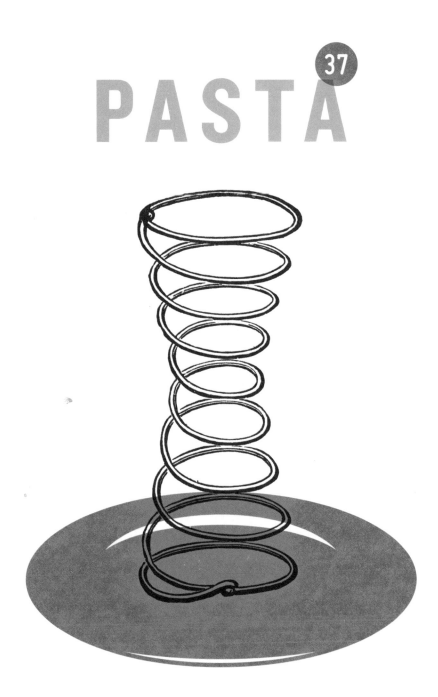

asta in Italy divides into the fresh egg pasta of the north and the equally delicious durum-flour-and-water pasta of the south, which is usually dried. The first kind is made of *grano tenero,* the relatively soft wheat also used to make most Italian bread, and the taste of egg is at least as important as that of the wheat. Probably more important than either one is the precise yielding but somewhat firm texture. All the best of this *pasta fresca* is made by hand, typically rolled out in a vast sheet covering an entire table. Any worthy restaurant in northern Italy makes its own, which used to mean that nearby housewives came in for a time each day. No Italian would ever claim that pasta from a machine of any sort is the same. The second kind of pasta is made of *grano duro,* hard durum wheat, mixed with only water and then commonly dried to make *pastasciutta* ("dried pasta"). The focus is on the taste of great durum wheat. When Americans eat pasta in Italy, we're often struck by the small quantity of sauce, but for Italians what's important is the pasta. At quick everyday family meals, pasta may be the main item, but otherwise pasta in Italy is a *primo* (a first course, which at other times might be soup, risotto, or gnocchi) and not a *secondo,* like fish or meat. In no other country is there such widespread critical admiration for pasta. An Italian friend wrote to me not long ago, "Pasta is one of those subjects I consider infinite . . . Like wine. Or cheese."

Pasta is made from ingredients other than wheat, and of course it's made in other countries. And the divide between fresh-egg and dried-durum isn't really that simple. Egg pasta is sometimes dried, and durum pasta is sometimes eaten fresh. And soft-wheat fresh pasta doesn't invariably contain egg (Tuscan *pici* are made with water). Pasta belongs to the cooking of Spain (*fideos*), Greece (whose *trahana* is fermented), and North Africa (whose couscous was originally made by Berbers). Egg noodles are part of the cooking of Germany, Hungary, and other European countries. The first people to make pasta were the Chinese, at least four thousand years ago, and they were the first to make filled pasta. Noodles are important in Japanese, Korean, and other Asian cuisines. Judging by the roots of various Italian words for pasta, it might have been brought to Italy by Greeks or by Arabs.

All over Italy, not only regions but here and there individual villages make particular kinds and shapes. The flour is normally white but sometimes whole wheat, and sometimes wheat flour is mixed with buckwheat or chestnut flour. Counting kinds is like counting French cheeses: how many you end up with depends on how hard you look and where you draw the lines. The historian Oretta Zanini De Vita, in her *Encyclopedia of Pasta,* describes 310 kinds, from *abbotta pezziende* (durum-flour lozenge shapes from Abruzzo) to *zumari* (durum-flour strips from Puglia, almost extinct). But even hers isn't the last word.

The region of Emilia, which includes Parma and Bologna, has by some accounts the best, and certainly the richest, traditional cooking in Italy, and it may be the world center of appreciation for egg pasta. The various filled shapes, often served in rich broth—ravioli, *tortelli, cappelletti,* and more— might contain well-cooked tender meat, ham, sausage, or mortadella, alone or mixed with greens or rice or ricotta along with breadcrumbs and grated cheese. And there are more fillings in other places. From Mantova, in the Veneto, comes *ravioli di zucca,* filled with winter squash. One of the great pleasures of the Langa area of Piedmont is *agnolotti,* typically filled with meat but also sometimes greens. Filled pasta in the north is often served simply with butter flavored with fresh sage. And beyond the traditional fillings, now almost anything is possible.

Pasta, especially dried, is part of the everyday diet all over Italy, but a few generations ago that wasn't true. Most Italians lived in the countryside, worked in agriculture, and were poor. Pasta took time to make; bread was the everyday starch. For most Italians, pasta was only a feast-day food—and all the more highly valued. In large areas of Italy, it was eaten only once or twice a year. The big exception was Naples and the surrounding towns, where by the sixteenth century family businesses were making and selling pasta. In Naples, *maccheroni,* dried pasta, was the archetypal street food of the poor, who lowered the strands into their mouths with their fingers. Pasta was equally a food of the city's nobles but with more luxurious sauces and condiments.

The first European pasta was probably made from durum wheat, and in Italy it spread north from Sicily. *Grano duro* contains less starch and more protein than other wheat. It grows in arid places, giving higher yields there than *grano tenero* does. In the durum-wheat region of Puglia, the heel of the Italian boot, the bread, too, is made of *grano duro* (above all the outstanding hemispherical loaf of the ancient town of Altamura, where the bread of certain bakeries is as good as any I've ever eaten). The quality of the raw material—the wheat itself together with the milling—is extremely important. Some varieties and strains of durum wheat are more flavorful than others. The best-known older one is called Senatore Cappelli, a specialty of the pasta maker Latini, in Abruzzo, and there are Mongibello, Quadrato, San Carlo, Varano, and more varieties.

One of the first places where pasta was made and dried commercially was the town of Gragnano, a short way south of Naples, called *la città della pasta.* As early as the seventeenth century, most Gragnanesi were already employed making dried pasta. The breezes from the Gulf of Sorrento were ideal for drying, and streams from the hills provided water to turn the grain mills, as well as to mix with the flour. Well into the twentieth century, racks of pasta were set to dry in the street. Today in Gragnano, three of the remaining companies are more industrial, about ten are more artisanal, and there are also some *microartigiani.* Recently, "Pasta di Gragnano" became a controlled appellation (Indicazione Geografica Protetta), which will help maintain quality. The packages I've bought held dark yellow-tan pasta with a dusty-, almost sandy-looking surface. The flavor was vastly greater than that of other dried pasta I've tried.

Better factories press the dough through plain bronze dies, *trafile,* rather than Teflon-coated ones. The bronze leaves a rougher texture that holds more sauce. Much more important is slow drying. Natural drying took two days to two weeks or more, highly dependent on the weather. Today most pasta is dried with hot air in a few hours. But the best small-scale Italian companies stayed with slower drying, using gentler sources of heat, a method that now is back in vogue. It takes one to two days, according to the shape and ambient humidity.

A few of the more common southern shapes are *strozzapreti* or *strangolapreti* ("priest stranglers" in varied shapes, often oblong and folded or twisted), *cavatelli* (indented so they curl inward and look a little like small hats), and *bucatini* (long, hollow tubes). *Spaghettoni,* fat "strings," hold their firm texture much better than the usual thin spaghetti, which even after they're drained tend to overcook before you have time to eat them. Some of the southern shapes are made particularly by hand. Once they all were; the hollow ones were rolled around a straw. In the old part of Bari, in Puglia, women sit outside their houses forming *orecchiette* ("little ears") by hand, leaving the impression of a thumb in each little disk. They sell them to restaurants or shops. In Abruzzo, fine spaghettilike strands are cut on wires *alla chitarra,* "guitar style"; they have rougher sides and a square cross section and therefore more surface area.

Two well-known kinds of pasta are really little dumplings. "The *gnocco,*" says Zanini's *Encyclopedia of Pasta,* "is the ancestor of almost all the Italian pastas." Gnocchi were made originally with breadcrumbs or flour and only later began to be lightened with potato. The other kind, *gnudi,* "nudes," are ravioli fillings without any pasta covering. They're mixtures of flour with cooked chard or spinach, ricotta, *pecorino* cheese, and a little spice. They sound like a playful modern innovation, but they go back to the 1200s. They seem hardly to be pasta at all, and yet in Italy they're always regarded as pasta and are considered the forebear of it.

A variation on the pasta theme is the excellent smoky kind made in various shapes in northern Puglia and part of neighboring Basilicata from *grano arso,* slightly burnt wheat. Once, after the great wheat fields had been harvested and burnt over in the old agricultural practice, the poorest peasants would seek the grains that had fallen to the ground. That wheat was ground into flour and then mixed with some regular flour to make bread and pasta. Today, *grano arso* is specially made, nothing at all to do with poverty. The pasta, eaten in the region with various vegetables and sauces in their seasons, has a gray cast and a delicious mild smokiness.

Doneness is a matter of taste and culture. As you head south in Italy into durum-wheat territory, the pasta is less and less cooked. It remains closer to flour and tastes more strongly of wheat. The pasta I ate in northern Puglia's main city of Foggia was very firm, sometimes so little cooked at the center that it was almost hard. It took chewing and had a raw-flour taste, which wasn't troubling. Once in a restaurant there, I was served pasta as soft as in northern Italy; feeling courageous, when the chef passed by, I complained. He removed the plate immediately with apology, and he soon came back with the usual firm *strangolapreti*.

HOW TO BUY PASTA, WITH A FEW THOUGHTS ABOUT MAKING AND COOKING IT: Better brands leap upward in flavor. Among more industrial producers, a point of reference is the Speciale Gastronomia line from Felicetti in Trentino. Look also for producers from Gragnano, especially the Cooperativa Pastai Gragnanesi, and small producers elsewhere, including Martelli from near Pisa, Latini in Abruzzo (with its single-wheat-variety pastas), Rustichella d'Abruzzo (including its Primo Grano pasta from heirloom wheats), and Benedetto Cavalieri, deep in *grano duro* territory on the Salentine Peninsula of Puglia. Freshness must matter somewhat with dried pasta, and yet, sealed in a plastic package, the good flavor seems to last indefinitely.

If you make pasta yourself, you control the ingredients and freshness. To learn the skill, nothing beats watching someone really accomplished or at least seeing a video. North American unbleached flour has good flavor, but it's higher in protein than Italian, and the dough isn't easy to roll thin. To arrive at the lower protein of Italian oo flour, you might think you could just mix higher-protein flour with low-protein unbleached pastry flour, but pastry flour has little flavor. For North Americans, it's simplest to buy *tipo 00* Italian flour in an Italian market. Otherwise, use our flour and make the dough more tender by adding a little olive oil and extra yolks (the latter, for richness, are sometimes added in Italy). Give the dough a rest of several hours so it can relax before you roll it out.

Strangely, the usual serving of pasta, whether fresh or dried, is the same size. I allow at least five ounces (125 grams) per person, depending on who's eating and what follows. Put the pasta into enough rapidly boiling water for it to move freely, and don't forget to salt the water well, a good tablespoon per gallon (about four liters).

It may be sinful to overcook pasta, but how much is too much? We all know we should cook pasta *al dente*, "to the tooth," but no one seems able to put in words just what that means, partly because it's a matter of taste. Especially with dried pasta, what's interesting is the gradation of texture from the soft surface to the firm core, which is more obvious in thicker shapes. Fresh pasta can never be as firm or have as much variation. The less you cook any pasta, the more flavor it will have. In order not to miss the moment when it's just the way you want it, start biting into samples a couple of minutes ahead. If you plan to mix the pasta with a sauce, drain it a minute or so early and mix it with the sauce to finish cooking in it and absorb its flavor. Use enough sauce to adhere to all the pasta, but not so much that a lot of sauce will be left on the plate. For maximum freshness, I wrap the grating cheese in a napkin and place it on the table with a grater.

COMPLEMENTS TO PASTA: Sauces containing larger pieces go with shapes of pasta of roughly the same size, so they're easier to eat together. Otherwise, the notion that a particular shape goes with a particular sauce is only a matter of old habit in different parts of Italy, as much as it gives pleasure to honor that history. The potential flavor combinations are almost as numerous as foods, starting with the suave noncompetitors—olive oil, butter, cream—and running through garlic, anchovy, and aged grating cheese before branching wide.

NOTES ON WINE: The wine for pasta depends on what you put on it, though the starch smooths things and enlarges the possibilities.

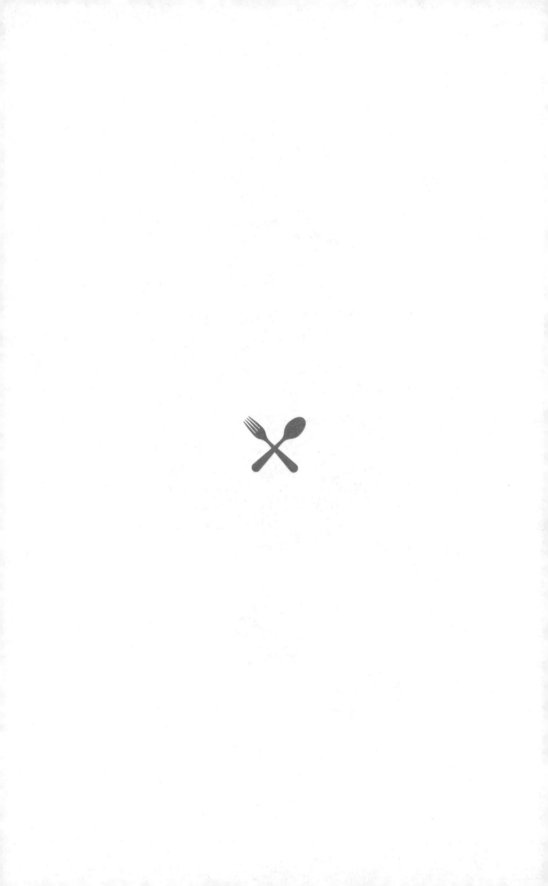

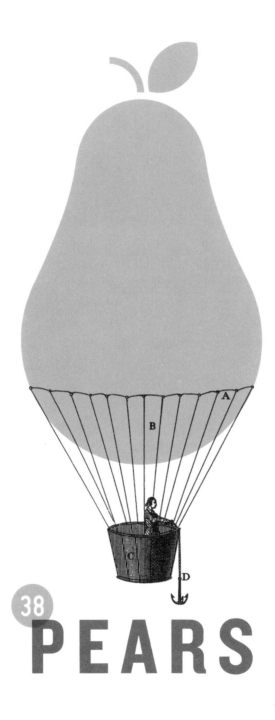

38

PEARS

There's no better ending to a meal, especially a long one, than ripe fruit. And nothing is more perfect than a pear, with its refined, often musky aroma, its sweetness, gentle acidity, juice, and gratifying melting texture. Edward Bunyard, the great English nurseryman and fruit connoisseur of the first half of the twentieth century, wrote in *The Anatomy of Dessert* (whose sole subject is fruit): "I begin with a confession. After thirty years of tasting Pears I am still unfurnished with a vocabulary to describe their flavour." He cited others who found almond, vinousness, rose, honey, walnut, and more flavors. None of those words is wrong, yet none describes the essential flavor of pear. (I mean the European pear, *Pyrus communis,* as opposed to the quite different round, crunchy Asian pears, most of which are *P. pyrifolia.*) The common US varieties—Bartlett, D'Anjou, and Bosc, plus, at a far distance, Comice and then Seckel—all date from the eighteenth and nineteenth centuries and are among the very best. A drawback in certain pears, including good ones, is the gritty cells concentrated around the core, a sort of botanic sand, which is more prevalent if pears are harvested too late. Where almost all fruits ripen on the plant, pears ripen only off the tree. Those raised in the Pacific Northwest, source of most US pears, can survive remarkably well in the not-necessarily-kind US supermarket distribution system. Because growers *must* pick hard fruit, it can be handled and shipped without damage. The rest of us can then buy pears, leave them out to ripen for a day or a week, as needed, and eat them tender and fully ripe. Perfect ripeness, when it finally arrives, may last only a day.

For that to happen, though, the grower must harvest the pears when they are "mature"—neither too early nor too late. Professionals judge by firmness using a penetrometer, which sends a plunger into the flesh, and for different varieties they seek somewhat different resistance. Home growers are told that a pear is mature when you twist it upward and it snaps off briskly, except for Bosc, which doesn't readily detach. Most varieties also subtly lighten in color. Pears left on the tree never develop full aroma; instead they turn coarse and mealy, and brown at the core, and then they rot. The first varieties are ready for harvest as early as July, the last in December. The later the pear, the longer it keeps in the cellar or in cold storage. Yet in order to ripen, all pears except a rare few need a period of chilling, from two weeks up to eight or nine, depending on the variety. The most effective temperature for both flavor and texture is 50 degrees F (10 degrees C), though pears are often kept much colder. After that essential period, they ripen well at cool room temperature. (My father, not someone who was generally interested in food, was always disappointed when the rest of the family, infallibly, ate all the pears in the bowl before any were completely ripe. Only years later did I realize how good a ripe pear could be and how many pears we had sacrificed.) Softness, juiciness, and aroma all come together at once, influenced by the usual agricultural factors of growing methods, soil and climate, the orchard's precise location, and the year's weather.

No one can say how many varieties of pear exist in the world, but a reasonable guess is several thousand. Many of the best were selected 150 to 250 years ago by breeders in France and Belgium. Any good eating variety cooks well, but in France you can still sometimes find special cooking varieties, requiring very long cooking. And tannic European varieties for making perry, the pear counterpart to hard cider, are undergoing a small revival and even spreading a little to the United States. Some mainstream varieties now take the form of patented sports—offshoots of the originals, with red color or perhaps another less obvious advantage.

Some of the most delicious pears are:

D'ANJOU (BEURRÉ D'ANJOU or NEC PLUS MEURIS) The original name in 1819 was Nec Plus Ultra Meuris, chosen by the Belgian breeder Jean-Baptiste Van Mons to honor his gardener, Pierre Meuris. (D'Anjou's full name, like that of some other pears with melting texture, begins with *beurré,* from the French word for "butter.")

With its full shape and little or no neck, D'Anjou is covered with a smooth green-yellow skin and sometimes shows a blush. The pears are slower to ripen than most, and then they remain longer at an optimum state. The aromatic flesh has a softness verging on slipperiness, which I find just slightly off-putting in an otherwise outstanding pear. Red D'Anjou, from a sport, is similar.

BARTLETT (WILLIAMS or WILLIAMS' BON CHRÉTIEN) The first tree of what is today the world's most common pear was found growing wild in about 1770 by John Stair at Aldermaston in Berkshire, England. Later the variety was distributed by a London nurseryman named Williams under his own name. Bartlett was the nineteenth-century Massachusetts farmer who spread the variety in the US. It's the standard choice for commercial canning, and with its strong perfume, as Williams, the variety is favored in Europe for pear brandy. But the aroma isn't always seen as positive. Bunyard, who liked the pears' "abundant juice and tenderness," said that they had too much musk. Bartlett is one of the rare varieties whose ripeness shows in an obvious change in color from green to yellow (and there's often a blush from the sun). Bartlett ripens more quickly than other leading pears and then more quickly overripens. A number of patented sports exist, including red ones. And some people say that the similar Beierschmitt, a seedling of Bartlett planted in Iowa in about 1900, tastes superior, but it's thin-skinned and bruises easily, so it's planted only in home gardens. (I've never had a chance to taste it.)

BOSC (BEURRÉ BOSC) Raised from a seed planted in 1807 by the Belgian breeder Van Mons, Bosc looks different from most pears. It has a long neck, and its skin is entirely or almost entirely russeted, an appearance like ground cinnamon, tinged at first with green and then, as the fruit ripens, with gold. (Russeting appears in many pear varieties, as well as in apples, if only as a patch around the stem.) Bosc pears are aromatic, and their somewhat firm, granular flesh holds its shape well in cooking. Bosc has more and larger grains of sand than other major varieties, but it's an excellent pear.

COMICE (DOYENNÉ DU COMICE) The first tree bore fruit in 1849, planted from a seed in a fruit garden in Angers in the Loire Valley, and almost immediately most connoisseurs considered Comice the finest pear. Its combination of flavor, juice, and tenderness is particularly refined. (Harry and David sells a version of it as Royal Riviera.) The compact pear shape is covered by yellow-green skin, and the fine-textured, sweet, juicy, perfumed flesh becomes as meltingly soft as that of any pear. Softness, however, is the variety's commercial limitation: the fruits are easily damaged. Yet Comice has so much appeal that it continues to be sold in American supermarkets, at least in small quantities. For the eater, the tenderness is a plus, and the only shortcoming is the moderately astringent, slight gritty skin. Comice tastes much better peeled. In cooking, despite the tenderness, if you use the pears before they're completely ripe and handle them with care, they aren't damaged. Among major US varieties Comice is my preferred choice for both eating and cooking. It's never imported but still confined to its old Northern Hemisphere season.

MAGNESS Developed by Howard Brooks at the USDA research center in Beltsville, Maryland, and released in 1968, Magness, a cross between Comice and Seckel, is at the top in flavor, but it's not a good producer and is very little grown. See "Warren" below.

SECKEL The original tree was discovered outside Philadelphia around 1760, and for years its location was kept secret. Seckel is a small pear with a pretty shape. The skin is sometimes green, sometimes blushed with red, sometimes entirely ruddy. Breeders like the variety's disease resistance. Picked at the right moment, chilled briefly and then fully ripened (I rarely find it at its best), Seckel has a soft texture and a superb sweet, spicy flavor.

WARREN The late amateur fruit grower T. O. Warren found this pear in about 1978; apparently, it was growing at an abandoned Mississippi State University experimental orchard at Hattiesburg. True European pears grow poorly in the South, normally being killed by fire blight. This variety, which undoubtedly originated elsewhere, has a strong resistance to the disease. Warren and Magness so much resemble each other that for a time they were thought to be the same, and some people still wonder. The skin of either one is green, somewhat russeted, and sometimes has a blush. The flesh is aromatic, soft, juicy, and almost free of grit. Warren is sold at a few California farmers' markets, and a number of US fruit lovers consider it (or Magness) to be the best pear. Not long ago I tasted Warren for the first time, and I can see the point, though I still prefer the delicacy of Comice.

WINTER NELIS (BONNE DE MALINES) Raised from a seed in about 1815 by Jean-Charles Nélis of Mechelen (called "Malines" in French) in Belgium, Winter Nelis was once the standard US winter pear. But it's small, has a somewhat unattractive russet-blotched skin, and takes a long time to ripen. It disappeared decades ago from the mainstream market, and I don't know it from experience. I include it here because it's raised a little by growers in northern California and it suggests the range of pear possibilities, and because U. P. Hedrick, in *The Pears of New York,* published in 1921 and still the best US book on pears, described it as "tender, melting, juicy, luscious, with a rich, sweet, aromatic flavor—one of the most delectable of all pears."

Cooked, the flavor of pears is too refined and they aren't tart enough to complement meat in the way that an apple or a prune, say, complements pork, but pears suit dessert admirably. You can make more ambitious things—soufflés, tarts, charlottes; pear makes one of the most elegant sorbets. But sliced ripe pears cook quickly, and several satisfying, homey desserts are easy to make. You can fry pears in butter (when they're nearly done, add sugar, let it caramelize, take out the cooked pears, deglaze with a little white wine, boil for a minute to a light syrup, optionally add coarsely ground black pepper, and pour the syrup over the pears). You can bake pears with cream (and sugar, in a buttered dish, finishing them under the broiler). You can poach pears in red wine (with an equal amount of water, some sugar, a little spice, removing the pears afterward and reducing the liquid to a syrup). All those are excellent complements to an aged sweet wine.

HOW TO BUY AND RIPEN PEARS: When you face a display of pears, it's frustratingly impossible to know whether any will turn out to be completely delicious. Some may already be ripe, or none. The simplest test for ripeness is to press gently on the shoulders to see whether they give a little as they should. But did the pear merely turn soft and mealy, or did it become luscious and jump upward in flavor and juice (or does it lie somewhere between)? You depend on the grower to have harvested at the right time, chilled the pears afterward to the right temperature for the right time, and not then held them for too long in cold storage. Inevitably in any batch of pears, some were picked at a less ideal state than others. The first varieties are generally ready in August, and the last disappear in March. (In North America, at times of year when we don't have our own pears, we get the same top three varieties from South America. Those pears may taste fine, but I avoid them, preferring to eat our own pears in season.) The longer a pear has been stored, the shorter the time needed to ripen it, and summer pears ripen faster than fall or winter ones.

If the pears you buy aren't ripe, leave them at cool room temperature—60 to 70 degrees F (16 to 21 degrees C). Warmer than that and the core tends to turn mealy. (You can speed the process by putting pears in a paper bag to trap the ethylene gas they produce and need for ripening, but the bag isn't necessary and doesn't allow you the pleasure of looking at them, and you don't notice the changes each time you pass by.) Look for color growing lighter, although the change is subtle in most pears other than Bartlett. The varieties that ripen slowest, such as D'Anjou, remain in a fully ripe state the longest. If you don't think ripe pears will be eaten before they become overripe, refrigerate them, and they'll hold longer.

Some people, including good growers, never peel a pear, not even Comice, with its distracting somewhat astringent, crunchy skin. But a peeled pear always tastes better. On the theory that some of the best flavors lie just beneath the skin, I peel thinly.

For cooking, use pears a day or two short of full ripeness, so they retain a little more acidity and don't become too soft in cooking. To prevent the peeled fruit from browning before you cook it, squeeze on some lemon juice or put them straight into poaching liquid (usually, I just work quickly). Keep pears whole for poaching by coring them through the bottom with a melon baller. If you halve pears, for whatever purpose, then when you core them also cut out the strings that connect the core with the stem. In the poaching pot, to keep from marring the tender fruit, rather than a metal spoon use a wooden one reserved for sweet flavors.

COMPLEMENTS TO PEARS: Pears make a good salad, dressed with lightly flavored walnut oil and lemon juice and combined with the crunch of lettuce or Belgian endive. Pears go with fresh cheese, and they soothe aged cheese—blue, Parmigiano, or *pecorino*—but together the flavors are merely all right. In dessert, the best pear complements tend to be obvious: sugar, butter, cream, custard, pastry, dry white and red wine, dessert wine, and vanilla. Lemon juice helps pears that need acidity. Almonds are in tune with pears, and an alternative to sugar is delicate acacia honey. Although spice can bury pear flavor, the alliance fundamentally works. To the wine for poaching half a dozen pears, add a small piece of cinnamon bark, two or three whole cloves, a vanilla bean, and, with red wine, a small bay leaf or juniper berries. Threads of saffron are good when you poach pears in white wine—with red they create a medicinal taste. Perhaps unexpectedly, pears are good with a distinct amount of ground black pepper (as I write this, I start to wonder about Szechuan pepper and the hard-to-find long pepper), such as in poaching liquid or a pear tart. I've never been convinced by the combination of pears with chocolate, as in the old-fashioned dessert *poires belle Hélène* (poached pears with vanilla ice cream and chocolate sauce)—

there's no dialogue between pears and chocolate, though there's a pleasant contrast. Old pear recipes often call for pear eau-de-vie, which overwhelms the pears' innate flavor, but Cognac added to the custard in a pear-custard tart heightens the pear taste. And although caramel eliminates the subtleties of pear flavor, it's extremely delicious in a pear *tarte Tatin*.

NOTES ON WINE: A ripe pear provides its own liquid refreshment. But cooked pears, when there's butter, sugar, perhaps cream, and preferably crisp browned pastry, are an excellent opportunity to drink an aged, fully sweet white wine.

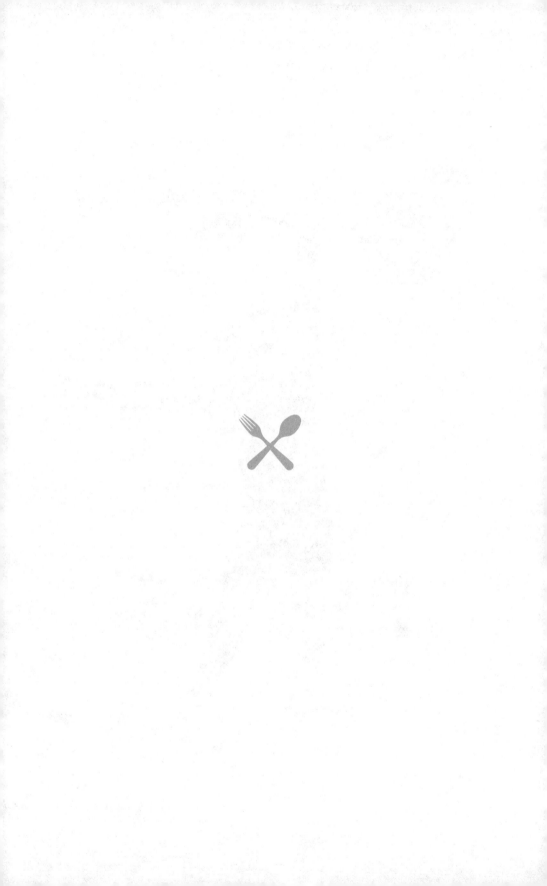

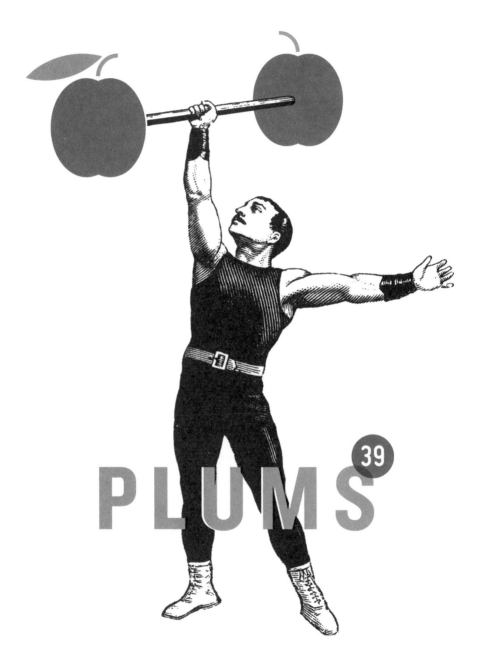

PLUMS ³⁹

39. PLUMS

A serious amateur apple grower I once knew turned at the end of his life to raising plums. He lived in Michigan and told me that the great varieties were so scarce the only way to have them was to grow them yourself and that, anyway, to have a perfectly ripe plum, you should pick it from the tree. But a plum is more durable than a strawberry or a fig, and particularly in California some small-scale growers produce excellent plums. Most US plums come from California, but they grow well in other states, and we all ought to grow plums if we can. (Over a period of ten years, I planted half a dozen trees, which had beautiful pale, highly scented blossoms, but the birds always ate the few fruits before they ripened. It seems to take both patience and skill to produce plums.) The essence of a delicious plum is sweet nectar contrasting with a sharp, flavorful, often astringent, elastic skin. A plum is luscious, though not melting like a pear; it's more fleshy. Plums come in yellow, green, red, dark blue, and black; some have blushed skins, and many show dots. Covering them is a waxy bloom, looking like fine powder. You rarely see many varieties, but there's a world of them.

Most are either European (*Prunus domesticus*), whose fruits are more oval and sweeter, or Japanese, also called Chinese (*P. salicina*), whose fruits are rounder and juicier and have tarter skins. The Japanese account for most of the eating plums and tend to be clingstone (the pit is bonded to the flesh). They arrived in the United States in the second half of the nineteenth century and were bred here into new varieties, some of which spread to other countries. The early-ripening Santa Rosa, once a leading variety (abandoned in favor of larger, firmer ones), is generally considered the most delicious Japanese plum. But there are Elephant Heart, Satsuma, and many more. Each has its peak during the long season.

The varieties of European plum, which tend to be freestone, not only are delicious when fresh, but cooks turn to them because the Japanese have more water. European varieties include the large Yellow Egg; the Italian prune plum (also called Fellenberg), excellent for fresh eating and cooking; such lesser-known ones as Mount Royal, from Quebec, and the group of nearly all-green or all-yellow plums known as the gages in Britain and in France as the Reines Claudes, after the wife of François I. Too fragile for commerce, the gages are at least five centuries old. Some of the more aromatic are Reine Claude de Bavay, Oullins Gage, Count Althann's Gage, and Transparent Gage (Reine Claude Diaphane: held up to sunlight, you can see into it). And among all the gages—and all plums—the variety commonly named as best is the true Greengage, or Reine Claude *verte* (or sometimes *dorée*).

The golden Mirabelles, from France, used especially for cooking, are considered a form of European. The two main varieties are Mirabelle de Nancy (known by the fifteenth century) and Mirabelle de Metz (known by the seventeenth century). Then there are damsons, usually put in their own subspecies of European, and so named because they came centuries ago from Damascus. Wild damsons are small and sour. The cultivated varieties, usually clingstone, are less astringent but still normally cooked with significant sugar. Known in France as Quetsche, damson is also used to make eau-de-vie. Other wild plums with edible fruit include native American species, such as the largely Midwestern American plum and the East Coast beach plum. Usually placed with plums are the many varieties of pluot, combinations of mostly plum with apricot—a reaction to the decline in flavor of mass-market plums.

Happily, even the varieties sold underripe in supermarkets—almost any whose skin is red or darker—produce good to excellent flavor in cooking, largely because of the tannic, acidic skins, which also produce beautiful, deep colors. They make ice cream and sherbet, ices, dessert soup, plum sauce for ice cream, as well as elaborately concocted desserts. Plums are very good cooked in a custard tart, they're my favorite fruit for a brioche tart, and they make excellent preserves.

Drying alters plum flavor completely. The high notes are replaced by deep ones, delicious in themselves and highly useful not just in dessert but in savory cooking. Prunes go with roast goose, roast pork, and braised beef.

The most famous prune, the *pruneau d'Agen,* from around the town of Agen in southwestern France, is made from the variety Prune d'Ente. In the US, Agen prunes cost nearly twice as much as those from the Central Valley of California, the world's largest producer of prunes. There, too, the quality is generally high. The US variety, called French Improved, is descended from mid-nineteenth-century imports of Prune d'Ente. From 1943 to 1949, French government researchers on bicycles, knowing that the variety embraced many clones, selected sixty outstanding trees and reduced those to the six best. One of them, number 707, now makes up roughly three-quarters of all French plantings of Prune d'Ente. (The 707 was tried in California in the 1980s and didn't do well.)

A main difference between French and California prunes comes from climate. The latitude line of Agen, followed around the globe to the New World, runs a little north of Toronto. The French trees receive significant rain during the growing season, and they're pruned to be open, so that the fruit is exposed to more sun. The Central Valley trees require irrigation and receive much greater heat, and they're pruned so the foliage will protect the fruit.

Besides the effects of clones and locations, a slight superiority in the Agen prunes may be due to slightly greater ripeness at harvest. The timing in California is determined by measuring the softness of the fruit, which is linked to sweetness. The French growers test sugar content directly with a refractometer, looking for 21 degrees Brix and sometimes achieving much more. Ripeness in France often used to be determined not by the grower but by the fruit itself, which, when it ripened fully, would fall to the ground. To prevent bruising, growers would spread straw beneath the trees as a cushion. Now, in nearly all the Agen plum orchards, the harvest is accomplished by machines that shake the trees and catch the fruit. They pass through the orchard four to seven times, as the fruit ripens. In California, similar machines, for economy, pass just once.

Long ago, the Agen plums were dried in the sun or, on farms, in cooling bread ovens. Today mechanical driers reduce the moisture of all prunes to 21 to 23 percent for keeping, and then before packaging they're rehydrated to 35 percent, to make them softer and more delectable. You no longer have to soak either French or US prunes before use. To ensure safekeeping, producers of *pruneaux d'Agen* now either add the preservative sorbic acid or its relatives or they pasteurize at 70 degrees C (158 degrees F), giving a slightly darker color and a more concentrated, caramel flavor.

Prunes are more common than plums in savory cooking, for instance in *porc* or *lapin aux pruneaux* (pork or rabbit with prunes, red wine, and *lardons*), cock-a-leekie (chicken, leeks, prunes), and sometimes a beef *daube,* including an oxtail one. The prunes go in toward the end of cooking, so they don't turn to mush. And prunes make excellent condiments: prunes in vinegar go with pâté de campagne, and prunes in red wine go with roast pork and goose. Either condiment improves when kept for a couple of weeks in the refrigerator, where it keeps indefinitely after that.

HOW TO BUY PLUMS AND PRUNES: At the right farmers' market in late summer, you may find genuinely ripe plums of a top variety. Plums always used to be considered one of the fruits that would ripen off the tree, but now it's recognized that some varieties do so much less than others. And all have more flavor if they ripen on the tree. There are famous names, including various gages and Santa Rosa, but don't be wary of unfamiliar ones. With experience of a particular variety, you can tell something by softness, or buy six or eight plums and try them over several days. Refrigerate ripe plums only if they'll spoil before they're eaten. A freestone plum is easy to cut in half by slicing it around the circumference from stem to blossom end and twisting. With a cling variety, you can cut away wedges or, messily, cut around the circumference, twist to partly open it, and then slip a sharp blade in the opening and cut the halves free of the pit. I've never been afraid of too much acidity, but if you're concerned, then peel the fruit to limit it. When you cook plums, for a bitter-almond note, crack the pits and add the kernels to the pot.

With prunes, you can feel the degree of softness inside a plastic package, but you can't tell anything about flavor until you taste, and not all brands are equal. Most California prunes are now pitted, but only about half the French ones are. Almost by definition, unopened prunes hold a little more flavor.

COMPLEMENTS TO PLUMS AND PRUNES: The acidity and tannic skins of cooked plums go with pork, lamb, duck, and goose; rosemary or thyme underlines the savory side of the combination. In desserts, plums go with almonds, walnuts, buttery pastry, and cream, including ice cream. I'm inclined to stick with those, because there's no danger of competition, but plums also go with lemon, orange, cardamom, and other spices.

Excellent with prunes are pork, rabbit, goose, and beef (especially oxtail), usually cooked in red wine with the prunes added near the end. Prunes are excellent on their own, cooked in red wine or soaked in Armagnac (the latter are good with fresh or ripened cream or ice cream). Prunes stand up to lemon or orange zest, spices, and walnuts. They aren't bad with chocolate. Prunes and custard have a poor reputation in Britain, but the combination is also French and, made well, it's good. To throw in something little known, the *pauchade aux pruneaux* of Auvergne, in southern France, is a custardy prune *clafoutis,* just prunes put into more or less the same batter as for Yorkshire pudding and baked in a very hot oven. (Beware that *prune* in French means "plum"; the word for "prune" is *pruneau.*) Prunes cooked in red wine (with a hint of sugar and no spice) are excellent with Roquefort.

NOTES ON WINE: With any savory food containing sweetness, such as from plums or prunes, the crux of choosing a wine is to find a bottle, usually white, that's just slightly sweeter than the dish or else a dry red wine big enough to stand up to the bit of sugar. With lamb accompanied by a tart plum sauce, or rabbit or pork with prunes, the choice might be a slightly sweet Chenin Blanc, such as a Vouvray *sec* or *demi-sec;* with a beef *daube* with prunes, the wine might be a red Châteauneuf-du-Pape, whose extra alcohol helps carry the wine's flavor. (I admit that out of every hundred wines I try with alcohol at 14 percent or more, however highly recommended, I might like two. In all the rest, the alcohol stands out and the flavors tend toward flat ones of overripe and cooked fruit.) With fresh plums at dessert, the usual suggestion is sparkling Moscato, but any wine risks competing. Cooked plum desserts have enough flavor that they need fully sweet wines, and the combination is always easier with pastry and cream. Prune desserts go with Banyuls, Bual Madeira, or another sweet oxidized wine, or a rich botrytized sweet one.

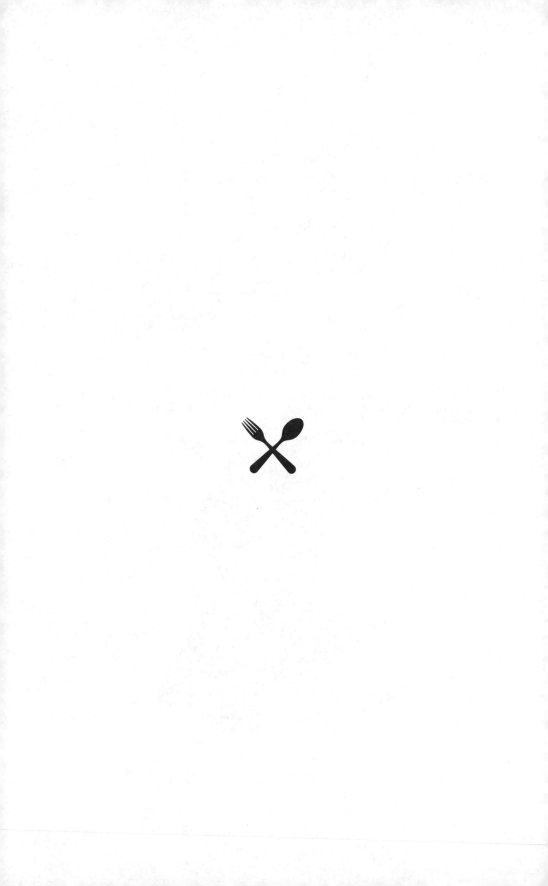

40. PORK AND WILD BOAR

Ninety-nine percent of the pork sold in North America is flavorless or nearly so. Even when carefully cooked, it's typically dry and rubbery. It comes from commodity pigs, produced by the inhumane, unsustainable, unhealthful, polluting methods embraced in the last quarter of the twentieth century by almost the entire US pork industry. The pigs are bred for leanness without consideration for tenderness, taste, or the animals themselves. In the interest of efficiency, they're kept in close indoor confinement, generating a powerful stench. Conditions are commonly so bad that the pigs are fed a steady low-level supply of antibiotics to keep them from becoming sick.

In stark contrast with that meat, juicy, marvelously tender, well-marbled pork comes from compassionately raised pigs—healthy animals raised outdoors with options for shelter and space to roam and indulge their instincts to root and nest. During the warm months, they eat prime pasture plants, as well as plenty of grain provided by the farmer. Fat is the main carrier of flavor in meat; fat marbling running through lean gives an impression of juiciness and usually coincides with tenderness. We value fat in pork, although more fat isn't the same as more flavor and marbling isn't essential. Good pork isn't all one thing. It's more likely to come from pasture and hay, sometimes wild forage, and it depends on breed. Pork can taste deliciously meaty, sometimes nutty, or it can be sweeter and more delicate, with lighter-tasting fat. Exceptionally, a pork loin has a silky tenderness recalling tenderloin. By nature, pork flavor is subtle and mild; it's often called sweet. A really big, meaty flavor comes from cooking pork with generous amounts of salt and from fat and browning. I bought my first *porchetta* sandwich long ago from a roadside stand outside the Tuscan town of Vinci. The freshly baked roll held thick slices of seasoned pork cut from a glistening mahogany creature set in the middle of the counter. In the sandwich, on top of the meat, was the only condiment offered or needed: a piece of the salty, luscious, crunchy skin. This was the apotheosis of pork.

The pig belongs to the same species as its ancestor the wild boar; the two readily interbreed. Both are *Sus scrofa,* the pig being distinguished by the added word *domestica.* Wild boars, lean and long-legged, thrive all too readily in the wild, damaging cropland and forests by rooting. The meat of a young wild boar is prized. Raw, it's darker and more pinkish-purple than pork. Cooked, it slightly resembles the darker muscles of a pork shoulder. But *wild* wild boar is like that only if it's less than a year old. As the animal grows, the meat becomes steadily tougher and stronger-flavored, and if it's eaten at all, it's braised for hours in wine and high-flavored broth. Besides, the meat of the mature males has a somewhat off-putting urine scent. Wild boar can be farmed, and when it is, thanks to the grain in the diet, the results are more tender and mild. The big contrast with pork is that wild boar isn't marbled—the fat lies outside the muscles—and overcooking quickly turns the meat dry. But when wild boar is cooked with the same attention we ought to give all meat, it's perfectly moist. I once had in my kitchen the whole carcass of a young, farm-raised wild boar, and it was some of the best meat I've ever tasted.

The pig, like the wild boar, is an omnivore. It will eat anything above- or belowground, although in practice pigs are fed mainly corn mixed with soy. In the US, pig production largely coincides with the Corn Belt, especially Iowa, and pigs raised in other regions of the country are usually fed grain from the Corn Belt, although milo (grain sorghum) may be gaining ground. Once, pigs were commonly taken to the woods in fall to fatten on acorns, and particularly in Spain they still sometimes eat acorns, which gives superior meat, notably for ham. Pigs that live outdoors and eat grass and other pasture plants, or what they find in the woods, are healthier and have better meat. (Good meat doesn't come from unhealthy, unhappy animals any more than delicious vegetables come from sick plants. We know, for instance, the scientific reasons why stress produces tougher meat.) Maybe pigs can be raised solely on pasture and hay without any grain and have delicious, tender meat, but I've yet to encounter that.

A number of old breeds are prized for taste, though a farmer warns that you have to get an old breeding line with good quality meat. Best-known in the US is Berkshire, originally from England and also called by the Japanese name Kurobuta ("black pig"). The meat is well-marbled, juicy, and tender, with an admired delicate flavor, but the litters are small, and the sows have a reputation for rolling over and crushing their young. The Duroc, golden to dark red, appeared in New York in the 1820s from uncertain origins; it may contain some Berkshire, which could explain its marbled meat. Tamworth, a red pig originally from Ireland, has a long body with a balance of lean and fat that gives it a reputation as a bacon breed; the flavor might be a little richer than that of Berkshire. Red Wattles, associated recently with East Texas, may have arrived in New Orleans in the 1700s from the South Pacific; they're large animals with a tassel on either side of the neck and lean meat. The small, feral Ossabaw, from an island off the Georgia coast (and descended from pigs brought from Spain four centuries ago), has a thick layer of back fat. The Gloucester Old Spots pig, supposed to be the oldest English breed, also has a high proportion of fat. The black Guinea hog, probably from the Guinea coast of Africa and once the most common kind in the Southeast, is small, hardy, and again fairly fat. The black Ibérico, also known as *pata negra* ("black hoof"), actually a family of related breeds, makes Spain's famous hams. Commonly, US farmers who raise more-natural pork cross breeds, for example, to combine the mothering qualities and reasonably good meat of a Chester, Large White, or Landrace sow with the marbled meat of a Duroc boar. Exceptionally, you can find pork labeled as coming from a particular breed.

We think of marbling as ideal, but you can have flavor, juice, and tenderness without it. They're directly linked not to fat but to the higher pH of darker meat, which occurs naturally in certain breeds, including Duroc and Berkshire. And despite the common view that pork should be very fresh and doesn't improve with hanging, aging in the cold for two weeks produces more tenderness, juiciness, and a little more flavor. It's better if the meat isn't sealed in plastic but instead is hung in large cuts in moderately dry air.

A very few of the most natural-minded pig farmers don't castrate their male pigs, something that's usually done within a week of birth. But as un-castrated animals grow older, their meat acquires the sometimes powerful, offensive aroma called "boar taint," the same thing that occurs in male wild boars. During cooking, a sweet, earthy funk can fill the kitchen. It comes from two compounds in the fat, one of which becomes a pheromone that attracts female pigs. Not everyone can taste boar taint, and I don't mind a little of it. Farmers in some countries, such as the United Kingdom and Ireland, avoid the problem by slaughtering pigs at a younger age, before the problem arises.

The loin is the most-valued cut, for its flavor and juice combined with at least moderate tenderness. The loin's single neat muscle is ideal for roast-ing or, separated into chops, for sautéing. If you want extra marbling and tenderness, choose the shoulder end of the loin, sometimes sold in the US as the "rib end of the pork loin" or "blade loin roast." (In France, where it's more appreciated as a separate cut, it's the *échine.*) The muscles of the shoulder get more exercise and have more flavor, but not all of them are tender. Shoulder is excellent when ground for sausage and pâté de cam-pagne, and it can be braised. (Marinating meat beforehand in wine or other acidic liquid, despite the old lore, doesn't increase tenderness, but it does introduce flavor to the surface of the meat, enough to make a difference in a braise that's cooked very slowly and gently, as it should be.) A fresh, un-brined ham is partly tough and almost hopelessly bland. The ribs are full of flavor, like the belly. One of the best belly preparations is *rillons,* a form of charcuterie from Anjou and Touraine, in France: large cubes of fresh belly are salted overnight, then cooked in a depth of fat, very slowly, until they're brown and tender. Unlike most charcuterie, they're served hot, reheated as needed. Among the pig's other, more diverse parts, one or two feet add gelatinous body to a braise, and the feet, tails, and ears all lend themselves to long cooking in winey broth.

Not everything delicious comes from a particular cut. Southern bar-becue, in all its variation from region to region, is an entire world. The very long, slow cooking depends on cool heat and smoke coming from hard-wood, and you can barbecue any part of a pig (as well as beef and other meats). Half an animal isn't unheard of. Barbecue is simple yet highly skilled cooking, and the degree of success depends on the pitmaster. From succulent barbecue comes pulled (shredded) pork, another great food. It's very distantly related to French *rillettes,* which are close to *rillons* in name but not so much in taste. They're usually made from a shoulder but can be made from half the animal (if you have a big enough pot)—you need a mix of textures. The cut-up meat is cooked extremely slowly, with just salt, until when stirred it falls apart. *Rillettes,* including their fat, are put up in pots and sealed under more hot fat for keeping, and later spread on bread. All this is not to get into the virtues of lard itself, the most important traditional fat almost wherever pigs are raised.

Pork's greatest affinity is for salt, whether in lightly brined fresh meat, sausage, or fully dry-cured and aged ham (see "Ham and Bacon"). You exchange the fresh taste for a stronger, meatier one. A brine is as easily made as a marinade and, like it, allows herbs and spices to be introduced to the meat. But even just sprinkling salt over the surface and leaving the meat in the refrigerator for a couple of days has a marked beneficial effect.

Some people today prefer their pork rare, but even if there's no danger of trichinae, pork gains in flavor with medium cooking, just to the point where the meat starts to lose the first drops of juice. Wild boar is the same, though there's more risk of dryness.

HOW TO BUY PORK AND WILD BOAR: For superior taste and every other good reason, buy humanely raised pork. That might come from an individual farm or a large group of producers (the largest and most widely available is Niman Ranch). Some farms are certified as humane. The Animal Welfare Approved and Certified Humane Raised and Handled programs have high standards, but not every certification has meaning, and most humanely raised pork isn't certified. In a store, no matter what cut you're looking for, notice whether the loins are well marbled, which suggests that the pork was well raised and all the cuts are good. A special fatty tenderness tends to come from particular breeds, but fat doesn't automatically coincide with juice, flavor, and tenderness. A more reliable sign is darker color, associated with breeds such as Duroc and Berkshire. For flavor and tenderness, it's also better that the meat has aged for at least ten days, though you may have no way of knowing that. Because methods and results vary, a first purchase, especially from a single small farm, can be an experiment. Wild boar, available in the US from some specialist suppliers, can also be an experiment.

HOW TO COOK PORK AND WILD BOAR: Aside from the long cooking of a braise, the best combination of juice, flavor, and tenderness comes with medium doneness—140 to 150 degrees F (60 to 65 degrees C). The juice is pink but runs clear, and for that wild boar may need to be at the top of the temperature range. In the high heat of most grilling (close to hot coals, no closed lid), all but the tenderest chop quickly toughens, and the surface especially becomes hard. The heat is easier to control when you sauté on a stovetop, and even then I lightly flour the chops to keep the surface from becoming tough.

Meat on the bone tends to be more succulent, but because bone heats more slowly than flesh, you can't get absolutely even doneness. It helps if, in advance, you spread out chops at room temperature to warm for an hour or a little more, or if you set out a roast for up to several hours. It further helps if you brown the meat first using high heat and then lower the heat, so the temperature rises more slowly and evenly throughout and you don't miss the doneness you're looking for. You can finish the meat, including chops, in a low oven, about 150 to 160 degrees F (65 to 70 degrees C). Especially if you roast in a hot oven, be sure to remove a roast before it reaches 145 degrees F (63 degrees C), because as the outer heat continues to penetrate, the center's temperature continues to rise, another dozen degrees or more if the oven was very hot and depending on the size of the piece. Allow the roast to rest for at least twenty minutes so the juices distribute themselves evenly and don't run out at carving.

COMPLEMENTS TO PORK AND WILD BOAR: The prime complements are rosemary, dried Greek sage (sold in whole branches in Greek groceries—very different from cloying rubbed sage), thyme, and, more unusual, Tuscan fennel pollen. Juniper and clove are good, though they cover some of pork's mild flavor. Spice is key to the character of pâtés and terrines. Exceptionally, milk complements pork in *arrosto di maiale al latte* (the loin, first browned in fat, is cooked slowly in milk, which is gradually reduced to a thick, golden, nutty sauce). Fatty pork benefits from the acidity of sauces with wine or vinegar, of sauerkraut, of sweet-and-sour onions. More powerful complements are anchovies, olives, and tapenade. Or serve a separately prepared *sauce piquante* (onions, shallots, vinegar, stock or *jus,* capers, and cornichons), which is also good with leftover meat.

Some of the best vegetables with pork are the most obvious. It loves onions, especially roasted in fat, and it loves all the wide cabbage family, from sweet young green heads to Brussels sprouts, kale, mustard greens, and broccoli raab. Pork goes with all the bitter or astringent greens, wild or cultivated, including spinach and chard. (Spinach can be simply buttered; the rest are good cooked with chopped garlic, first cooked to translucence in olive oil.) Pork goes with bulb fennel, lightly browned and cooked slowly with a little water and whole unpeeled garlic cloves (a recipe of the writer Richard Olney). Pork is excellent with a mixed purée of celery root and potato.

Like duck and goose, pork is at home with cooked fruit—apples, quinces (if they're tart), apricots, sour cherries, prunes. The apples can be cut in wedges and browned slowly in butter. Dried sour cherries, soaked beforehand for a few hours and drained, can be added to the red-wine sauce for a braise. Prunes excel in *porc aux pruneaux* from Touraine—better in a red-wine version than the old one with cream and currant jelly. In fall, pork or wild boar goes beautifully with red cabbage cooked with apples and goose fat.

Wild boar likes all the above, particularly tart fruit, celery root–potato purée, and sweet-and-sour tastes. It goes with chestnuts, spice, and red-wine sauces, including braises flavored with chocolate. If you have wild boar bones and trimmings to roast, you can turn them into a classic brown *sauce espagnole* (with a little vinegar, some juniper berries), and then with extra black pepper you have a *sauce poivrade* for your meat.

NOTES ON WINE: It seems odd as I write it, but it's true that most good wines are too flavorful for the typical mild flavor of pork, even quite fatty pork. And although pork is often said to have a subtle sweetness that responds to some sweetness in wine, the white wines from Alsace and Germany, which you might expect to go well, are often too sweet for the meat. In the opposite direction, completely out are very dry and acidic wines or tannic ones. To help pork stand up to a wine, brown the meat well and deglaze the pan with the same wine, so all ends up in a sauce. And there's more tie with a slightly sweet wine if the sauce, too, contains a touch of sweetness, such as from onions or fruit.

Among white wines, I'm drawn especially to a dry or slightly sweet Chenin Blanc from the middle Loire Valley (appellations including Montlouis, Vouvray, Touraine, Jasnières, Saumur, Anjou, and Savennières). Pork also goes with the lighter sorts of clean, aromatic Friulian and Slovenian whites (though not the more acidic versions of Ribolla Gialla). A simple rosé suits pork, though a light one has become harder to find (global warming hasn't helped).

Among light reds, I've had success with red Sancerre (Pinot Noir), red Jura (Pinot Noir as well as the local Trousseau and Poulsard), fresh, fruit-tasting Loire Cabernet Franc (from the appellations Bourgueil, Chinon, and Saumur-Champigny), and Gamay from the Loire and Beaujolais. Some of the many Italian red possibilities are light Nebbiolo, light Chianti without too much acidity, old-school light Dolcetto, Lambrusco, and wines from the slopes of Etna in Sicily.

Wild boar opens the way to stronger, more mature reds; the greatest, certainly from Burgundy, are at their best with game. Besides Burgundy, turn to spicier, gamier examples of Syrah, whether from Australia (Shiraz) or the northern Rhone (the appellations Crozes-Hermitage, Saint-Joseph, and Cornas up to costly Côte-Rôtie and Hermitage). Still in the realm of wines that suit game, wild boar goes with substantial traditional Nebbiolo, including great Barolo, traditional Brunello di Montalcino, traditional red Rioja, and old Bordeaux. More modestly, it goes with substantial versions of Chianti.

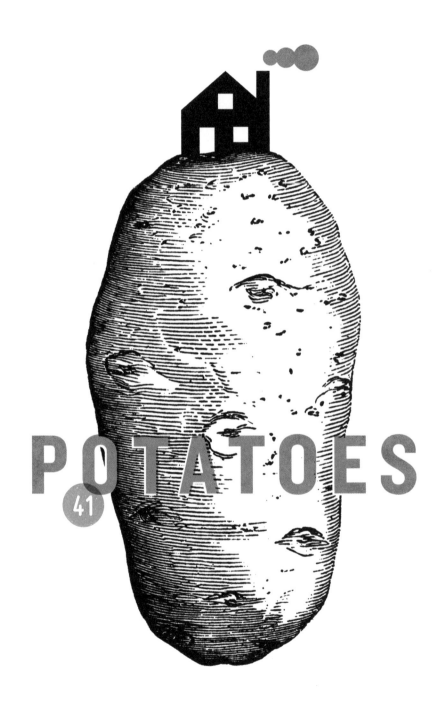

POTATOES

41

With their quietly rich, nutty flavor, potatoes flatter strong foods and are an unsurpassed carrier for delicious fat. Taking the options to an extreme, they can be fried very slowly in lard until they're nearly like candy. Perfection comes in multiple forms: just-dug new potatoes hot with butter and flavored with chives, sliced cold new potatoes in salad with crunchy lettuce and again chives, potatoes mixed with celery root in purée and eaten with wild boar, potatoes deep-fried in duck fat, potatoes baked with cream and a hint of garlic in a gratin, or mashed with truffle juice (in a kind of subterranean sympathy).

The potato originated high in the Andes of southern Peru and northwestern Bolivia, and the Andes still hold the greatest number of species and varieties—three thousand by one estimate. The skins can be almost any color—brown, red, yellow, blue, purple—and some of the last have deeply pigmented blue or purple flesh that remains strong in color after cooking. The best-tasting potatoes are dry-farmed in high, dry, cool territory resembling their original home. These high-altitude potatoes are smaller, but they keep better, are more nutritious, and have much more flavor. Most US potatoes, in contrast, are irrigated, and the potatoes contain much more water.

New potatoes appear underground at the same time that the plants flower. To me, new potatoes are not much bigger than an inch in diameter. (You can harvest them by digging under the plant, but the disturbed plant never really recovers. I uproot the whole thing.) New potatoes are creamy and light; some of the creamiest, most flavorful I've ever eaten were from the variety Irish Cobbler, sent to me by a farmer in Pennsylvania. The most delicious new potatoes I've grown in my own climate were Urgenta. Steaming preserves new-potato freshness, lightness, purity, and creaminess. The only danger is overcooking, which turns them sodden. To underline the freshness, some cooks put a couple of mint leaves in the pot; more to the point, when the potatoes are done, are butter and thinly sliced chives.

Flavor accumulates during the season, and as the potatoes mature, their texture becomes more definitely waxy—dense and moist—or more mealy—dry, crumbly, and detectably granular on the tongue (turning fluffy when whipped with liquid into purée)—or somewhere in between. You get to know the varieties best if you grow them yourself and have a surfeit throughout the summer. (They're no fun, though, when they attract Colorado potato beetles, with their fat, lurid-orange grubs.)

I've planted a number of varieties whose flavor I had heard about or that I chose from catalog descriptions. More often than any other, I've grown the creamy, flavorful French La Ratte, a fingerling, meaning it's small, long, knobby, tender, and waxy. La Ratte achieved fame when the chef Joël Robuchon made it (or sometimes the prosaically named BF15) into purée using two parts potato to one part butter, a combination so innately flattering that you had no awareness of the amount of fat. I've grown other fingerlings—Banana, Caribe, Bintje, Rose Finn Apple—and there are many more possibilities. Mostly, though, I don't find fingerlings to have special flavor. Early on, you eat their thin, tender skins, but as the season wears on, the skins grow tough and the potatoes are tedious to scrub and peel.

There are middle-ground potatoes, too, between waxy and starchy, which some people like best for mashed potatoes. Among those I've grown are Island Sunshine, German Butterball, Carola, and Yellow Finn, besides which there are Red Norland, Kennebec, Katahdin, Red Gold, and plenty more.

Of the frankly starchy varieties, the famous one is Burbank Russet, dry and floury—the model starchy baker—selected by Luther Burbank out of the thousands of plants he grew from seed in the 1870s. Russet Burbank became the Idaho potato. I once grew its relative Green Mountain, which dates from 1885. The potatoes were the size of bricks and had a strong russet flavor. With all their starch, russets make a nutty purée with perceptible granules of starch and an innate dryness, badly in need of butter and liquid, which are easily supplied. There's no genetic tie between russeting and starch, but consumers expect them to go together, and so breeders keep breeding starchy russets. One of the good nonrusseted starchy potatoes is the widely available Yukon Gold.

As I looked into varieties for this book, I realized there was considerably more to know. In *100 Vegetables and Where They Came From,* the cook-gardener-historian William Woys Weaver writes, "I am inclined to believe that serious potato lovers will agree with me in calling Arran Victory the ultimate potato." It was bred on Scotland's Isle of Arran in 1912. I've never grown it or the other flavorful potatoes Weaver cites—All-Red, Lumper, Négresse, Peach Blow, Roseval, and the Yam (the last is neither a yam nor a sweet potato but a variety of regular potato).

Before baking, coat the skins of potatoes with oil or butter to make them crisper. Peeled potatoes lose some flavor to boiling water (some turn tough unless you start them in cold water), while baking concentrates the flavor. The best mashed potatoes are made from baked potatoes. Whether you like starchy mashed potatoes or waxy or in-between is a matter of taste. However you cook them, a ricer, compared with other ways of mashing, gives a lighter, more even texture. A food processor produces an inedibly glutinous one.

The best fried mashed-potato cakes are also made with potatoes baked for the purpose, then mashed and fried before they have a chance to cool. They're especially delicious mixed with bits of fat-cooked onion or dry-cured ham. A wide, flat potato cake, starting with raw potatoes and fried or baked slowly in some fat, is one of the simpler-sounding yet more difficult preparations. *Rösti* potato cakes, from switzerland, are made of grated potatoes, originally cooked in lard and now commonly butter, usually with added cheese or onion and, these days, many other things. French *pommes Anna* is a skillet cake of sliced potatoes browned slowly in a generous amount of butter until cooked through and crusty. A *paillasson* is a cake made of straw-thickness potato sticks or shreds. Too often these cakes come out gummy or else fall apart. You need just enough surface starch to bind them together. Sometimes you rinse some or all the starch from the potatoes beforehand; it depends on the variety.

Gratin dauphinois is scalloped potatoes made carefully with cream and infinitely better than scalloped potatoes with milk. *Pommes lyonnaise* are home fries well browned in fat and served with fried onions plus parsley on top (optionally, a little vinegar in the onions). From the Aubrac region of France comes the emblematic *aligot,* a dish made of fresh Laguiole or Cantal cheese melted with mashed potatoes and often a little garlic; it's beaten theatrically in the pan with a wooden spoon to produce a loose elasticity.

One of the best and oldest ways to cook potatoes is disappearing for lack of the needed pot. Ceramic potato "devils"—really stovetop ovens—have become difficult if not impossible to find, unless perhaps you know a potter. They were made in various countries, sometimes of earthenware. (One brand that may still be available is the German Kartoffelteufel.) The covered pot holds in steam, while the bottom gives an attractive rustic char, like baking in ashes. You shake the pot from time to time to rotate the potatoes. They're especially good cooked with whole cloves of unpeeled garlic.

The best french fries are made by cooking the sliced potatoes twice: once at a medium temperature to cook them through and dry them and again, after cooling, at a slightly higher temperature to brown them outside and give a much crunchier surface. (A single frying gives soggy fries.) Even better are raw potatoes cut into small, thin rectangles and twice-fried to make souffléed potatoes; steam from the center inflates the envelope of crust to make crunchy pillows. But are any of these really better than well-seasoned, deep-fried potato fritters?

HOW TO BUY AND STORE POTATOES: New potatoes, just dug, are available only at the start of the season; small potatoes aren't necessarily the same thing. Apart from any question of type, bigger potatoes have more starch than littler ones, simply because they're more mature. The best potatoes at any stage look as if only enough time has passed since they were unearthed for any clinging soil to have dried. They show no cuts or bruises, no sprouts or wrinkles. But potatoes do store well; even sprouting ones taken from the cellar at the end of winter can taste good. Yet the potatoes for sale in supermarkets often have off-flavors, and I don't know the cause. Mass-market organic potatoes almost always taste better.

Potatoes keep better when they're unwashed, still dusty with soil. Refrigeration causes some of the starch to turn to sugar; left long enough in the cold, they taste strangely sweet and brown quickly in the pan before they cook. Most of the sugar turns back to starch when potatoes are again stored at warmer temperatures. If they've been exposed to light, they accumulate poisons; cut away and discard any green parts. New potatoes don't keep.

COMPLEMENTS TO POTATOES: Potatoes love fat—goose, duck, olive oil, tallow, lard, butter, cream, and cheese (Cheddar, Gruyère, Munster, blue). They go with the entire onion family—leeks, chives, garlic (including raw garlic, finely chopped and sprinkled over fried potatoes along with parsley). Potatoes like cream and leeks in vichyssoise. They love grilled steak with its juices—they love meat juices in general. Their earthiness is complemented by boletes. Boiled and mashed potatoes go with sausage and cured pork in all its forms and with corned beef. Potatoes go with smoked salmon and other cured fish, including pickled herring. In salad, they like rocket, watercress, lettuce, Belgian endive, Dijon and other mustard, and capers.

NOTES ON WINE: Champagne and other dry sparkling wines are excellent with the fat of french fries. But generally with potatoes, of course, the wine depends on what else is on the plate.

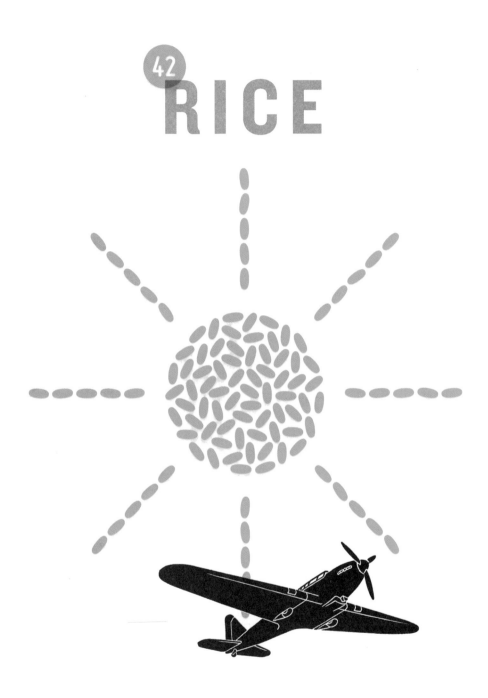

42
RICE

I once watched a Venetian in a good restaurant order *riso burro,* simple rice with butter, which at the time amazed me. Only years later did I realize how good rice in northern Italy can be and how delicious that bowl of buttered rice must have been. Rather than standing on its own, rice normally sets up other flavors, in the way that pasta, bread, potatoes, and dried beans do. It moderates strong sauces, provides relief from powerful spice, and absorbs flavor, such as broth or saffron in pilaf or risotto. The French, with all their focus on technique, manage to cook rice badly; the raw material is rarely special, and the outcome is rarely light or right. The Western countries that care most about rice have the longest history of cultivating it: Spain and Italy. In Asia, it's hard to separate rice from the very idea of eating, and the kinds and uses are deeply developed. I'm a rice tourist in the sense that I've only skimmed most of the possibilities. Rice is *Oryza sativa,* a grain, and when it hasn't been heavily processed for the mass market, it has a clear grain flavor. I've heard of a kind of rice, not grown for sale, that has a nutty earthiness so strong as to be barnyardy and distasteful. In good rice, I sometimes taste an echo of that power but reduced to mere grainy nuttiness.

The big divide is between long- and short-grain, *indica* and *japonica* (also called *sinica*), though there are also the smaller categories of aromatic (basmati, jasmine) and sticky (glutinous) rice. Short-grain rice was one of the earliest crops to be domesticated, in China. Long-grain came later. Sticky rice, partly translucent when cooked, is a tradition in many countries but especially in Laos, where two-thirds of the rice eaten may be sticky. (It's not a clear category but a spectrum, from more starchy to highly sticky.)

There are various natural colors of rice—brown, black, red, green— but white rice is valued everywhere above all. After harvesting, the bran is removed from most rice, leaving it white, and in the worst cases of factory processing, rice is parboiled. The darkest kinds retain all the bran, which keeps the grains from sticking together. White rice is often rinsed before it's cooked to remove any starch dust, so the grains stick less.

In the West, the short-grain starchy types are presented at a peak of flavor and texture in Italian risotto. First the grains are cooked in butter or butter and oil to ensure that they won't give up too much surface starch. Then broth is added a little at a time, traditionally with steady stirring, each addition being completely absorbed before the next. At the end, butter and Parmigiano go in, and the risotto is eaten immediately. For risotto, you need rice that gradually absorbs the flavor, releases starch to thicken the surrounding liquid (however little remains at the end), and yet, when it's done, retains a nutty core. (So-called risotto made with other grains makes no sense—only certain short-grain varieties accomplish the goals. But barley "risotto" looks better on a menu than barley "porridge.")

Better rice for risotto takes longer to cook; it contains more starch of a kind that doesn't break down in cooking and retains that firmer core. The top varieties are Vialone Nano, Maratelli, and Carnaroli, which are grown, like most Italian rice, in Lombardy and Piedmont in the Po Valley of the north. Arborio, also used for risotto, is a more everyday variety. Starchy short-grain Italian rice is, in a seeming paradox, graded by length; *fino* and *superfino* are the longest.

Short-grain rice also makes Spanish (originally Valencian) paella and other Spanish rice dishes, in which, as in risotto, the individual grains remain separate and retain a nutty firmness in the center. Similarly to risotto, the grains are briefly cooked in fat, then cooked in liquid in the wide, shallow *paelles* or *cassoles,* without covering, so the cook can watch closely as the liquid evaporates. If the rice were pressed together in a deep pot, the individual grains wouldn't remain as separate. And the rice is never stirred, so the grains don't release starch. A Spaniard once said to me, "When I first saw risotto being cooked in Milan, I thought it was a sacrilege." In Spain, rice is grown in the Ebro Delta, in the south of Catalonia, next to Valencia. The best variety, although harder to grow and rare, is the old one called Bomba, which holds its resistant center much longer.

Supplì, street food from Rome (the name is derived from the French word *surprise*), are breaded, deep-fried balls of rice; commonly the rice is mixed with *ragù,* egg, butter, and Parmigiano with mozzarella in the middle (the melted cheese is the surprise). The strings of cheese connecting the halves led to the name *supplì al telefono.* Especially in Sicily, you find similar *arancini* (named because they're fried to the color and shape of "little oranges"), in diverse versions without mozzarella. *Sartù,* from Naples, is a more *alta cucina* (haute cuisine) dish: a timbale of rice with additions such as chicken livers, onion, pancetta, peas, and mushrooms. *Risi e bisi* from the Veneto is just what the name says, "rice and peas," the peas going first into a flavorful broth, followed by the rice—it's a soup, not a risotto.

Any list of rice dishes must be superficial. *Risotto alla milanese* includes saffron, marrow, red wine, and beef broth; rice enters stuffings for grape or cabbage leaves. Rice is colored black with squid ink (called *arroz negro* in Valencia and *risotto nero* in various parts of Italy). The many dishes of the Indonesia *rijsttafel* ("rice table") make a book in themselves. *Jollof* rice from West Africa is an umbrella name for one-pot long-grain dishes containing onions and spices, including hot pepper, and almost whatever meat, fish, or vegetables you choose to add. The base of Vietnamese *phở* is broth and rice noodles. The essence of sushi isn't fish but vinegared rice.

The long-grain rice favored in North America probably arrived with slaves from rice-growing areas of West Africa, and the habit, especially in parts of the South, remains the African one of cooking the rice to a relatively firm state. Today in the US, large commercial crops of rice are grown in Louisiana, Texas, and California. For any sort of rice, in order to get the right texture, something that isn't quite agreed upon, there are countless methods and various kinds of automatic cookers, which many people who love rice prefer. Lately, I've been cooking mine in a heavy ceramic Japanese *donabe,* with excellent results, assuming you like tender, perfectly separate grains (which with short-grain varieties are also somewhat cohesive and sticky). And for separate grains and clear flavor, it helps to wash the raw rice several times before you cook it.

The famous old US variety, which a few decades ago nearly disappeared, is Carolina Gold. In Louisiana, Cajun "pecan rice" comes from a flavorful variety milled so it retains some bran (no pecans in it). "Rice and beans" is the name of a dish in many parts of the world. In New Orleans, it's specifically "red beans and rice," often with some form of pork. Hoppin' John, also from the South, is rice with cowpeas or black-eyed peas, ham bone, onion, and sometimes hot pepper. Cajun "dirty rice" is made with white rice, chicken liver, and giblets with bell pepper, celery, garlic, and onion.

North American wild rice is a wholly different grain (*Zizania palustris*), and the only sort worth buying is completely *wild*. Much of the flavor comes from the "parching"—toasting—used to loosen the grain from its hull (followed originally by treading in soft moccasins to free it completely). Even today the rice is harvested by hand, often by Indians working from canoes. The thin bran coating is streaked tan-green—very different from the thick, hard, black coating of cultivated "wild" rice, grown in paddies and specially bred so it can be harvested by machines. The paddy kind is devoid of interest; the wild one is delicious.

COMPLEMENTS TO RICE: Almost anything, but perhaps especially, with the risk of a tilt toward the West, onions, beans, many kinds of fresh and dried mushrooms, shrimp and other shellfish, ham, sausage, broth and stock of all sorts, butter, milk, Parmigiano, white truffles, saffron, chile pepper, herbs and spices of all kinds, and fermented soy.

NOTES ON WINE: None.

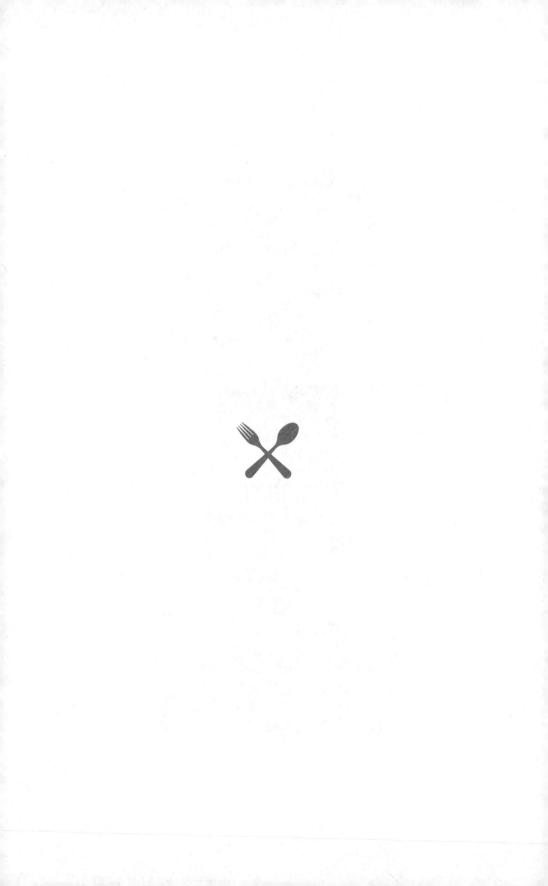

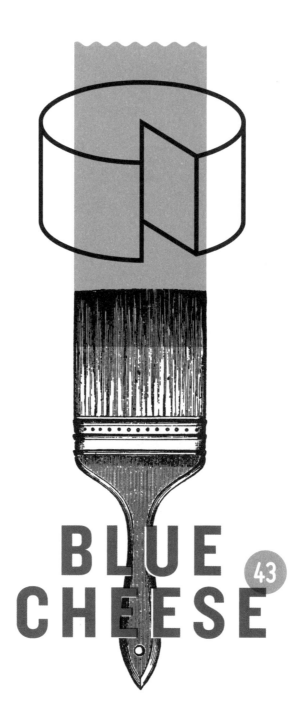

BLUE CHEESE 43

43. ROQUEFORT AND OTHER BLUE CHEESES

Roquefort, the classic blue cheese from ewe's milk, aged in the caves of the village of Roquefort-sur-Soulzon in the South of France has been made since at least the eleventh century (although it isn't clear that it was always a blue cheese). A well-made Roquefort offers an unusual combination of intensity and refinement, a sweet piquancy mingled with spice. Compared with cow's and goat's milk, ewe's milk is higher in protein and much higher in fat, and it gives a lighter texture to Roquefort. And ewe's milk contributes its own different flavors as the cheese ages. The appellation—the first for any food or drink in France, established in 1925—embraces a vast area. The heart of it, closest to the village, consists of limestone plateaux ringed with cliffs and covered in shallow soil; summers are hot and dry. Very little will grow there; almost the only activity is raising sheep. Nearly two thousand farms milk a total of 750,000 ewes, of the native Lacaune breed, in a season that commonly runs from mid-December through mid-July. The cheeses are aged in caves built into the fractured rock beneath the village at the edge of the Combalou Plateau. By way of fissures called *fleurines,* a continuous supply of moist, cool air passes through the caves. In most of them, the temperature remains between 46 and 50 degrees F (8 to 10 degrees C), varying hardly more than a degree or two year-round. The best caves are the most humid. Roquefort today has seven producers, the largest of which is Société, responsible for multiple brands and more than two-thirds of total production. All the cheese is made in dairy plants, eight of them, from small and manual to large and industrial, located from about five to thirty-five miles (ten to sixty kilometers) outside the village. The total area that produces milk for the cheese is so large and geographically diverse—some is more mountainous, cooler, and wetter—that any uniqueness compared with other blue cheeses can come only from the caves and the particular blue molds found there: strains of *Penicillium roqueforti.*

Six hundred strains of it have been identified in the caves, though I believe just four (it's not information the producers readily share) are currently used to ripen the cheese. To ensure that the cheeses turn sufficiently blue, the producers have long propagated and added mold. The old way was to take big round loaves of rye bread, poke holes in them, and leave the loaves in the caves for weeks until, when they were broken open, the interior was solid blue and filled with powdery spores. Before the 1970s, when the strains currently in use were identified, the bread used to capture variable wild molds, and the range in quality of the cheeses was wide. Some were powerfully odorous, some were badly off in taste, but the best, however few, were better than any of today's. Two producers still use rye bread, but they introduce a chosen strain of mold into the loaves. The moldy loaves are ground into powder, which is mixed with the whole milk or curd.

The curd, when set, is cut into cubes, drained, and packed loosely in the molds so as to leave tiny air spaces between the fragments, openings where the blue mold will grow. The cheeses are drained without pressing, unmolded, and the surfaces are salted. Each cheese, so it will turn more evenly blue throughout, is then pierced with thirty-two stainless-steel needles to provide oxygen for the mold to grow. In the cave of at least one producer, the cheeses still rest directly on oak or chestnut shelves. Under the current rules, Roquefort must be aged from the day it was made for a minimum of ninety days, of which at least two weeks must be in the caves, and some cheeses spend three weeks or a little longer. Then the cheeses are wrapped in a square of tough tinfoil to keep out air and prevent the mold from growing so much that it entirely dominates the flavor. A balance between white and blue is essential for taste. The slow maturation continues at separate facilities outside the caves, where the air is refrigerated to a degree below freezing.

There's a link between temperature and taste, and in 1925 the mandatory period for aging in the caves was three months. Compared with a cave, a modern installation makes it easier to move the cheeses in and out, monitor them, control the temperature, humidity, and exchange of air. (In the original caves, the air currents rise or fall through the *fleurines* according to the wind and often change direction in the course of a day.) Does the modern short time in the caves followed by months of deep chill obscure or bring out the individuality of the milk and cheese? Longer, colder aging produces a stronger, more complex flavor, and with the seasonal production of milk, slowing down the evolution allows a more consistent taste year-round. But at cold temperatures, one main part of aging—the one in which proteins are broken down—is slowed almost to a halt, while the part in which fats are broken down continues, and those altered fats are responsible for a more aggressive blue flavor. Toward the end of cold aging, a peppery sharpness can appear and build, a problem that can be reduced with care and the right strain of *P. roqueforti.* Above 50 degrees F (10 degrees C), however, protein breakdown naturally dominates and gives sweeter, nuttier, perhaps more delicious flavors.

France has other blue cheeses, some thirty of them, and nearly all are made of cow's milk. (Persillé de Tignes is goat.) Roquefort is one of the world's few blue cheeses made from pure ewe's milk. Spain and Portugal are the center for blues made of mixed milk, cheeses such as Cabrales, Gamonéu, Picón Bejes-Treviso, and Valdeón, some of which can be intensely blue.

Each of the following has its particular characteristics and the potential to be great:

STILTON (PDO) The tall, unpressed cow's-milk drums were already famous in the early eighteenth century when Daniel Defoe passed through the village of Stilton, in the east of England. Today the cheese comes from an area of three counties around Melton Mowbray, and especially from the Vale of Belvoir. Some Stiltons tend to be moister, sweeter, and fruitier; others are drier, more caramel and nutty. Even the drier examples shouldn't be dense but instead buttery in consistency. Unfortunately, to qualify for the name, today the milk is required to be pasteurized, which doesn't prevent some Stilton from being very good. (PDO is the EU's

Protected Designation of Origin, the English translation of AOP and DOP.)

GORGONZOLA (DOP) Italy's celebrated blue cheese probably originated in the Lombard town of Gorgonzola, now part of the eastern suburbs of Milan. It's mainly an industrial cheese these days, and most is made west of Milan in Novara, from milk produced in a wide area of Lombardy and Piedmont. Sadly, like the milk for Stilton, it's now required to be pasteurized, and most of the cheese doesn't excel. Originally, the cheeses were transported for aging to natural caves in alpine valleys. The drums of Gorgonzola come in two distinct types. The more traditional *piccante* cheeses are firmer, drier, and bluer, are aged longer, and taste sharper and spicier. The modern *dolce* (mild) style is creamy, and those cheeses are much younger, though with time they can become stinky. The *dolce* cheeses are more popular, but the *piccante* have more complex flavor. Gorgonzola is fine on its own and makes a compelling sauce for gnocchi or pasta.

CASTELMAGNO (DOP) In a small area of the mountains of Piedmont in northeastern Italy, just three communes, including the scarcely inhabited one of Castelmagno, high in the beautiful Valle Grana, turn raw cow's milk into an ancestral blue cheese. The earliest mention of Castelmagno cheese by name dates from 1277, and in its region it has long been famous, yet during the mid-twentieth century so many farmers left the mountains that the cheese nearly disappeared. Fortunately, it has somewhat rebounded. Castelmagno is made of finely broken dry curd pressed into a rustic drum shape, roughly as high as it is wide and weighing anywhere from about 4½ to 15 pounds (2 to 7 kilos). Although Castelmagno is usually classified as blue, the cheeses often didn't used to be blue at all, and many still aren't. The bluing occurred spontaneously only when a crack allowed an opening to air. A slice of a Castelmagno that's just a few months old shows a dry, crumbly white center, and the taste is lightly acidic, even lemony, pleasing but not special. Much more interesting, though rare, are moister cheeses aged for a year to a year and a half, by which time the center has turned a pale, dirty yellow. The taste is rich and complex; any blue portions are creamier and stronger than the rest, making an extraordinary cheese.

CABRALES (DOP) The strong, rustic Cabrales, produced in and around the Spanish village of that name in the mountains of Asturias, near the Atlantic Coast, is usually very blue. It can be made with raw cow's, goat's, or ewe's milk or any mix of the three. At least some of the cheese is still aged on wooden shelves in natural caves, ventilated by Atlantic winds, where once the bluing occurred spontaneously. The yellowish background color of the Spanish blues, depending on their age and the kind of milk, tends to be darker than that of any of the French blues. Cabrales used to be wrapped and sold in the leaves of the sycamore maple (*Acer pseudoplatanus*); now it is wrapped in foil. (Some of the related blue Valdeón is still wrapped in leaves.)

As a group, the moister blue cheeses, and perhaps especially Roquefort, are vulnerable to age and mistreatment. Roquefort is usually at its best when it's shipped by the producer, and further aging only does harm. (When a blue cheese is too old, off, or mistreated, the taste can be sharp, salty, and aggressive, and the flavors can be harsh and ugly.) After you've bought a good piece, eat it promptly to see just how delicious blue cheese can be.

HOW TO BUY BLUE CHEESES: Taste first, if you're allowed; the cheese may have been kept too warm, too dry, or too long. It's best that a piece be cut to order from the whole drum. (Any cheese loses flavor more rapidly after it's sliced and exposed, and Roquefort deteriorates more quickly than most cheeses. The big producers would surely argue for the advantages of their vacuum-packed pieces, and they would be somewhat right.) In blue cheese of whatever kind, neither darker mold nor more mold is necessarily better.

It's important to have a balance between white and blue, and the mold always grows poorly near the outside, because early on that's the saltiest part. Where ivory is the background color of Roquefort, the cow's-milk blues, such as Stilton, are yellowy and become more so with time.

Some advice specifically for Roquefort: At four months, it's new, and after eight to ten months most drums decline and off-flavors appear, although exceptional cheeses improve after that. Fall is typically the best season, as for other cheeses, because the ones for sale then (barring delays in the export pipeline) were made from spring milk, which is typically the best milk of the year. With Roquefort, look for a background color no darker than ivory and mold that's blue or green, not gray, which indicates that the cheese is old. (The color rule doesn't automatically apply to other blues.) And look for a cut surface that gleams, suggesting a richer, more tender cheese. Good flavor includes the faintest hint of something like nail-polish remover (which is more pleasant if you think of it as recalling tarragon), but certain cheeses acquire a strong smell of it, especially those made with a particular strain of penicillium, when they're too mature or kept wrapped for too long. Nowadays Roquefort is less likely to be too salty, although the saltiness of any cheese increases as it ages and loses moisture.

The best Roquefort producer by general consensus is Carles, the second smallest in size, still cultivating the blue mold in rye bread and still working by hand. But Coulet, Papillon, and Crouzat Constans are all very good, and when, for lack of choice, I've bought Société, no one has complained. The best Stilton comes from Colston Bassett Dairy (a cooperative of four farms in the village of that name), especially the drums it makes for the specialist dealer Neal's Yard Dairy. Stichelton is a sometimes-excellent raw-milk take on Stilton; it's the proprietary name of a cheese first made only in 2006, on Welbeck Estate in Nottinghamshire, outside the Stilton area. The best Castelmagno I've tasted came from the *stagionatura* (cheese cellar) at Valcasotto in Piedmont, part of the Beppino Occelli cheese business. Other things being equal, choose Castelmagno marked *di alpeggio,* which comes from animals on mountain pasture.

HOW TO STORE AND SERVE BLUE CHEESE: A piece of moist blue cheese can change quickly, so try to eat it on the same day you buy it. If more than a few hours will pass, keep the cheese wrapped and in the refrigerator, but be sure to take it out several hours before you serve it—earlier for a larger piece. Unwrap it, set it on a plate, and cover it with a clean cloth or inverted bowl. Only when cheese warms to 50 to 60 degrees F (10 to 16 degrees C) does it show all its flavor. As a moist blue warms, a little whey will flow. At the table, slice the cheese parallel to the radius of the original wheel, so everyone gets some of the tender, flavorful center.

COMPLEMENTS TO BLUE CHEESES: The number-one complement to cheese is bread, and for Roquefort and most other blue cheeses the bread should be a white or mostly white "country" loaf or a very good, fresh baguette. Some people like rye or walnut bread—walnuts themselves are a near-certain success with blue cheeses. With a great blue, I find it hard to do anything other than eat it with fresh bread. But if you do cook with blue cheese, for instance making a sauce for pasta or a savory custard tart, then the sweetness of a moister, fruitier blue is pointed up by tarragon; a few finely chopped celery leaves are also good. Cooking turns the creamy texture of blue cheese into a grainy one. It helps if you minimize the cooking or do no more than melt blue-cheese butter on a steak (mash equal weights of cheese and butter, and mix in finely chopped chives, tarragon, and black pepper). Blue cheeses, crumbled, go well in a salad (such as of Boston lettuce and mâche dressed with heavy cream, white-wine or cider vinegar, olive or walnut oil, and salt and pepper with, again, chives). Most fresh fruits distract from a great blue, although the sweetness of grapes or ripe pears soothes a strong, sharp one. Also delicious with Roquefort are prunes, such as those from Agen, not far away, cooked briefly in red wine with a touch of sugar and served cool.

NOTES ON WINE: "Roquefort is a wine killer," wrote Richard Olney, who cared about great wine as much as anyone. The difficulty with blue cheeses comes from their strong flavor, sharpness, and salt, which swallow up a large part of the fruit of wine. (Alternatively, water is an impeccable choice with cheese.) But many people enjoy red wine so much that with Roquefort they drink a good red Burgundy or, more often, Bordeaux. The red wine works better if it is less tannic, usually meaning older, but don't waste a really good bottle; a better option may be a lushly fruity young red without much tannin. That might be a Zinfandel that isn't high in alcohol or, more or less from the region of Roquefort, a Marcillac. (Rather than a red, though, among dry wines I prefer a rich white, such as from Pinot Gris.) The wine most often recommended with blue cheeses is Sauternes, whose sweetness soothes the cheese, but Sauternes can be too concentrated and sweet: one bite of cheese and one sip of wine are enough. A younger blue cheese, of whatever sort, takes a younger wine, and among the many sweet choices are a young *moelleux* Jurançon, for its freshness. In fact, if there's a best wine for blue cheese in general, it may be Jurançon. A very different sweet option is the oxidized wine Maury or the closely related and often recommended Banyuls. But Jean-Michel Parcé of Domaine du Mas Blanc, the great producer of Banyuls, once told me that Roquefort doesn't have enough sensation of fat for Banyuls, that Muscat goes better. He does like drier bottlings of Banyuls (which from Domaine du Mas Blanc can be identified by the 18 to 19 percent alcohol on the label) with other blue cheeses, such as Fourme d'Ambert, Bleu d'Auvergne, and Stilton. The classic British accompaniment to Stilton is of course vintage or tawny Port. The possibilities with Spanish blue cheeses include Port, Spanish cider, and sweet, dark Pedro Ximénez sherry. With Gorgonzola *piccante,* some varied sweet Italian options are Picolit, Malvasia delle Lipari, and Moscato di Pantelleria. And with blue cheeses, especially the nuttier ones, it's not out of the question to drink a strong Belgian ale or a big oatmeal stout.

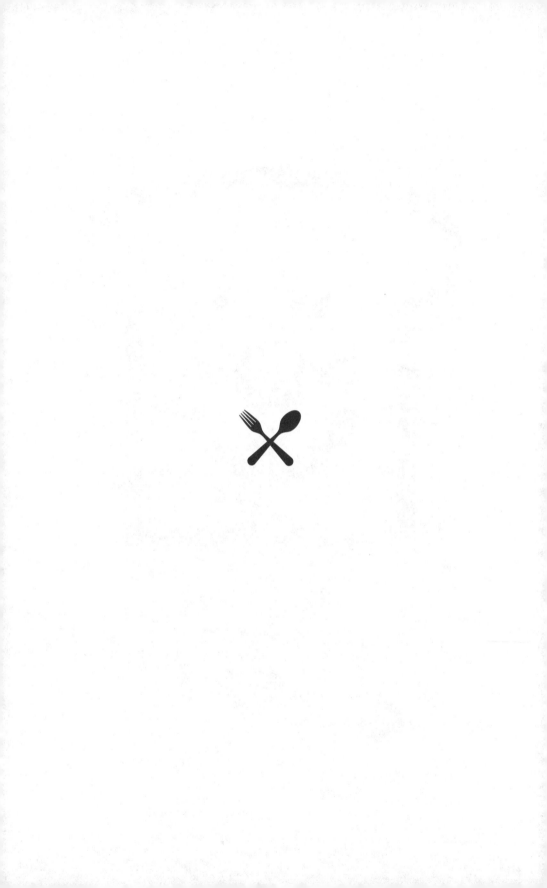

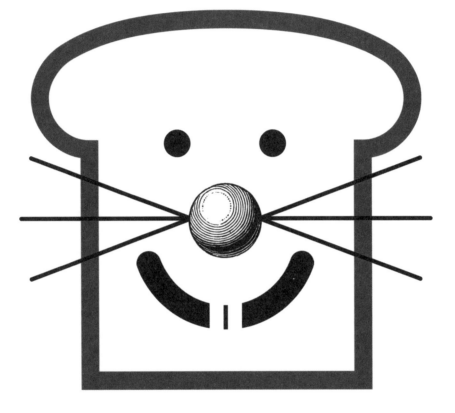

RYE
BREAD

44

Dark, close-textured all-rye bread, raised with a sour leaven as it almost must be for good texture, has a particularly intense flavor that's wonderful on its own and with other foods. In German, it's commonly called *Schwartzbrot*, "black bread," although in some regions the word is applied to mixed-grain loaves, and there are other specific sorts of German rye, including pumpernickel. Once, the loaves of dark rye were enormous—five, ten, twenty-five pounds. A slice of *Schwartzbrot* shows an even distribution of tiny holes. The flavor runs in the earthy direction of grain, malt, nuts, mushrooms, coffee, dark molasses, and bitter chocolate. But in North America, our rye bread commonly contains no more than a quarter or a third rye and tastes nothing like that. (I wish it weren't necessary to add that I mean caraway free. The seeds, often ground, undercut the rye taste; they're so common that some people think caraway is the taste of rye. To me, its flavor in bread is almost abhorrent.) In North America, if you don't live near an exceptional artisan or bake it yourself, good rye is hard to find.

Rye tolerates cold and poor soil better than wheat does, and rye bread remains the typical kind in a large portion of mostly northern Europe, running from Russia through Scandinavia and Germany into the Südtirol, the small German-speaking slice of northern Italy. Within that area, the farther south you go into climates more hospitable to wheat, the more wheat a loaf of rye is likely to contain. In Germany, to be called "rye," loaves must be 90 percent rye (as wheat loaves must be 90 percent wheat). Other loaves are called "rye with wheat" or "wheat with rye," depending on which is in the majority. In much of Western Europe, rye has long been in retreat, and for lighter texture and milder flavor rye flour is commonly diluted with large amounts of wheat. When both grains are whole, the combination is good, but all-rye belongs to a higher category. The French, who make such good wheat bread, make almost no dark rye and only a small amount of mixed rye-wheat bread, which isn't especially good, even in Alsace, where the traditions are Germanic. Compared with wheat bread, the taste of rye comes less from fermentation than from the quality of the grain itself. A problem in North America is that we grow rye mostly for cattle feed, not for flavor in bread. The kind of rye also affects the color; darker varieties were common in the past. A lighter color and taste can also come from separating out part or all of the bran from the rest of the rye flour at the mill, and for some people removing part of the bran gives the best taste and texture. (You can't make white rye flour, because the center of the seed isn't white but light gray.) In a good loaf, a strong rye taste and sourness are in balance. Rye bread holds its moisture and keeps much longer than wheat, remaining fresh for four to five days and holding good flavor long after that.

But rye is a temperamental, technical bread. Wheat mixed with water forms elastic gluten, which allows the dough to retain the gas of fermentation and thus expand and rise, but rye doesn't do that. On its own, it creates a limited, fragile rise. (I've made a successful, nonsour loaf from fresh rye flour, handling the risen dough very gently. The baked bread was sweet and delicious.) Even a rye-wheat loaf doesn't swell that much in the oven; the dough is slashed on top, but the marks hardly open. One way to introduce some lightness to all-rye is to use meal rather than flour. Meal is grain broken into pieces, and larger pieces have more air space between them. Any further lightness comes from the rye sour, meaning the starter. But any such leavening is unpredictable with wheat and more so with rye.

The sour, made of just rye flour and water, as it's used up, is regularly refreshed with more flour and water. A German baker once commented to me about a big covered plastic bucket of rye sour, "When you open it, it should give you a good wake-up smell." The rye cultures are variable, a selection of the same yeasts and most of the same acid-producing bacteria that appear in wheat sourdough. The precise culture doesn't seem to affect rye flavor the way it does wheat. With a rye sour, it's more that an experienced baker can tell the fruity smell of a regularly used and refreshed one. An all-rye dough needs no commercial yeast, but some bakers add it anyway.

It's hard to explain the difficulties of leavening rye without throwing in a little science. Two key components of rye, starch and pentosans, when they're mixed with water to make the dough, will hold some gas and lighten the bread. Compared with wheat, rye contains twice as large a quantity of pentosans, which absorb six to seven times their weight in water and form a dense, jellylike gum. Rye also contains more enzymes than wheat—the same ones that turn barley starch to sugar to make beer. The enzymes break down the starch and pentosans and diminish the firm viscosity of the dough. But in some years, especially with older varieties of rye, the quantity of enzymes is too great, and they can go too far and make the bread wet and gluey. The acidity of the rye sour slows their activity and makes the dough more elastic. More often now, with current varieties of rye, the problem is too few enzymes, and bakers must add some enzyme-filled barley flour. Making rye bread is a balancing act. There's a fine line between too little enzyme activity and too much. With the right amount of it and the right acidity, the crumb is more moist, loose, and open.

Bakers glaze the loaves with a mix of water and starch, often potato starch, brushing on the mixture before the loaves go into the oven or as soon as they come out. The combination of starch and heat creates the shine. The initial heat and steam help to swell the loaves, but after that the dense bread must be baked slowly, so that the heat penetrates fully and the enzymes have time to finish their work. The danger in a high-enzyme dough is that the enzymes will turn so much starch into sugar, before they're stopped by heat, that beneath the top crust there's a soupy pudding. Even an ideal rye loaf, when you slice it, leaves a slight smear across the knife.

Part-rye loaves are certainly good as well as traditional; they were once commonplace in much of Western Europe. The English name for a half-rye, half-wheat loaf is maslin; it's *pain de méteil* in French. One of the best combinations is equal parts rye, corn, and wheat, which made up the one-time everyday loaf of the northeastern United States (its nearest surviving relative is sweet Boston brown bread). Rye also goes with sunflower seeds, linseed, pistachios, barley, oats, and other grains. An old alternative to caraway is charnushka (*Nigella sativa*), to use its Russian name, a much less fragrant seed that's sometimes confusingly called black caraway in English.

Pumpernickel—all-rye, heavy, dense, sour—originated in Westphalia. About a century ago it became the professionally made bread we know today, baked in covered molds in special steam chambers. It's made with only water, salt, sour starter, and medium-sized meal, so it has slightly smaller openings than *Schwartzbrot*. The loaves remain in the steam oven for a minimum of sixteen hours and up to twenty-four. Steam keeps the bread from drying out during that time. The temperature starts at a moderate 200 degrees C and falls to 100 (about 400 to 212 degrees F). The slow heating of the dense loaves allows the enzyme activity to continue for a long time, turning a significant amount of starch to sugar. The innate rye darkness is increased by the enzymes and browning reactions. Pumpernickel has only small mechanical openings and no lift from yeast. The slightly malty taste from the enzymes is enhanced by the roasting effect of the steam chamber's heat. On the outside, there's almost no crust. A loaf must be thoroughly cooled before it's sliced, and its taste is intense. For good reason, the slices are thin.

HOW TO BUY RYE BREAD: It's hard to tell much about the taste of rye bread from its appearance. A darker brown-black suggests a stronger taste, though there might be added coloring. You can check the ingredients on a label or ask questions, hoping to hear that there are only rye, water, salt, and sour culture. The taste should be complete and balanced, with a tang but without sharp acidity or distracting bitterness. When the bread is completely cool, keep it wrapped in plastic.

COMPLEMENTS TO RYE BREAD: With all its strong character, dark rye comes to the foreground. Although it's not as adaptable as wheat bread, it goes well with many things. It's hugely complemented by dry-cured ham and other cured meats, especially smoked, and by cheeses, from fresh to aged, including stinky. It goes with smoked salmon, gravlax, pickled herring, and sauerkraut, as well as mustard or horseradish and lettuce in a sandwich.

NOTES ON WINE: The smoky, slightly spicy, vegetal flavor of rye, particularly when matched with cheese or cured meats, goes with beer more than with wine—a range of kinds of beer, though very dark ones are too much for the cheese and provide little contrast with the bread. If you prefer wine, look to a light red or an aromatic white, optionally a white with a little sweetness.

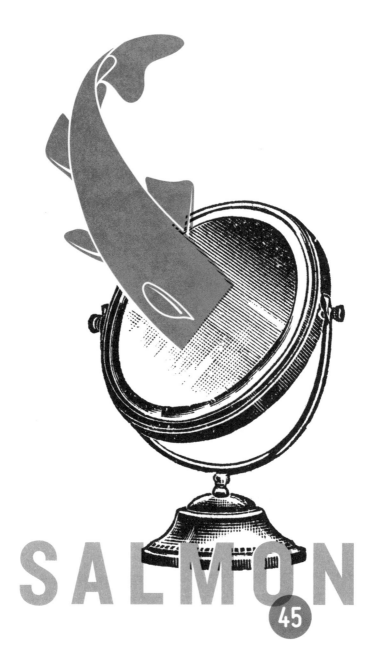

SALMON

45

The salmon is a leaper. From the ocean it swims up the river of its birth, sometimes hundreds of miles, to spawn; it's capable of leaping ten feet. The salmon was designed for speed, agility, and endurance. Its life centers on that journey, including gaining the strength and fat it requires to succeed. The fish are fattest at the start of the run, when they leave salt water and enter a river's mouth. They used to be found in every river of their huge territory, until they were overfished, blocked by dams, suffered loss of water to irrigation, and lost other habitat, sometimes to pollution. The Atlantic salmon, *Salmo salar,* which was once found as far south as Long Island Sound, survives on the American side of the ocean in only a few rivers of northernmost Maine, though in many more in maritime Canada. The total numbers, however, are small, and efforts to revive them have met with limited success. Wild Atlantic salmon in North America are commercially extinct. All the fresh Atlantic salmon sold here, apart from a few wild fish flown in from Europe, are farmed, in North or South America or Europe. On the European side, although they have disappeared from certain rivers and are badly diminished in most, salmon are found from the Portuguese-Spanish border northward, and some populations remain strong. On the Pacific Coast, five salmon species, all in the genus *Oncorhynchus,* are found from central California northward, and so far they persist in healthy abundance in Alaska. Many fish have little flavor, but not salmon, thanks partly to the fat. (In slices of smoked salmon, it's easy to see the pale fat between the rings of pink muscle.) Salmon is firm, meaty, and flavorful. It's something of a chameleon fish in that its flavor is distinct yet delicate enough that it goes with both mild and fairly strong flavors—butter and cucumber as well as dill, onions, lentils, salt pork, red wine, and smoke.

We're biased toward the kind we know. The Paris chef Alain Senderens once described all Pacific salmon as "second-rate." I first came to know the Atlantic salmon, but the best Pacific salmon are at least as good. If you compare them with wild Atlantic, the wild Pacific are perhaps a little stronger in flavor and firmer-fleshed. Three Pacific species are most valued. The King, or Chinook, is the most prized and the largest, with an average size in Alaska of twenty pounds. It's high in fat, and the color can be a brilliant orange-red; exceptionally, it's white, though there's no difference in taste. Next comes the Sockeye, or Red, with its strong red color; it's also high in fat. The Coho, or Silver, the second-largest Pacific salmon, weighs a dozen pounds on average and has a bright red-orange color and not quite as much fat. Less well-regarded are the Chum, or Keta, and the small Pink.

The color of the flesh reflects not only the species but the time of year and diet. (In farmed salmon, the color is carefully calculated and determined by what's added to the feed.) There are fattier and leaner wild salmon, according to the species and when and where they were caught, as well as fattier and leaner cuts, the leaner meat being more subtle. Farm-raised salmon tends to have too much fat, enough to taste oily, though many people like the richness. However fat salmon are, after they are caught their fat seems to be more stable than that of other fatty fish, such as mackerel and bluefish, which quickly turn fishy.

The very idea of eating a wild fish rather than a farmed one is appealing: it's more authentic in taste, more romantically tied to nature, and cleaner-tasting (if it comes from clean waters). But we've lost most of the great supply of wild fish that, with a little care, we ought to have had forever. They've been partly replaced by a much smaller but ever-increasing supply of farmed fish. The big, troubling question is how much damage the farming does to the oceans. Farm-raised salmon and other fish are concentrated in undersea cages or surface pens, where they eat and defecate in profusion. They're also bred for yield and speed of growth, perhaps losing other valuable qualities (and there will be steady pressure to allow genetically modified stocks). The Monterey Bay Aquarium's Seafood Watch advises us to avoid all farmed Atlantic salmon unless they were raised in inland tanks in closed systems, because of the amount of other fish the salmon require as feed, the diseases that can spread to wild fish, and the inevitability that escaping salmon will breed with nearby wild fish and weaken them.

The salmon caught during the wild runs have always been preserved by salting and often by both salting and smoking. Modern smoked salmon receive no more than a token cure, so the taste is more like that of Scandinavian gravlax or even sashimi than of traditional smoked fish. The modern cure uses just enough salt to complement the delicious combination of raw fish, aromatic flavorings, and light smoke. There's a hint of sugar, usually dill, perhaps mustard seed, juniper berries, white peppercorns, anise or fennel, which individually are so subtle as to be indiscernible. As with the fresh fish, the loin (the best part of the filet, toward the tail) is the thickest and best part; the belly is fattest and sweetest, and the tail is leanest. Good fresh smoked salmon is completely unfishy. Its texture is buttery, not oily. It's wonderful to have a whole side to cut with a very long, narrow blade, in slices so thin you can see your fingers through them.

For gravlax, the fresh salmon is covered with a mix of salt, sugar, dill, sometimes white pepper, juniper, or spices, and while it cures it's weighted to make it more compact. Lox is also in theory unsmoked, although most of what's sold as lox in New York City today is lightly smoked. Lox used to be cured in very salty brine, but that kind seems to have almost disappeared. Salmon roe is brined, too, and keeps for a time.

Still popular on the Pacific Coast is traditional hot-smoked salmon, which is cooked through and contains enough salt and smoke to fully preserve it. (The only ingredients of the real thing are salmon, salt, and smoke.) The perfect amount of salt is just enough to preserve the fish without refrigeration. The texture should be firm but not tough, and the fat should give an impression of moisture. The flavor is straightforward but not at all simple.

These days salmon, like tuna, is often seared outside and left rare inside. To my taste, it has the most flavor and moisture when it's cooked just to the point where it ceases to be translucent. It's delicious grilled, sautéed, or roasted, but its delicacy is shown when it's poached or slowly baked in parchment. In the heat of summer, no meal is more satisfying than a whole cold poached salmon (preferably protected by a coat of the now very retro-seeming aspic, as little as it may enhance taste, and decorated with the blue stars of borage flowers).

HOW TO BUY SALMON: The broad season for fresh wild salmon is summer and fall. King salmon is available in small quantities through the winter from small boats. The season for Sockeye is mid-May to mid-September, and for Coho mid-June to mid-October. Salmon holds its freshness longer than some fish, but seek it at its very freshest. It should look just caught, or just fileted; it should feel firm and show no sign of drying. The smell, if you can pick it out among the odors of a fish store, should be unfishy and clean—*very* fresh salmon has an uncanny cucumber odor. Cook any fresh fish on the day you catch or buy it. Meanwhile keep it as close to freezing as you can: put it directly on ice in the refrigerator.

Keep cold-smoked salmon deeply chilled, and eat it promptly. It's at its peak about twenty-four hours after smoking, and it keeps only a matter of days, unless it's vacuum-sealed in plastic (the small packages holding slices are never quite as good). Traditional hot-smoked salmon will survive warm temperatures, but I refrigerate that, too. (Beware that some hot-smoked Alaska salmon tastes like hot dogs. Read the ingredients to see that nothing more has been added than salt and smoke.)

COMPLEMENTS TO SALMON: Freshly squeezed lemon is enough, but salmon likes the flavor of dill, tarragon, parsley, chervil, and fines herbes (parsley, chives, tarragon, and lots of chervil). Salmon especially likes cucumber salad (peeled, seeded cucumbers sliced in half-moons, salted, drained, mixed with crème fraîche, and flavored with dill). It likes accompaniments of peas, new potatoes, new onions, lentils (cooked, for instance with carrots and onions and served with *lardons*), leeks, shallots, sorrel, spinach, asparagus, salt pork, and bacon. Hot poached salmon, especially from leaner fish, goes with *beurre blanc*. Cold salmon goes with many of the same things as hot—cucumber salad, cold peas, cold new potatoes, dill, chervil, fines herbes, borage, watercress, and mayonnaise. Cold-smoked salmon goes with pickled or salted capers, black pepper, cold boiled potatoes, rye bread, bagels and cream cheese. Both cold- and hot-smoked salmon go in scrambled eggs and omelettes.

NOTES ON WINE: Poached fresh salmon with a rich sauce such as *beurre blanc,* goes with richer examples of Chenin Blanc (maybe especially from Anjou, where the sauce probably originated), of Sauvignon Blanc, of white Burgundy, including *premier* and *grand cru* Chablis, and with the mineral quality of Savennières (an Anjou Chenin) and the sweet wine of Coteaux du Layon (again Anjou Chenin). The same wines, as well as Riesling, suit cold poached salmon.

Roasted or grilled salmon and preparations with cured pork or a red-wine sauce go with full-flavored rosé or a light red with little tannin and no oak. The prime candidate is Pinot Noir, the reflexive red choice with salmon, but one that's not too strong. Reds especially require very fresh salmon (the wine brings out any fishiness). And salmon, like lobster, when served with a rich sauce, can suit *vin jaune* and other strong *sous voile* Jura whites. Salmon with a tomato sauce goes with rosé, and salmon with lentils goes with rosé or Pinot Gris.

The fat and flavor of smoked salmon makes a good textural match with the acidity of Chablis, Riesling, and Champagne, though only a more concentrated bottling really stands up to the salmon flavor. For novelty, turn to Alsace Gewürztraminer.

Salmon, fresh or smoked, has a particular sympathy with Sancerre, which is pure Sauvignon Blanc from the upper Loire Valley appellation that includes prime territory for the variety, though high quality is spreading in Touraine and other parts of the Loire. But Sauvignon has an ambiguous nature. Is it an herb and vegetable wine, a salad wine, a fish and raw-oyster wine, a goat-cheese wine, a charcuterie wine, a wine for roast chicken? Harvested at the usual ripeness, Sancerre is more acidic and herbal. Harvested very ripe from a top vineyard, it can be so rich that the grape variety is hardly recognizable; it's excellent in a completely different way. To me, the optimum, most complex Sancerre comes from a top vineyard, but the grapes have a middle ripeness that conveys some of both sets of characteristics.

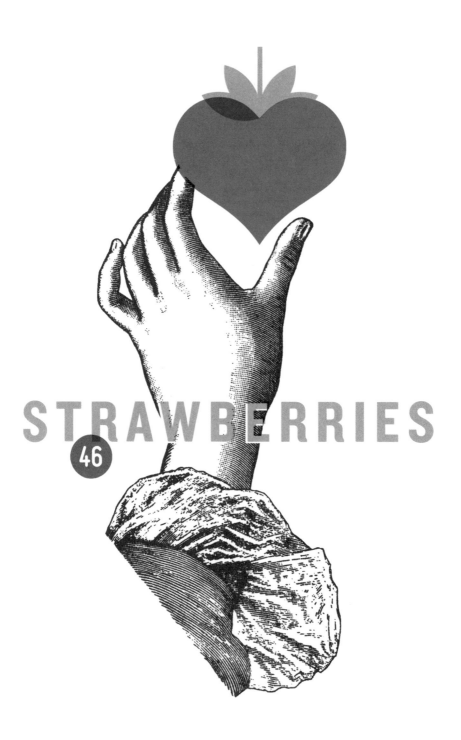

STRAWBERRIES

46

46. STRAWBERRIES

To be perfectly delicious—sweet with a hint of sharpness, tender, full of essential strawberry perfume, which often veers in the direction of pineapple—strawberries must be completely ripe. I hesitate to say it, for fear of discouraging anyone, but ripeness lasts just one day. And the more aromatic the variety, it seems, the narrower the gap between ripe and overripe. The most aromatic varieties are typically smaller, softer, more vulnerable. Once on a hot June day, during the short time it took me to drive home from a pick-your-own place, the flat of ultraripe strawberries sitting beside me half-melted into juicy mush (I made jam). The vulnerability of strawberries may explain the English name: *straw* likely refers to the old and still-current practice of raising the plants in a bed of straw. That protects them from winter frost and, when the season arrives, holds the fruit above the damp, decaying earth, keeping the berries dry and preventing rain from splashing them with dirt. It's no help to pick the berries underripe, because once off the plant, they don't gain in sugar or flavor, they only soften and rot. All strawberries belong to the genus *Fragaria,* from the Latin for "sweet-smelling, fragrant," but the words don't apply to current mainstream varieties. Those have been bred for disease- and pest-resistance and for large fruit, which reduces the labor cost of picking. But too high a yield means less flavor, because there are proportionately fewer leaves sending the precursors of aroma to the fruit. Supermarket strawberries are now sometimes eerily red clear through, while their texture is firm, almost crisp, and unchanging, so the berries remain intact for days. In taste, they can be hard to distinguish from a kiwi. Superior varieties are generally older, and their fruits are smaller, less durable; today in North America they are grown only for local markets. Besides those older conventional types, two particular strawberry species have small fruits that are especially high flavored.

The finest perfume probably belongs to the tiny alpine, or wood, strawberry, *F. vesca,* often called the *fraise des bois.* It's the common wild strawberry of Europe, and it was cultivated in France by the 1300s. The alpine strawberry was carried to North America, where it quickly escaped into the wild. In my lawn it struggles against the mower and trampling feet. The berries are tiny; you need patience to pick even a few dozen, and they can be dry and seedy. Yet the taste is exquisite. Alpines are easy to grow, and the best cultivated varieties—if you can get them—are somewhat larger, have better texture, and retain a nearly wild flavor. They are almost never grown for sale in North America, although they are raised a little here and there in Europe. In Sicily, for instance, the cultivated *fragolina di Ribera* is believed to have been brought from the north of Italy by soldiers returning from World War I. Like most other alpine varieties, it has red fruit, but certain varieties bear fruit that remains creamy white even when ripe.

Some people prefer another species: the musk strawberry, *F. moschata.* I admit that I've never tasted it. Just a few fruits are said to fill a room with their perfume, a cloying intensity that puts some people off. Native to Central Europe, the musk strawberry is also known as the hautboy or hautbois ("high wood") strawberry, maybe because it holds its flowers and fruit high above the leaves. Musk strawberries are bigger than alpine but smaller than conventional and too soft to ship well. They're also less cold hardy than many other kinds of strawberry. For all these reasons, they're hardly grown commercially in North America.

The conventional modern strawberry combines two different New World species. One is the Virginia, *F. virginiana,* the common strawberry of eastern North America. (Where the alpine usually holds its flowers and fruits above the leaves and its seeds are flush with the fruit surface, you can tell the Virginia because its flowers and fruits are below the leaves and its seeds are in pits.) The other parent of the modern strawberry is the Chilean, *F. chiloensis,* also called the pine or beach strawberry. It's native to the Pacific Coast from southern Alaska to California, and it grows in coastal Chile and Argentina, as well as in Hawaii. Both the Virginia and Chilean species were carried to Europe, but the Virginia was little grown in its new surroundings, and the Chilean succeeded commercially only in the coastal climate of Brittany around the village of Plougastel, whose reputation for strawberries continues today. There, in the mid-1700s, growers found that the Virginia and Chilean had formed accidental hybrids with higher yields. The Virginia contributed, says the present-day American fruit connoisseur David Karp, cold-hardiness, red color, and acidity, and the Chilean contributed larger size and firmer texture. Breeders from the start headed in different directions, he explains, "with examples evoking raspberry, apricot, cherry, and currant." Today's commercial varieties are ever-more-complicated crosses, impossible to sort out. Breeders are working to address their taste shortcomings, even to add musk flavor.

Low-acid varieties taste sweeter, but some acidity is needed to offset the natural sugar, and in strawberries, as in many other fruits, stronger acidity seems to coincide with the finest aroma. Fully ripe northern strawberries are generally more acidic and have that high-pitched aroma. As with other fruits, too much cool, gray weather inhibits ripeness, rain fills the fruit and dilutes flavor, and more and stronger sun gives more sugar and flavor.

Nearly all strawberry desserts call for raw fruit, whether simple strawberries and cream or mousse, Bavarian cream, frozen soufflé, ice cream, or ices. As good as the cold desserts can be, the cold mutes flavor. A freshly baked tart shell lined with pastry cream and raw strawberries, served at room temperature, conveys the full flavor. (Brushing with melted raspberry jelly helps berries with weak taste. Another prop is equal quantities of raw strawberries and raspberries, pressed through a strainer to strain out the raspberry seeds and poured over the fresh strawberries.) Jam and jelly capture a superb strawberry flavor not far from the fresh, if the fruit is cooked for the shortest necessary time. Then there are warm desserts, such as a soufflé of alpine strawberries or raw strawberries covered with sabayon (zabaione) and gratinéed. They're delicious, but for a light, satisfying dessert, nothing beats great ripe strawberries on their own.

HOW TO PICK OR BUY STRAWBERRIES: At the beginning of the season, the berries are relatively huge; first to ripen on each plant is the king berry, much larger than the fruits that follow. As strawberries ripen, they become redder and softer. Within a variety, the darkest individual fruits are the ripest, although darker red varieties aren't better. (You may see some strawberries that are "cat-faced," with seedy unformed tips. When they were tiny, they were stung by tarnished plant bugs and paralyzed at that spot. They're edible but not as good.) Because ripeness is fleeting, you have to pick through the rows daily. After a few dry, sunny days, the taste is more concentrated. Strawberries keep better if they're picked with the green cap on; to do that, you have to pinch the stem carefully between your thumbnail and forefinger and pull to break the stem. If you don't have the luxury of your own patch, look for a grower who plants flavorful varieties. While the best kinds are June-bearing (their fruit benefits from the longest days), some are "everbearing" (providing a smaller, steadier supply) or day-neutral (giving most of their fruit in spring and fall). I once planted an everbearing kind with low expectations, and though the berries weren't on the level of the best, I was surprised at how good they tasted.

Some flavorful varieties to look for: in the northeastern US, Sparkle (the conventional variety I grow, introduced in 1942 and sold at some farmers' markets); in California, good though not tip-top varieties are Chandler, Gaviota, and Seascape (introduced in the 1980s and 90s by the University of California); in the Pacific Northwest, look for the everbearing Quinault (1967, Washington State University); in Florida, look for Oso Grande and Selva (1980s, University of California). A modern French variety with an excellent reputation is the early, somewhat small-fruited Gariguette, created at Avignon in the 1970s. From it has come the fine four-way cross Mara des Bois (though in my garden, Sparkle beats it), which is raised by a number of US market gardeners. Besides all those, you may be lucky enough to find a grower selling good alpine or musk strawberries, at a price. In the future keep an eye out for a revival of Fairfax (1933, USDA, a parent of Sparkle), which has a top reputation but has been out of commerce, and of Marshall (1890, Massachusetts), which not long ago was all but extinct. Marshall was raised on a commercial scale in Oregon into the 1960s and in the US was widely considered the best strawberry ever grown, which didn't prevent it from being replaced by higher-yielding varieties with more durable fruit.

Strawberries last longer if you pick them in the cool of the morning and keep them in a shady spot until you're ready to eat them. Because they so readily absorb water, which dilutes flavor and speeds deterioration, rinse them only if there's dirt and only just before you hull them (if they need to be hulled at all). Pass them under the tap quickly and immediately roll them gently on a towel. Avoid refrigeration, because they pick up off-flavors and the cold may harm the taste. If you have to keep utterly ripe strawberries until the next day, sprinkle them with sugar, cover them, and then do refrigerate them.

HOW TO PRESERVE STRAWBERRIES: To carry the wonderful taste of ripe strawberries through the year, the simplest thing, especially if the berries are clean and don't have to be rinsed, is to slip them into plastic food storage bags and freeze them just as they are. Similarly, freezer jam keeps all the fresh flavor: you just mix crushed raw fruit, sugar, and commercial pectin following the package recipe and freeze it. (Like that jam, low-sugar jam isn't jam in the traditional sense; it requires added calcium to set and has too little sugar to act as a preservative. And the reduced sugar offers no superior balance in taste.) You can capture a bright color and a strong, nearly fresh flavor in regular cooked jelly, jam, and preserves, but only if you boil the fruit very briefly in a shallow layer in a wide pan, so as to evaporate just enough water to allow the fruit to set. You can achieve gorgeous flavors and elegant textures—a cut piece of jelly should be soft enough to sag and swell outward yet hold its sharp edges.

To gel, any fruit requires acid and pectin, its own or added, plus added sugar. Most recipes prescribe a fixed ratio of fruit to sugar—a lot of sugar—plus, usually, a fixed ratio of lemon juice, and they call for pectin almost no matter what. And most instructions still call for extended boiling, although the short-time, shallow-layer method is gaining ground. The books cite one or more of about five ways to test whether the boiling jam or jelly will set. Yet they rarely if ever talk about desirable texture or taste—the things anyone who loves great jam and jelly really cares about.

Not just each kind but each batch of fruit varies enough to completely trump any cookbook formula. Less-ripe fruit is higher in pectin and acidity, for example, and rain just before harvest gorges fruit with water. The difference in strawberries can be dramatic. Berries bloated by rain end up as little balls floating in juice unless you boil them far too long or kill the taste with sugar. If you can, pick berries for jam only after a couple of dry days.

Sugar fixes color and flavor and acts as the main preservative. To prevent the finished jam or jelly from spoiling, you need about 65 percent sugar. But if you're going to properly can the jam (processing the filled jars in boiling water) and eat it fairly quickly after it's opened, then what do you care? (You can seriously discourage mold by keeping the jam in the refrigerator, but then you end up eating cold jam . . .) You need only enough sugar to get the fruit to gel. Adding more sugar, though, means not only a sweeter result but also shorter cooking and better flavor. For the very brightest color and flavor, add most or all the sugar at the start of cooking, not later, even though you will throw away some of it if you strain out seeds and skins.

I take the purist approach and avoid adding commercial pectin. I suspect almost no fruit requires it. If a fruit lacks its own pectin, then do as cooks have always done and combine it with a high-pectin fruit, such as apple, currant, or quince. (The shallow layer–quick boiling method doesn't apply to quince, which requires long cooking no matter what.)

Acidity is needed not only to form a gel but also to balance sugar and help preserve and hold flavor. Avoid adding acidity if you can (much easier with cool-climate fruit), because it may never fully mesh with the taste of the fruit. Strawberries are low in both acidity and pectin, but you don't have to add either one if you boil off the extra water quickly.

Rather than worry about the sugar concentration, which is reflected in the temperature reading on a thermometer, check the ability to set by tipping the liquid off a spoon. At first it runs off one drop at a time; as it concentrates, it falls in two side-by-side drops; after that it sheets (falls off in globs), when it has perhaps gone too far! Whether that's so depends on the pectin and the acidity in the fruit.

Unfortunately, none of this lends itself to a standard formula. After you have a little experience with fruit from a particular source, though, you can find a sugar-to-fruit ratio and use it from year to year, adjusting only a little for the particular batch. It's hard to get just the same tenderness each time, but with the shallow-layer, short-boiling method it's easy to make impressively fresh-flavored jam.

COMPLEMENTS TO STRAWBERRIES: Number one is rich cream or a freshly made, luscious cream cheese, which I admit is almost impossible to find in North America unless you make it yourself. Vanilla underlines the ripe fruit flavor of strawberries, as it does with most fruits. It's perhaps more a cooking tip than a complement, but fresh strawberries short on acidity benefit from a squeeze of lemon juice, and dull ones can be heightened with raspberry. Strawberry and rhubarb are harmless together but to my mind no more than that. And mint leaves, however cheerful, have no special affinity for strawberries. Many people like to pour freshly squeezed orange juice over strawberries. Sliced bananas and strawberries go together. So do almonds and strawberries, both the nutty side of the nuts and the aromatic bitter-almond side (like almond extract). You might expect chocolate to compete, but instead it sets off the fruit flavor of strawberries. It's *very* delicious to mash the berries, roughly, with a little sugar and then add some of the red wine in your glass (Beaujolais, the wine most often named, is good); the sugar forms a bridge between fruit and wine. Alternatively, pour over the berries some lightly sweet sparkling Moscato, such as Moscato d'Asti, which needs little or no additional sugar, or add a small stream of syrupy, sweet, intense Muscat wine. From an entirely different realm, black pepper is excellent on fresh strawberries, as are, separately, drops of luxurious true balsamic vinegar from Modena or Reggio.

NOTES ON WINE: With superb strawberries, there's no need for a glass of wine. But if the fruit falls just a little short, sparkling Moscato goes well— even better if there's rich cream on the berries. When a strawberry dessert includes cream or, preferably, both cream and buttery pastry, opt for a fully sweet wine, such as Sauternes, Coteaux du Layon, or Mosel Beerenauslese.

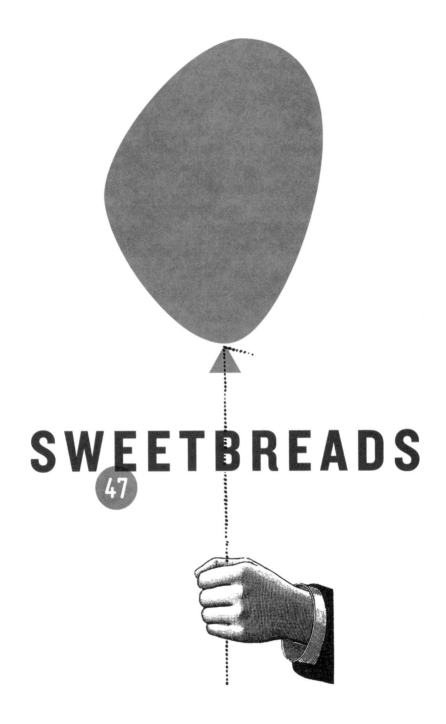

SWEETBREADS

47

47. SWEETBREADS

L ike brains, sweetbreads have a rich, delicate sensuality—carefully
cooked, they offer a fragile texture not so far from custard (the description often applied to brains). Very Old World, maybe not for everyone.
Also like brains, for contrast, they're sometimes dipped in egg and breadcrumbs and sautéed to give a surrounding crust. French haute cuisine has
many recipes for them. In contrast, Italian sweetbread recipes are scarce,
today almost nonexistent. Larger sweetbreads come from veal (*ris de veau*
in French); much smaller ones come from lamb (*ris d'agneau*) and kid (*ris de
chevreau*) and are used more in *ragoûts.* The traditional season is spring,
some weeks after the animals were born. The sweetbread is the perishable
thymus gland, which all but disappears as an animal matures. It comes in
two parts. The "heart," which is located near the heart, is preferred for its
larger, more compact shape and tenderness. It's connected to the longer
"throat" sweetbread, which, when a cook removes the surface cartilage
along one side, tends to fall into pieces. The curious English name explains
nothing—we can only guess where *sweetbread* comes from. (Once, as a
child with my family in a restaurant, I ordered sweetbreads, expecting
something like dessert for a main course. No one stopped me. I ate them
and said nothing.) I've cooked sweetbreads only once, never having lived
where I had easy access to them. (You may have to order them specially.)
The way they're prepared may tell a lot. They must be very fresh. These
days, they're sold already quite pale, but they always used to be soaked in
cold water for several hours, or overnight, to draw out remaining blood and
whiten them. Then they're gently poached (better than the old boiling), just
long enough to firm them and make them easy to handle (they remain raw
in the middle), and then they're chilled in cold water. They used to be
pressed overnight as they chilled fully, to give an even thickness, but the

redoubtable cook Richard Olney believed that this deprived them of "succulence," and it's his advice I follow. (He wanted to serve me sweetbreads once, but he could only find brains.) Once the sweetbreads are thoroughly chilled, you remove only the fat, cartilage, and outer membrane, carefully leaving the skin beneath so they hold neatly together. Only then are they ready for a recipe. They're sometimes braised whole but more often sliced. Or they're turned into *ragoût* (sometimes presented in puff pastry) or a terrine or even grilled. Overcooking produces an almost entirely different, coarser, meatier item. The whole point is delicacy; a sign of it is the pale color.

In late spring, *ris de veau* are served with the vegetables that excel at that time—green peas, spinach, sorrel, sometimes asparagus—the sweetbreads and cooked vegetables being put together only at serving so the contrast in flavor is sharp. Rich and relatively mild and neutral, sweetbreads go well with many sorts of things. Acidity, such as from spinach or sorrel, counters the rich blandness—bland in the old positive sense of "suave."

Green peas are the outstanding complement. The old-school French dish is *ris de veau à la Clamart.* (The town of Clamart, outside Paris, was known for its green peas, and "Clamart" on a menu refers to peas.) The whole "heart" is braised on a bed of carrots and onions with veal stock. For freshness, sweetness, and greenness, the *petits pois* are cooked very quickly with butter in a few spoonfuls of water. The braising liquid is reduced to a syrup and poured over the sweetbread, which is then surrounded with peas, an emblem of spring. Any simple sweetbread preparation is excellent with peas.

COMPLEMENTS TO SWEETBREADS: They go with spring vegetables—peas, sorrel, spinach, asparagus. They go with butter, cream, bacon (smoked or unsmoked), lemon, mushrooms (especially morels) with cream, black truffles, tomato, dry or sweet white wine, onions but not garlic, the perhaps too-predictable Madeira (or has it fallen so far out of fashion that it seems new?). Some chefs like a counterpoint of vinegar, such as an interesting flavored one or a sweet one like Banyuls.

NOTES ON WINE: Sweetbreads call for a somewhat refined wine. Depending on what goes with them, that might be a white Burgundy (a Meursault, for example) or a light, refined red, which could be a young, somewhat lesser Burgundy (such as Mercurey). If the dish includes green peas, then the wine needs a suggestion of sweetness, in aroma or from very subtle sugar, found in a Loire Chenin, for instance, or in the rich juiciness of a substantial white Bordeaux. The white wine for sweetbreads should be clean, focused, somewhat complex, and could come from many places. Especially if there's cream, it could be more emphatically sweet, up to the richness of a Sauternes or Coteaux du Layon (but those wines make a very rich combination, and where do you go from there?).

TRUFFLES ⁴⁸

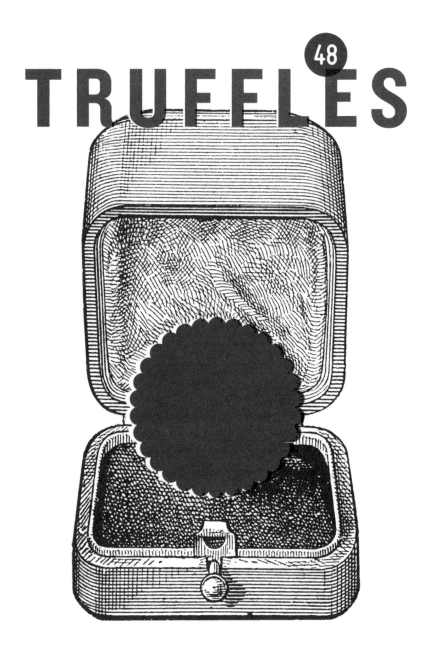

48. TRUFFLES, WHITE AND BLACK

The little agglomerations of bulbs, tan, brown, or black, especially when the soil is still clinging, look like nothing you'd want to eat. And the interior of a truffle, sliced open, is strangely veined. Nothing appears aboveground. The permanent part of the fungus is a network of filaments, the bulbs being merely the spore-bearing part. Like many fungi, truffles live in symbiosis with the roots of trees, each giving benefits to the other. Then, in the woods in autumn and early winter, the aroma from the buried ripe truffle rises up through the soil, sometimes strong enough to draw truffle flies (which eventually lay their eggs in a truffle, with the side effect of spreading the spores). Like some other wonderful, rich aromas, and some distasteful ones, this one comes from forms of sulfur. It has a suspect quality; it might be garlic and cheese, and it has been called cabbagey. But mainly it's truffle, and the kinds have their own characters. For finding truffles, nothing beats the nose of a dog or, better, a pig, because the truffle contains a sex hormone that attracts the female pig. But you need a new pig each year, because they grow too big to handle. Most truffle hunters prefer dogs, which also attract less attention to the secretive hunt. Of the various truffle species, just two have outstanding aroma and really count: the white Alba truffle of northern Italy (*Tuber magnatum*) and the black Périgord truffle of southwestern France (*T. melanosporum*), which also grows in certain other areas of France, as well as Spain, Italy, and some other countries.

Italians see the white truffle as obviously superior, and the French appreciate it but find it less subtle and gratifying than the black. Both are superb and different; it's not really a question of one being better. Sadly, as truffles have become scarce and prices have risen higher and higher, both kinds have fallen deep into the realm of luxury. There do exist other European species at a fraction of the cost, but they have little or no aroma. And none of the canned products capture the flavor. A better option is white truffle salt: ground truffle mixed with the crystals, at a moderate price, with genuine flavor, and a little goes a long way. White truffles are eaten raw. Usually, a shower of thin slices, with the crispness of an extra-firm nut, goes on hot food. The main experience is of aroma, and it's lost in real cooking. In contrast, black truffles require heat, though not much cooking, to bring out the full flavor. I first tasted them mixed with mashed potatoes, and the person I was eating with, having no idea what the flavor might be, said, "These are the best mashed potatoes I've ever eaten." The best way to appreciate either kind is with simple foods. Often, sliced or slivered, they're added to scrambled eggs, and in particular the white are shaved over hot egg pasta with just butter and Parmigiano.

The white truffle grows wild, especially under the basket willow. The reduced supply is due to overharvesting, loss of land to development, wild boars that uproot and consume them, and truffle hunters who, like wild boars, dig holes and leave them unfilled, so frost enters and damages the underground network.

In Italy, I once had the extremely good fortune to eat a multicourse meal so thickly layered with sliced white truffles that when I left the powerfully truffle-scented air of the small restaurant, the outdoors smelled strange. That was extreme, but it's important to have enough truffles, good ones, that you don't have to search for the flavor or regret that it disappeared so quickly. Until the middle of the twentieth century, black and white truffles were much more plentiful and affordable. In Piedmont, the region of Italy that includes Alba, two or three generations ago truffles were eaten by the rural poor, because they were free to those who could unearth them. (They weren't rare, the price wasn't high, and access to markets wasn't necessarily easy.) Truffles went into the Piedmontese *bagna caoda,* the warm anchovy-and-garlic-filled sauce for dipping bell peppers and cardoons.

Black truffles prefer oaks, and the supply has been reduced for reasons similar to those that have diminished the whites. Of the remaining black truffles, a good portion are cultivated, as they have been for more than a century in France and now Spain and Italy. (There are also efforts in the US.) The underground network takes years to become established and produce. Both species are sensitive to soil and climate, and in the wild no one can predict just where they will be found. Recent more aggressive efforts at cultivation have met setbacks, and some plantations have been badly contaminated with the inferior, similar-looking winter truffle, *T. brumale*. But there has been some success, and it seems inevitable that cultivation will be mastered.

In North America, certain truffles found in the Pacific Northwest have enthusiastic admirers: the Oregon black truffle and especially the two Oregon whites, which are much less expensive than the great European truffles. They grow under Douglas fir. The black (*Leucangium carthusianum*) is found from fall to early winter. And there's both a spring Oregon white (*T. gibbosum*) and a fall one (*T. oregonese*), with the seasons barely overlapping in winter. But even some of those who know the Oregon truffles well feel ambivalence. The chef Greg Higgins, of Higgins in Portland, says, "Both the Oregon white and black have the intensity of a typical European summer truffle. Under perfect conditions they're both capable of being quite savory. The whites with notes of musk and sweet spices and the blacks aromatic of chocolate, port and tropical fruits . . . Neither is at all as pungent as European whites or blacks. The whites need to be picked near full ripeness or you might as well shave a wine cork over your food. The blacks can be ripened if stored properly in rice at room temperature till perfectly ripe." That method keeps the surface of any sort of truffle dry and flavors the rice, which captures the escaping aroma. Truffles are also stored with eggs, which become the basis of a truffle omelette, along with actual truffle. (Overripe, the black Oregon truffles are dominated by ammonia.)

Much worse than no truffles at all is truffle oil. Every brand I've tried has tasted fake, and the cloying aftertaste can linger for an hour or more. The oil is commonly flavored with 2,4-dithiapentane, the main natural flavor compound in white Alba truffles, which isn't present at all in other truffles, or not in significant quantities. I once made my own oil by immersing five grams of paper-thin top-quality white Alba truffle slices in 100 milliliters of excellent mild olive oil, and I put the covered jar in the refrigerator. (The cold inhibits botulin, and there's a small risk of botulism in the anaerobic conditions of moist food submerged in oil. I also cleaned the outside of the truffle well and, as a further precaution, added salt.) The next morning, the oil had congealed in the cold, and it tasted distinctly of truffle. A week later, the flavor was at its peak. Tasted alongside my natural oil, even supposedly honest commercial oils were cloying and chemical. The homemade was far superior, though not the same as fresh truffle, and the good flavor lasted only two weeks. Apart from any use in oil, the aroma of a whole fresh truffle gradually changes and diminishes, and once truffles are cut open, breaking the cells, the aroma compounds change more rapidly. It's hard to see how there can be any such thing as a good, long-lasting truffle oil.

As a rule, you eat truffles with other food, but often black truffles used to be prepared on their own. *Truffes sous la cendre*—"truffles under hot coals"—sounds deeply rustic, but a recipe appears in the cookbook *Les Soupers de la Cour* ("Suppers at Court") of 1755: "Being well-cleaned, wrap them in a number of sheets of paper without any seasoning; moisten the outer layers; cook them for one hour buried in hot coals." By the twentieth century, truffles were instead more often wrapped in puff pastry and baked in the oven, and sometimes still called *sous la cendre.* There used to be and maybe rarely still are *ragoûts aux truffes,* such as a small potful with only salt and pepper and a little white wine or broth, possibly herbs and aromatic vegetables, covered and cooked for ten minutes to half an hour, the whole finished with Madeira or Port and a little butter. (Sometimes the truffles were thoroughly cooked, which apparently changes the flavor to something less strong but possibly no less good.)

Most uses call for fewer black truffles. As a rule, they're first peeled. They go into terrines and stuffings for beef, pork, game, and chicken; they can be inserted in advance in slits in the meat. Not least they're put with foie gras (which is possible to produce by humane methods in fall, when the birds naturally fatten themselves for winter). The food needs time to absorb the truffle flavor before it's cooked; the perfume enters, and afterward not much of the flavor may be left in the truffle. The best-known classic is *poulet en demi-deuil* ("chicken in half-mourning"), with round slices of truffle, like giant polka dots, slipped under the skin before the chicken is poached.

Especially suited to black or white truffles are scrambled eggs, with the sliced or slivered truffles barely cooked along with the egg. Or you can add the black to the eggs ahead of time to perfume them fully. Either truffle goes on fresh egg pasta with Parmigiano. In a restaurant, the white are rapidly shaved onto the hot pasta as it sits before you. The black, requiring more heat, are very gently cooked first in butter with salt and pepper, timed to be done at the same moment as the pasta.

WHERE AND HOW TO TASTE, BUY, AND STORE TRUFFLES: An excellent place to encounter truffles is in a good restaurant in season in their native territory, in northwestern Italy or southwestern France. The white are available from October to the end of the year and the black from late November to mid-March. If you decide to invest in a truffle or two for yourself, beware that inferior examples and species are sometimes passed off as good ones. (In the future, a database of genetic markers may allow black truffles to be verified and even sold by place of origin.) Turn to a reputable dealer, which might be small and local. (Big names are Plantin in France for the black and Urbani in Italy for the white.) The truffles should be neither too firm nor too soft and have a marked odor. They don't ripen further but only lose aroma once they've been unearthed, so after you acquire them, consume them promptly. From the time they're unearthed, with the dirt on, they might last ten to twelve days. Professionals clean them just before sale, and then they must be used within a few days.

Use a stiff, dry brush to clean away dirt and a knife point as needed, and finish with a damp cloth or a quick, thorough rinsing in water. The black are normally peeled. I've never owned a proper truffle slicer. You can use a plain vegetable peeler, and I've used a sharp knife. Truffle slicers, razor-sharp, with adjustable blades for thickness, produce a quick, efficient shower of shavings.

COMPLEMENTS TO TRUFFLES: Once upon a time, when black truffles were plentiful, they became the most common flavoring in haute cuisine, put indiscriminately with almost everything. It's true that the truffle is so deep in its own category of taste that it doesn't conflict with other foods. If only to make that point, today truffles are sometimes used in dessert. Flattering to either black or white is the simplest background—scrambled eggs, risotto, egg pasta (either of the last two with butter and Parmigiano). Parmigiano goes especially with white truffles. They enter a Piedmontese *fonduta* (melted Fontina cheese with egg yolks). In season, black truffles go into the classic cervelas sausage of Lyon (which is sometimes taken a further step and baked inside brioche). Truffles are complemented by butter, cream, and meaty sauces.

NOTES ON WINE: Probably any decent wine will go harmlessly with truffles, but a rare lucky choice of an earthy, animal red Burgundy makes a special combination. You can find similar complementary aromas in great Barolo and Barbaresco, northern Rhone Syrah, and Châteauneuf-du-Pape (though the last in recent years tends toward distracting high alcohol). And truffles go with the Merlot-dominated wines of Saint-Émilion and Pomerol in Bordeaux. If you insist on white wine, then a refined Burgundy. And white truffles make perfectly good combinations with lesser Piedmont reds such as well-made Barbera, Freisa, and Dolcetto.

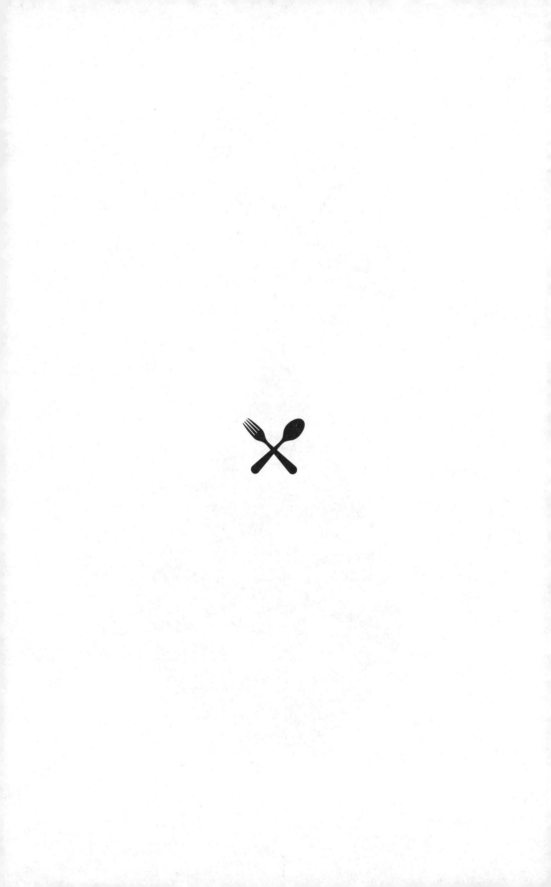

VINE⁴⁹GAR

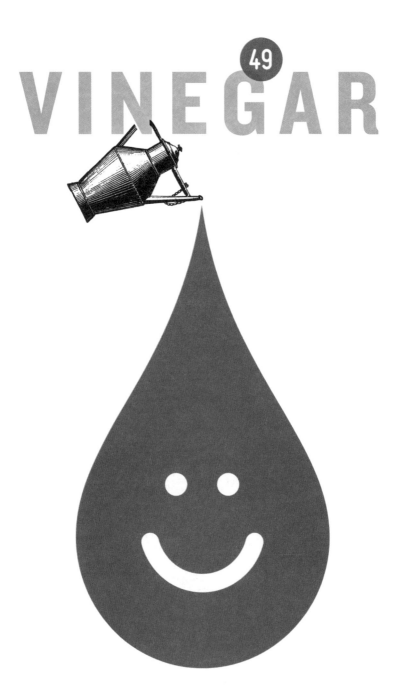

49. VINEGAR

Vinegar—*vinaigre* in French, "sour wine"—is primordial, the inevitable product of wine, one of the most important and least thought about components of good food, at least in Western cooking. You can make vinegar from any sweet substance that will produce an alcoholic liquid, not just wine but cider, malt, rice, honey, pineapple. And unless the liquid is so extremely sweet that sugar remains mixed with the alcohol, nature won't allow the vinegar to be sweet. Yet good old plain, nonsweet vinegar, especially from red wine, has been largely displaced on store shelves by concocted sweet vinegar, especially "balsamic." Not that sweet vinegar is bad by nature. Rarely, it's sublime, above all in the form of luxurious traditional *aceto balsamico,* which lives on its own higher plane. The problem with sweet vinegar is that it has limited use: it competes with the natural sweetness of whatever food it's added to. Apart from real *balsamico,* to me the most interesting vinegar is regular red-wine vinegar. White-wine vinegar has more neutral flavor, though it's useful, too, mainly because red gives a dingy color to pickles and cream sauces. The tannin of red-wine vinegar brings with it more depth, more nuance, more flavor, to balance sheer acidity and the particular strong flavor of acetic acid, the acid that defines vinegar. The more aroma and flavor vinegar has, the less its acidity is apparent. Up to a point, the better the wine, the better the vinegar. Good red-wine vinegar brings strong aromas of fruit, like the best fruit in wine, usually in the realm of small red fruits (strawberry, raspberry, red currants), occasionally accompanied by flowers.

Whatever its kind, vinegar is an essential preservative. Beyond pickles, it makes marinades, condiments, all the sweet-and-sour tastes. Before refrigeration, people were used to more acidity in food than we are today.

Fresh meat was wiped with or immersed in vinegar to allow it to keep for a short time; smaller amounts of vinegar were added to certain cooked foods to do the same. Yet vinegar takes a leading role in very few dishes. Two of them, in France, are *poulet au vinaigre* and *sauce piquante.* (A sweet-and-sour taste was common in medieval and Renaissance French cooking, but it hardly exists today in France. It disappeared in the seventeenth century, after the aristocracy switched to a simpler, more modern cuisine in which sweetness was confined to dessert.) Yet scattered sweet-and-sour dishes survive in the north of Italy and a larger number in the south. There's broadly Italian *lepre in dolceforte* (sweet-and-sour hare); specifically Venetian *saor* for vegetables, fish, or meat; and certain Sicilian dishes (usually attributed to Arab influence but possibly older), of which the best known is *caponata* (sweet-and-sour eggplant). For some of us, vinegar continues to play a subtle role in balancing and lifting dishes that might otherwise be flat—a stew, a soup, a sauce. Any of those can sometimes be nicely pointed up by a discreet addition of vinegar, like a seasoning, almost like salt; a few minutes' cooking takes away the rawness and melds the flavors. At the table, vinegar enhances cooked greens or beets. But its greatest role is surely in vinaigrette. Containing no sugar itself, the vinegar respects the natural sweetness of fresh produce. It's irreplaceable with ripe tomatoes, and when the vinegar in vinaigrette is very good, the tomato enhances the vinegar and not the other way around. The effect is uncanny.

Most commercial wine vinegar doesn't taste like much, because it starts with cheap wine, which can give a muddy taste and off-flavors. And the industrial process doesn't help. Enormous vessels continuously circulate and aerate the liquid, sometimes producing vinegar in less than a day. The best-known device, the Acetator, made by the German company Frings, has the particular shortcoming that it employs a "submerged" fermentation, in which only one important species of *Acetobacter* is present, which gives a narrower flavor. And before bottling, most commercial vinegar is pasteurized or sterile-filtered to eliminate bacteria, which mutes what little nonacetic flavor there is. Depending on the amount of alcohol in the original wine, wine vinegar ends up with around 7 percent acetic acid. In the US, however, wine vinegar usually tastes watery, because it's cut with water to as little as 4 percent acidity, which is legal as long as that's indicated on the label. It's better value to step up and pay $10 to as much as $20 for half a liter of something interesting.

Like nearly all wine, vinegar often contains added sulfur as a preservative. But vinegar is itself a preservative, and, made well, it doesn't need to be preserved! Some producers may worry about microbiological problems, which can happen if the fermentation wasn't complete. Sulfites, being antioxidants, also protect certain good flavors, but vinegar has already been exposed to air during the making, so there isn't that much to protect. And sweet vinegar, without sulfur, pasteurization, or sterile filtration, isn't entirely stable: a small alcoholic fermentation may start in the bottle, followed by a further acetic one.

Better vinegar is fermented more naturally—more slowly and by a wider range of *Acetobacter* species; the liquid lies still in its vessel, so it doesn't lose as much flavor to air and oxygen—and is often made or aged in wood as opposed to stainless steel. The very best red-wine vinegar may be the one you make yourself from the remains of excellent bottles. That's simple enough to do. Mainly you just expose the wine to air in a dark, warm place, and you wait. Specifically, you can half-fill a glass jar with dry wine containing no more than about 13 percent alcohol, and cover it with a piece of loosely woven cloth held in place by a rubber band, to keep out vinegar flies, which are the same as fruit flies. The optimum temperature is the low 80s F (around 28 degrees C). It's even easier to make cider vinegar, starting with particularly rich, freshly pressed apple juice (US sweet cider) that hasn't been pasteurized, if you can get it; it first turns hard and then becomes vinegar. When the wine is left open to air, a "mother" forms on the surface, at first a thin veil, scarcely visible. Sometimes it becomes powdery; often it turns into a thick mat—whitish, translucent, slippery, and tough, like an aberrant form of gelatin. In fact, it's harmless cellulose, though it's better that the bacteria's energy goes into producing acid. The mother is the sign that acetic bacteria, present in the environment and often already in the wine, are gradually turning alcohol and oxygen into acetic acid and water. Unless too much sulfur or another, less desirable preservative was added at the winery, that automatically happens when wine is exposed to air. And that's why wineries keep their barrels topped up. In a few months—sometimes just two or three weeks—your vinegar is ready.

With one possible catch. The bacteria responsible for turning alcohol into acetic acid are unpredictable and sometimes veer off in the direction of a smell like nail-polish remover. To be precise, it's ethyl acetate, and it's a much worse defect than sugar. It may not be detectable if you add just a touch of vinegar to something, but enough ethyl acetate in vinegar makes salad inedible. It's difficult to prevent, and even certain high-end vinegars suffer.

Often superior is vinegar labeled as coming from a particular grape variety, such as Cabernet Sauvignon, or from a particular kind of wine. Sherry vinegar can be a bargain. One of the more interesting and uncommon vinegars is made from sweet Banyuls wine. The flavor of vinegar can be boosted by macerating fruit in it, such as fresh raspberries, or an herb, such as tarragon, and later decanting (or leaving the herb).

Probably every vinegar benefits from age, whether in a full wooden cask or in a sealed bottle. Lesser vinegars might improve for a year, while better ones might benefit from several years or more. Although the bottle you buy may already have aged in the distribution pipeline for months or longer, it may be worth setting aside for more time on a shelf. There's no perfect way to know, although with regular wine vinegar, a whiter or redder color suggests more potential (and a more golden or orangy one suggests the bottle is at least old enough).

The most exalted form of vinegar comes from the historic Italian region of Emilia: *aceto balsamico tradizionale di Modena* (and its close relative *aceto balsamico tradizionale di Reggio Emilia*), which is one of the world's most expensive condiments. A bottle holds just 100 milliliters (about 3⅓ ounces). That's the only size available, and in the US it often costs $100 or more—much more for older bottlings. This true balsamic vinegar has nothing in common with supermarket knockoffs, which range in taste from harmless to markedly crude and unpleasant, and their defects are only half tamed by sugar. These "balsamic" vinegars are made by mixing boiled-down grape juice with generally iffy regular wine vinegar and sometimes caramel, sometimes molasses, and only occasionally some genuine, young *aceto balsamico.* The real thing has been made for centuries in what today is a legally defined zone in and around the affluent city of Modena (and in a separate zone around nearby Reggio) on the wide, warm Po River plain. Traditional balsamic vinegar contains roughly 6 percent acidity, in the same range as regular wine vinegar, but in balsamic vinegar the sharpness is masked by sweetness and mellowed by time. Years of aging have concentrated and thickened the liquid, turning it a dark reddish-brown. *Balsamico*'s profound, long-lasting flavors are mainly of prune, maple syrup, caramel, and the deep meatiness (*umami*) found in soy sauce and the brown juices in a roasting pan. There are also hints of flowers, fresh fruit, and Port wine, with a shadow of astringency in the aftertaste.

Balsamico used to be made only in well-off families by the woman at the head of the household. The single ingredient was and is *mosto cotto,* "cooked must"—the freshly pressed juice of ripe grapes, boiled down to a sweet syrup. The grapes used in Emilia for *mosto cotto* are late-ripening and rich in sugar, mostly white Trebbiano but also red Lambrusco and several minor varieties. *Mosto cotto,* more often called *sapa* in Italian (*saba* in Modenese), is an ancient, delicious sweetening of the poor in wine-growing areas. *Sapa* gives a sweet-and-sour note to a few traditional Emilian dishes and is an ingredient of certain sweets.

To make *balsamico,* you pour the *mosto cotto* into barrels placed in an attic, and then, as with regular vinegar, you wait—but in this case for a very long time. The barrels rest on their sides with a small opening facing up and covered with a square of white cloth, held in place with a flat stone or a wooden block. A producer has one or more series of barrels, which may be more than a century old. Each of these *batterie* is composed of at least three, often five, and up to a dozen barrels, arranged in descending sizes. A large first barrel of oak might be followed by one of chestnut, then cherry, ash, mulberry, juniper, and more oak, each species contributing its own qualities to the *aceto.* At least a few producers believe that oak is best and use only that. No barrel is ever completely filled or emptied. Each fall, a little of the most aged vinegar is drawn from the last, smallest barrel, and that little may go into a *tragn,* a ceramic jug, for still more aging. The quantity removed is replaced with *aceto* from the next-larger barrel beside it, and so on from barrel to barrel until the largest barrel is replenished with new *mosto cotto.*

The transformation in the attic is complex. Within that first large barrel, an exceedingly slow and partial alcoholic fermentation takes place as the yeast struggle to turn just some of the *mosto cotto*'s sugar into alcohol. A second fermentation soon joins in as bacteria transform the alcohol into acetic acid. The liquid is exposed to air and to seasonal extremes of heat and cold. Certain elements oxidize, adding that dimension to the taste, while enzymes contribute many of the subtlest and most desirable flavors. As the vinegar moves from barrel to barrel, the changes become slower and slower. After a dozen years, evaporation has reduced the volume by roughly 90 percent, leaving a dense, precious liquid. I've tasted forty-year-old *aceto balsamico* that was thicker than honey, too thick to pour. It wasn't the best I've had, but it was the most concentrated, with a small edge of blackstrap molasses. Even from the same attic, no two *batterie* yield quite the same taste.

Balsamic vinegar wasn't traditionally used in cooking. A thimbleful was and sometimes is taken by itself after dinner as a *digestivo*—a balsam. But today *balsamico* is certainly used in cooking, and with its three-way balance among tartness, sweetness, and intense flavor, it seems to go with almost everything. A few calculated drops or more are an excellent culinary resource. Because cooking eliminates some of *balsamico*'s fine aromas, it should be added only just before serving or placed on the table as a condiment.

HOW TO BUY AND STORE RED-WINE VINEGAR AND *ACETO BALSAMICO:* Avoid wine vinegar with added sulfites, and beware that when you try an unfamiliar bottle, it may have the defect of tasting like nail-polish remover, which shows up even in some ostensibly good brands. One reliable French producer, which exports, is Martin Pouret, of Orléans, where the Pouret family (who later married into the Martins) has been making vinegar since 1797, the only longtime French producer to have adhered continuously to traditional methods. In blind tasting I can usually pick out Martin Pouret because of a slight flavor of old wood, which must originate in the *vaisseaux,* the barrels in which the wine ferments. A quarter of the vinegar is drawn off every three weeks and then aged in wood for a year before it's bottled. Two reliable Italian producers are Badia a Coltibuono and Castello di Volpaia. Both are known primarily for wine and are coincidentally located near the same town in Chianti; both age their vinegar in wood. When I compared a bottle of each side by side, the Badia a Coltibuono was pale red, the color of the palest young rosé wine; its taste was clean and good, with fruit flavor running into the aftertaste. I somewhat preferred the Castello di Volpaia, which had a more mature brick-red color, tasted older, and included slightly more fruit. An unopened bottle of good red-wine vinegar kept in the dark at indoor temperatures will hold its fruit flavors for several years or more and will improve during at least part of that time. Once opened and exposed to air, even special wine vinegar loses its best flavors in a few months.

If you can't easily get good red-wine vinegar, then try sherry or cider vinegar, both of which can be very good, and they are considerably less expensive. Sherry vinegar, like sherry itself, has none of the bright fruit notes of the best red-wine vinegar; in their place is a base of deep oxidized flavors. Hard cider, having about half as much alcohol as wine, makes vinegar that's about half as sharp and seems to avoid the nail-polish problem. Cider vinegar tastes of neither fresh nor cooked apple but of what I can only describe as fermented apple.

As for costly real *aceto balsamico,* to be sure you have the real thing, check that the label displays the complete phrase *"aceto balsamico tradizionale di Modena"* and that the bottle is the specially designed, globular 100-milliliter one. (*Aceto balsamico tradizionale di Reggio Emilia,* in just those words, comes in its own particular long-necked bottle holding the same quantity, but generally the Modena *balsamico* is better.) Real *balsamico* also comes in much less expensive young versions, too young to qualify for the label, though I haven't found a brand to recommend. Most *balsamico* is a blend with an average minimum age of twelve years, and the *extra vecchio* ("extra old") has an average age of at least twenty-five years; beyond that are special older versions, which cost considerably more. A few producers that stand out are del Cristo, Pedroni, and Malpighi. Even after it has been opened, a bottle of *balsamico,* tightly recorked, lasts indefinitely.

COMPLEMENTS TO RED-WINE VINEGAR AND BALSAMIC VINEGAR: The number-one complement to red-wine vinegar is olive oil, in vinaigrette for salad, and in that regular red-wine vinegar nearly always tastes better than *balsamico,* which is too heavy for lettuce and most other raw ingredients. (Still, for variety now and then, it works to add drops of real balsamic vinegar to a regular vinaigrette.) Red-wine vinegar, by itself, goes well on cooked carrots, beets, spinach, and other greens. Traditional *balsamico* will stand up to nearly everything and tends to complement rather than compete, though it's so complete in itself that perhaps nothing really complements it in return. Nonetheless, it matches a number of cooked vegetables, including bitter greens, such as dandelion and broccoli raab, especially cooked with olive oil. Tiny amounts of *balsamico* go with lobster and other flavorful seafood and fish, and with grilled poultry and red meats. Real *balsamico* underlines the meatiness of Italian *stracotto* (beef, usually, braised in wine), and it can enter other meat sauces, such as *ragùs. Balsamico* competes with very good tomatoes, but it can help weak ones. Drops are excellent on pieces of Parmigiano-Reggiano, a natural marriage of related flavors. Drops complement ripe cantaloupe and ripe strawberries, the latter mixed at the last minute with the *balsamico* and ground black pepper. Drops on vanilla ice cream have a mysteriously delicious effect, like a tart version of caramel sauce, and they go equally well though differently on custard.

NOTES ON WINE: No vinegar is friendly to wine unless the quantity is very small and, still better, has been well cooked with the food, and even then the dominant ingredients in the dish determine the wine. Drops of *balsamico* are more adaptable, and when they appear on lobster, I've liked a *sous voile* white from the Jura (and logically a rich mature white Burgundy would be good). With *balsamico* added to a red-wine sauce or a sauce made from braising liquid, or a rich *ragù* for pasta, either opt for a merely refreshing light red or echo the food with a rich, even powerful, red wine, such as Valpolicella and even Amarone della Valpolicella. With *balsamico* on Parmigiano, rather than risk the flavor competition of a rich red wine, try a good Lambrusco.

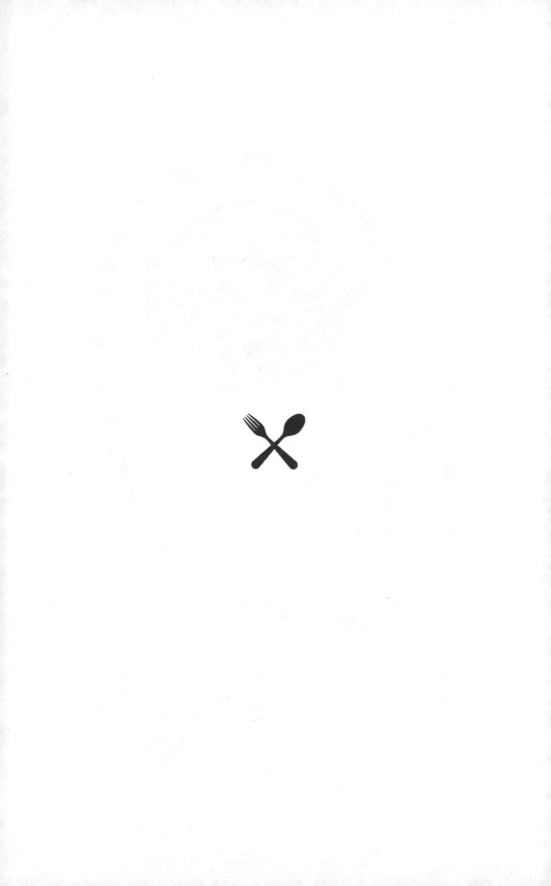

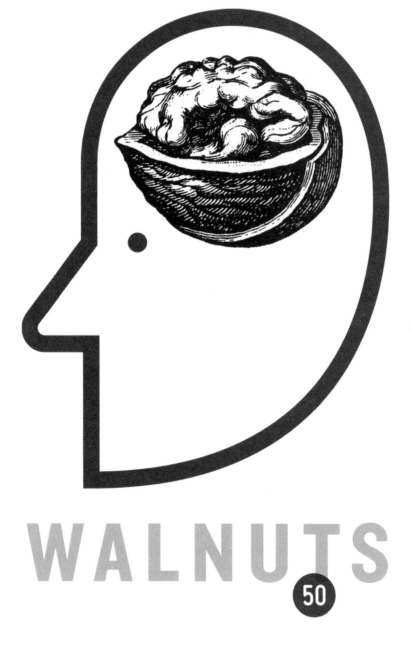

WALNUTS

50

50. WALNUTS

L ike most foods, walnuts are intimately tied to their season. Nearly all US walnuts, and a large portion of those on the world market, are grown in California's Central Valley. Toward the end of September, when the nuts have matured fully, their thick green outer husks split from the bottom upward, revealing the shells. The husks are high in tannin, which up to that point keeps out insects, protecting the kernels. (The acid is hard on your skin and stains it black.) The timing of the harvest counts, because during the last part of ripening the tree is still filling the kernels with flavor. The nuts used to be knocked down with sticks, or the growers waited until they fell. Now machines shake them free from the branches. The husks are removed mechanically, and the remains are washed off with powerful jets of water, leaving the thin, hard shells almost perfectly clean. If you harvest too early, though, you can't get all the husks off. Then the clinging, gritty, blackish material, which tastes awful, gets into the shelled nutmeats—a huge defect. To prevent the walnuts from molding they're dried while still in the shell. Sometimes that's done in the old way, in the sun, though the weather doesn't always cooperate, but usually it's done mechanically. If you've tasted walnuts in the fall at their ephemeral best, they're so much more delicious that you may think there's no reason to eat them at any other time.

Inexplicably, the nuts for sale then in US supermarkets taste as though they've been stored since at least the previous harvest, which must be true or they wouldn't taste so old. Apart from the loss of fresh flavor, the oil in the nuts gradually turns rancid, some nuts going much more quickly than others. The shells give some protection from air, light, and physical damage. For longer-term keeping, walnuts are commonly fumigated against insects and put into cold storage. Shelled walnuts are sometimes vacuum-packed. The crevices of the shell naturally have dark discolorations left by the husk, and in the US walnuts sold in the shell are commonly bleached to an even tan color. They may look more attractive, but the bleach can get inside the shells, and its use is prohibited in Europe and in organic production. Blotchy-looking in-shell organic nuts are likely to be much fresher and much better tasting, full of true walnut flavor.

One common name for walnuts is Persian walnuts, after the part of the world where the trees originated. In North America, we usually call them English walnuts, because the first ones arrived here on English ships and were different from native species, such as the curiously flavored black walnut (I'm one of the many people who recoil from it, almost as if it were rancid).

Superior—especially bigger and sweeter—Western varieties began to be selected in France in the eighteenth century. The oldest may be Franquette, which perhaps dates from that time and is still the most common walnut in France. Mayette, though, has the most admired flavor and is perhaps as old, and the still-popular Parisienne comes from an uncertain early date. The French varieties dominated in California until they were supplanted by their descendants, including Hartley (from a seed planted near Napa in 1892; one parent may be Franquette) and the now-dominant, high-quality Chandler (released by the University of California in 1979 and containing Mayette). Some of the newer varieties may be a little more bitter, because they were bred not primarily for taste but for such qualities as yield and good pollination. Among flavorful older varieties, the little-known Poe walnut, from Lake County, California, is less astringent than usual kinds and has a butterscotchlike flavor. In Italy, the most widespread kind is the well-regarded Sorrento, which is less a strict variety than a group of closely similar cultivars. In any case, vanishingly few walnuts are ever sold by variety. Some, however, bear geographic names, including the Noix de Grenoble, from southeastern France (from any of the three varieties Franquette, Mayette, and Parisienne), and the Noix du Périgord, from southwestern France (from Franquette, Corne, Marbot, or Grandjean).

The shell keeps out light and air, but mainly walnuts keep better in the shell because it protects the papery skin covering the kernel. The skin's antioxidant polyphenols are important in preserving the kernel. Varieties are selected for lighter-colored skins, which are more appealing to customers, although contrary to what you might think, lighter-colored skins tend to be more tannic—more astringent and bitter. And all skins darken slowly after harvest. Now and then in cooking you may want to avoid the strong taste of the skins in order to have the sweeter, blander taste of the *peeled* nuts. Most of the skins come off if you bake the shelled kernels at 325 degrees F (165 degrees C) for ten minutes—go too long and you'll get a strong toasted flavor—and then rub the kernels vigorously in a kitchen towel.

I sometimes fill a tart crust with whole walnuts and honey mixed with egg and bake it. Or I make a taller walnut-honey cake, for which I lightly toast the nuts and rub off most of their skins; the mashed nuts replace all the flour.

Very different in taste from the nutmeats are the few items made from immature nuts harvested in June or July before the shell has formed. The nuts are still so soft then that you can push a needle right through them. You wear rubber gloves to prevent the juice from irritating and staining your skin. Macerated in alcohol, these green walnuts make the Italian and French walnut liqueurs *nocino* and *vin de noix*. With their main component of husks, the drinks don't taste like the kernels, and yet they have a mysteriously deep, nutty taste. In England, the green walnuts, husk and all, are pickled—first brined and then put up in vinegar, to make black, decayed-looking objects, eaten especially with cold roast beef.

Among common nut oils—almond, hazelnut, walnut—the most useful in flavor is walnut. It adds a flattering nuttiness when it's used to sauté beef—the oil's smoke point is high, similar to that of other nut and vegetable oils. Whisked with lemon juice, it makes a superb dressing for lettuce and other greens. Dried walnuts are more than half oil, and once in large parts of France the primary cooking fat was walnut oil. In Italy, some were, and a little still is, made in places where olives don't grow; it was used by the poor, for whom olive oil was too expensive. Now walnut oil is a luxury fat. A little excellent walnut oil is made today in California.

Wherever the oil is made, the shelled nuts are first reduced to a paste, traditionally beneath turning stones, and then the paste is heated to increase the yield of oil and, as a side effect, give more flavor. The more heat, the greater the yield and the stronger the toasted flavor in the oil. Because walnut oil is less saturated than olive oil, it's even more healthful and it doesn't congeal in the refrigerator; it's also more susceptible to turning rancid. Strong-flavored walnut oil grows tiring, but lightly toasted walnuts give relatively light-flavored, light-textured oil.

In savory cooking, walnuts make sauces, such as Ligurian *salsa di noci* for tagliatelle or cheese-filled *pansotti*. Less familiar is the *aillade* of Toulouse, in southwestern France; it's a garlic mayonnaise, like aioli, but instead of being held together by egg yolk, the emulsion is made with mashed walnuts (the oil itself is walnut, olive, or a mix), and it sometimes contains parsley. The sauce goes on grilled fish and meats (veal, duck breast) and can be stirred into vegetable soup, like Ligurian *pesto* and Provençal *pistou.* In the country of Georgia, walnut sauces are common. *Fesenjān,* from northern Iran, is a stew of chicken, duck, or other meat in pomegranate juice with ground walnuts; it's made either sour or sweet-and-sour.

HOW TO BUY AND STORE WALNUTS AND WALNUT OIL: If you can find them, buy organic walnuts in unbleached shells just after the harvest, when the nuts are freshest and best. The shell helps to preserve the freshness, but even so, store the nuts in the cold. Shelled nuts, because the delicate nutmeat easily picks up off-flavors, are best sealed in a glass jar and frozen. Buy walnut oil, for freshness, in a container that blocks light and from a seller with high turnover. Try to determine from the label that the oil comes from the most recent harvest. Keep it refrigerated (the oil won't congeal), and use it within a few weeks of opening (as the best flavor declines, the oil is still useful for frying meat).

COMPLEMENTS TO WALNUTS: Walnuts go beautifully with garlic and parsley, as in *salsa di noci.* In Middle Eastern dishes, they go with yogurt, dill or mint, and cold raw-cucumber soup. Walnuts cracked at the table go with soft-ripened goat's-milk cheeses and with hard cheeses, such as French Comté, Swiss Gruyère, and Pyrenees ewe's-milk cheeses. Blue cheeses are a near-certain success with walnuts, which soothe them. Walnuts go wonderfully in bread, which in turn goes with soft goat's-milk cheeses. At serving, walnut oil goes well in a meatless cabbage soup or a spring-vegetable one; it goes with red meat. Walnut oil in vinaigrette enhances watercress, endive, thinly sliced raw cabbage, and green beans (though it hides the innate nuttiness of young *filet* green beans). One of the great taste trios is walnut oil with goat's-milk cheese and Sauvignon wine. (Whisk the oil with lemon juice to dress lettuce; accompany it with the goat's-milk cheese Crottin and a glass of the wine. All three—oil, cheese, and wine—are associated with the village of Chavignol, in the Sancerrois, though excellent examples come from other places.) *In sweet contexts,* walnuts go with autumn fruits (apples, pears), but they're perhaps better with cooked fruit (cherries, plums, berries) in pastry and plated desserts and with dried fruit (figs, dates, prunes), as in the dense traditional Italian Christmas cake *panforte.* They go with honey, as in baklava. Walnuts go perfectly with maple syrup on vanilla ice cream.

NOTES ON WINE: Walnuts suit fortified, intentionally oxidized wines, usually ones that are somewhat sweet. Classic with walnuts at the end of a meal are Port, sherry, and Madeira. Walnuts (and Roquefort) also go with the somewhat-related dark *vins doux naturels* from Catalan France (from the appellations Banyuls, Maury, and Rivesaltes). The intentionally oxidized wines often have pleasant *rancio* flavors, described for better or worse as "rancid walnut," which speak to the nonrancid flavor of walnuts. Another of the great taste trios is walnuts with Comté cheese and *vin jaune,* which is the superb dry oxidized wine that always has a *rancio* component and like Comté comes from the Jura Mountains of eastern France.

Acknowledgments

So many people have helped me so generously over time that I hesitate to name anyone in the certainty I will leave out so many others. I'm grateful to all who have taught me about these foods: the farmers, fishermen, cheesemakers, bread bakers, beekeepers, cooks, scientists, retailers, as well as winemakers (without whom the advice about wine would have had much less meaning). In many cases, they have spent hours patiently answering questions, and a few of the conversations have continued on and off for years. Nearly all the initial research took place in connection with writing for the magazine *The Art of Eating,* beginning in the 1980s.

Feeling the impossibility of gathering a fair list, which might run to several hundred names, I offer the names of some of those who have helped me the most, with an inevitable bias toward those who have helped recently. For his understanding of many topics, I'm first of all grateful to my friend James MacGuire, an outstanding chef, a living encyclopedia of French cooking, and one of the world's finest bread bakers (he has the rare combination of a disciplined mind and a sensualist's intuition for the state of fermenting dough). For generously sharing insights and prime information on many topics, I thank Harold McGee. For reading parts of the manuscript, I thank Winnie Yang. For holding me to a high standard in writing and thought when I first approached some of these foods, I thank Nina Maynard and Wendy Ruopp. For the pleasure of many conversations and for answering diverse questions, I particularly thank Bénédict Beaugé, Sebastiano Cossia Castiglioni, Mitchell Davis, and Nancy Harmon Jenkins.

For help with vegetables and fruits, I thank Anthony Boutard, Eliot Coleman, Keith Crotz, Barbara Damrosch, David Karp, Antoine Jacobsohn, David Sugar, Ram Fishman, the late Lewis Hill, Glenn Roberts, and the late Roger Way. My debts to bakers were built over many years. Among others, I thank the late Raymond Calvel, Hubert Chiron, Walter Koehn, the late Lionel Poilâne, Max Poilâne, Chad Robertson, and Steve Sullivan. For help with wild terrestrial foods, including fungi, I thank Boris Assyov, Paul Clemons, Doris Grazulis, John Grossmann, and Hank Shaw. For help with fish and seafood, I thank John Bil, Jeff Cox, Suzanne Taylor, Richard Hall, Mats Engstrom, Matt Ogburn, Jon Rowley, Brent Petkau, and John Finger. For help with chocolate, I thank Colin Gasko, Chloé Doutre-Roussel, Vincent Lebrun, Ed Seguine, and Alex Whitmore. For help with olive oil, I thank Mannie Berk, Franco Boeri, Sophie Denis, Ridgely Evers, Fiammetta Nizzi Grifi, Jean-Benoît Hugues, Maurizio Castelli, Mauro Marranci, Ilias Moutzouris, and Christian Pinatel. For help with meats, I thank Jude Becker, Mark Fasching, John Jamison, Mark Honeyman, Bill Niman, Ken Prusa, Russ Kremer, Lee Ranney, and Paul Willis.

For help with the vast and complex topics of cream, butter, and cheese, I owe thanks to Jean Berthaut, Robert L. Bradley Jr., Delphine and Jacques Carles, Luciano Catellani, Frère Christophe of the Abbaye de Cîteaux, Philippe Goux, Ihsan Gurdal, Jacques and Virginie Haxaire, Jean-Marie Henry, Randolph Hodgson, Andy and Mateo Kehler, Paul Kindstedt, the late Patrick Rance, Georges Risoud, the Robbe family, and Soyoung Scanlan.

To all those left off this list, I can only apologize.

Small and occasionally large errors easily creep into writing. For any that occur in this book, I take full responsibility.

I'm further grateful to Scott Moyers, who as my agent first opened the door to this book. I'm grateful to Ann Godoff of the Penguin Press for being convinced of its value. And I'm grateful to Ginny Smith Younce, who gave endless patience and support (and no criticism over lateness).

I thank the artist Mikel Jaso for his extraordinary illustrations. I thank Kim for her insights and support, and Kim, Max, and Zane for their patience.

Further Reading

A sampling of useful works.

Beach, S. A. *The Apples of New York,* volumes 1 and 2. Albany, New York, New York State Department of Agriculture, 1903. The enduring reference on varieties, with color plates.

Behr, Edward. *The Artful Eater,* second edition. Peacham, Vermont, The Art of Eating, 2004. Eighteen chapters on ingredients.

Benoit, Félix and Henry Clos-Jouve. *La Cuisine Lyonnaise.* Paris, Solar, 1980 (first published 1972). Traditional Lyon recipes, in French.

Boisard, Pierre. *Camembert: A National Myth.* Translated by Richard Miller. Berkeley, University of California, 2003. A full consideration.

Boni, Ada. *Italian Regional Cooking.* New York, Bonanza Books, 1969. Recipes and beautiful photographs of dishes against town and country landscapes.

Bourguignon, Philippe. *L'Accord Parfait.* Paris, Éditions du Chêne, 1997. The best book on matching French wine with French food.

Brooke, Justin. *Dessert Pears.* London, Hart-Davis, 1956. An English nurseryman's presentation of varieties and ripeness.

Bunyard, Edward. *The Anatomy of Dessert.* London, Chatto & Windus, 1933, and New York, Dutton, 1934 (first published in a small edition in London in 1929). Highly discriminating views on the taste of old varieties of fruit from another great English nurseryman.

Chanot-Bullier. *Vieilles Recettes de Cuisine Provençale / Vieii Receto de Cousino Provençalo,* fourth edition. Marseille, Tacussel, 1988. If I could own just one Provençal cookbook, this would be it, in French and Provençal.

Clark, Eleanor. *The Oysters of Locmariaquer.* New York, Pantheon, 1959. The classic account of oyster culture in Brittany.

Crane, Eva. *A Book of Honey.* Oxford, Oxford University Press, 1980. For the honey lover, by a British scientist.

Croze, Austin de. *Les Plats Régionaux de France: 1400 Succulentes Recettes Traditionnelles de Toutes les Provinces Françaises.* Paris, Montaigne, 1928. The real thing from long ago when automobiles were first transforming French tourism.

Curnonsky. *Recettes des Provinces de France.* Paris, Les Productions de Paris, 1959 (originally published in six volumes 1950–1952). Recipes collected by the great twentieth-century French gastronome.

Darrow, George. *The Strawberry: History, Breeding and Physiology.* New York, Chicago, and San Francisco, Holt, Rinehart and Winston, 1966. The definitive strawberry book of its time and still, to a great extent, of ours.

David, Elizabeth. *French Provincial Cooking,* revised edition. London, Michael Joseph, 1960. A strong portrait of French cooking.

Davidson, Alan. *Mediterranean Seafood: A Comprehensive Guide with Recipes,* third edition. Berkeley, Ten Speed, 2002. Essential sorting out of species with carefully chosen traditional recipes.

———. *North Atlantic Seafood: A Comprehensive Guide with Recipes,* third edition. Berkeley, Ten Speed, 2003. The same for the North Atlantic.

Del Conte, Anna. *Gastronomy of Italy.* New York, Prentice Hall, 1987. A handy reference by a native of Milan.

Dornenburg, Andrew, and Karen Page. *The Flavor Bible: The Essential Guide to Culinary Creativity, Based on the Wisdom of America's Most Imaginative Chefs.* New York, Little, Brown, 2008. Flavors that go together, the collated views of top US chefs.

———. *What to Drink with What You Eat: The Definitive Guide to Pairing Food with Wine, Beer, Spirits, Coffee, Tea—Even Water—Based on Expert Advice from America's Best Sommeliers.* New York, Boston, and London, Bulfinch Press, 2006. The collated views of top US sommeliers.

Farr, Ryan. *Whole Beast Butchery.* San Francisco, Chronicle Books, 2011. Practical meat cutting for anyone.

Francesconi, Jeanne Caròla. *La Cucina Napoletana.* Rome, Newton Compton, 1992. More than 700 pages of recipes and information.

Gaertner, Pierre. *La Cuisine Alsacienne.* Paris, Flammarion, 1979. If you could own only one Alsace cookbook, this would be it.

Gedda, Guy. *La Table d'un Provençal,* fourth edition. Paris, Roland Escaig, 1995. Recipes, almost entirely traditional, from a Provençal-speaking chef.

Gerken, Jonathan. *Apples I Have Eaten.* San Francisco, Chronicle Books, 2007. Photos of forty-seven varieties eaten in the fall of one year.

Gho, Paolo. *Dizionario delle Cucine Regionali Italiane.* Bra, Italy, Slow Food, 2008. A highly useful reference, in Italian.

Goldman, Amy. *Melons for the Passionate Grower.* New York, Artisan, 2002. And for the passionate eater.

Gonnet, Michel, and Gabriel Vache. *Analyse Sensorielle Descriptive de Quelques Miels Monofloraux de France et d'Europe.* Paris, Syndicat National d'Apiculture, 1998. Excellent on the taste of diverse kinds of mostly French honey, in French.

Gray, Patience. *Honey from a Weed.* London, Prospect Books, 1986. A cookbook of Tuscan, Catalan, Cycladic, and Pugliese food that is a prime candidate for best book ever written about food.

Hamelman, Jeffrey. *Bread: A Baker's Book of Techniques and Recipes,* second edition. Hoboken, New Jersey, Wiley, 2012. Excellent how-to and insights.

Hazan, Marcella. *Essentials of Classic Italian Cooking.* New York, Alfred A. Knopf, 1992. If there's one indispensable Italian cookbook, this is it.

Imhoff, Daniel, editor. *The CAFO Reader.* Healdsburg, California, Watershed Media, 2010. Discouraging but important information about "concentrated animal feeding operations."

Jacobsen, Rowan. *A Geography of Oysters.* New York, Bloomsbury, 2007. The best book on oysters, for the eater.

Jenkins, Nancy Harmon. *The Essential Mediterranean: How Regional Cooks Transform Key Ingredients into the World's Favorite Cuisines.* New York, HarperCollins, 2003. A deep look into selected raw materials.

Kamman, Madeleine. *When French Women Cook.* New York, Atheneum, 1983. Evocative accounts of regional food, starting in 1939.

MacGuire, James. "The Baguette." *The Art of Eating* no. 73+74, 2006. A fine presentation by a great bread baker.

———. "Pain au Levain: The Best Flavor, Acidity, and Texture and Where They Come From." *The Art of Eating,* no. 83, 2009. A complete understanding of great sourdough, starting with the flour and milling.

Masui, Kazuko and Tomoko Yamada, with photographs by Yohei Maruyama. *French Cheeses.* London, DK Publishing, 1996. (Originally published in Japan in 1993.) A hunger-inspiring visual record of more than 350 French cheeses.

McCalman, Max, and David Gibbons. *Mastering Cheese: Lessons for Connoisseurship from a Maître Fromager.* New York, Clarkson Potter, 2009. Just what the title says.

McClane, A. J. *The Encyclopedia of Fish Cookery.* New York, Holt, Rinehart and

Winston, 1977. Hard to beat, by a former fishing editor of *Field and Stream* magazine.

McGee, Harold. *On Food and Cooking: The Science and Lore of the Kitchen,* revised edition. New York, Scribner, 2004. The first place to look for answers to many questions.

Médecin, Jacques. *La Cuisine du Comté de Nice.* Paris, Julliard, 1972. One of the ten or so essential Provençal cookbooks, in French.

Olney, Richard. *Simple French Food.* New York, Atheneum, 1974. Perhaps the best cookbook of all, at least in the West, impeccably written, full of instruction.

Persano Oddo, Livia, Lucia Piana, and Anna Gloria Sabatini, editors. *Conoscere il Miele: Guida all'Analisi Sensoriale.* Bologna, Avenue Media, 1995. The taste of diverse kinds of Italian honey, in Italian.

Pitte, Jean-Robert. *Terres de Castanide: Hommes et Paysages du Châtaignier de l'Antiquité à Nos Jours.* Paris, Fayard, 1986. The role of the chestnut in France, in French.

Pomés, Leopold. *Teoria i Practica del Pa amb Tomàquet.* Barcelona, Tusquets, 1985. The best account that may ever be written of "bread with tomato," the great Catalan snack.

Rance, Patrick. *The French Cheese Book.* London, Macmillan, 1989. This remains the most thorough exploration of French cheese, by a passionate, purist British cheesemonger.

Reich, Lee. *Uncommon Fruits for Every Garden.* Portland, Oregon, and Cambridge, UK, Timber Press, 2004. Advice on growing but also on best varieties, such as of alpine and musk strawberries.

Risoud, Georges. *Histoire du Fromage d'Époisses: Chronique Agitée d'un Fromage Peu Banal.* Précy-sous-Thil, France, Armançon, 2000. The essence of the cheese Époisses, in French.

Roden, Claudia. *A Book of Middle Eastern Food.* London, Nelson, 1968, and New York, Knopf, 1972. A highly readable cookbook.

Roussel, Philippe, and Hubert Chiron. *Les Pains Français: Évolution, Qualité, Production,* Maé-Erti, Vesoul, 2002. An outstanding scholarly presentation of French bread from a professional baker's point of view, in French.

Rubino, Roberto, Piero Sardo, and Angelo Surrusca, editors. *Italian Cheese: A Guide to Its Discovery and Appreciation.* Bra, Italy, Slow Food, 2009 (a newer edition, in Italian, was published in 2009 as *Formaggi d'Italia: Guida alla Scoperta e alla Conoscenza*). Traditional cheeses in 293 varieties.

Saffron, Inga. *Caviar.* New York, Broadway, 2002. A fine account.

Salvatori de Zuliani, Mariù. *A Tola co i Nostri Veci: La Cucina Veneziana.* Milan, Franco Angeli, 1971. Traditional recipes, in Venetian.

Schneider, Elizabeth. *Vegetables from Amaranth to Zucchini: The Essential Reference.* New York, Morrow, 2001. Excellent information from a fine researcher.

Simon, Joanna. *Wine with Food.* London, Mitchell Beazley, 1996, and New York, Simon & Schuster, 1996. What goes with what.

Steingarten, Jeffrey. *It Must've Been Something I Ate.* New York, Alfred A. Knopf, 2002. Serious, entertaining investigations of varied foods.

Thiers, Harry D. *California Mushrooms: A Field Guide to the Boletes.* New York, Hafner Press, 1975. (Available online at www.mykoweb.com.) A highly practical resource.

Thorne, John. *Mouth Wide Open.* New York, North Point, 2007. Thoughtful explorations by a fine writer and cook.

Verdier, Ernest. *Dissertations Gastronomiques.* Paris, La Société des Cuisiniers de Paris, 1930s (first published in perhaps 1916). Observations about raw materials from the perspective of a late nineteenth-century Paris restaurateur, in French.

Waters, Alice. *Chez Panisse Fruit.* New York, HarperCollins, 2002. Insights into taste from the California restaurant that first began to pay close attention to raw materials.

———. *Chez Panisse Vegetables.* New York, HarperCollins, 1996. The same for vegetables.

Weaver, William Woys. *100 Vegetables and Where They Came From.* Chapel Hill, North Carolina, Algonquin Books, 2000. Fascinating views on chosen varieties by a gardener and cook.

Wolfert, Paula. *The Cooking of Southwest France.* Garden City, New York, Dial Press, 1983. Revised edition, Hoboken, New Jersey, Wiley, 2005. A key work on some of France's best food.

Zanini De Vita, Oretta. *Encyclopedia of Pasta.* Berkeley and Los Angeles, University of California, 2009. Three hundred and ten kinds of pasta, not dishes, from the perspective of the eater.

———. *Popes, Peasants, and Shepherds: Recipes and Lore from Rome and Lazio.* Translated by Maureen B. Fant. Berkeley, University of California, 2013. An outstanding new cookbook.

Index